Advanced
Health Assessment
of Women

Helen A. Carcio, MS, MEd, ANP-BC, has been involved in women's health care, both educationally and clinically, for the past 20 years. She was an associate clinical professor at the University of Massachusetts at Amherst in the nurse practitioner program for 10 years, where she was awarded the distinguished teaching medal. During that time she wrote a column for the *Hampshire Gazette*, in Northampton, Massachusetts, titled "Women's Health Matters." The column addressed the health care needs of women in the community and offered a forum for women to address their concerns.

She has written books on pathophysiology, infertility, and health assessments and she received the national award Nurse Practitioner Entrepreneur of the Year from *Advance for Nurse Practitioners and Physician Assistants.*

Ms. Carcio practices independently, is the director and founder of the Health & Continence Institute of New England, and offers workshops on launching continence care programs. She has established multiple bladder health centers nationally and continues to offer consultation services to other centers with the same focus. In addition, Ms. Carcio is a highly sought-after lecturer on women's health, bladder health issues, and incontinence. She has written 11 feature articles in the nationally recognized publication *Advance for Nurse Practitioners and Physician Assistants*, where she was a member of the advisory board. She is currently a member of the editorial advisory board for *Women's Health Care: A Clinical Journal for NPs*. Ms. Carcio was also the winner of the National Association for Continence (NAFC) Continence Care Champion Award.

R. Mimi Secor, MS, MEd, FNP-BC, NCMP, FAANP, is a family nurse practitioner (NP) specializing in women's health at Newton Wellesley Obstetrics and Gynecology, Inc., in Newton, Massachusetts, and a visiting scholar at Boston College William F. Connell School of Nursing. She is a national speaker and consultant, and president emerita and senior advisor for Nurse Practitioner Associates of Continuing Education (NPACE). Ms. Secor's 37 years of clinical experience as an NP have included emergency care, college health, private practice, prison nursing, and rural medicine. Before working for 7 years at Bethel Family Clinic, in Bethel, Alaska, she operated an independent Boston-area NP practice for 12 years. Among other credits, Ms. Secor is a nationally certified menopause practitioner (NCMP), a national radio host on ReachMD, and has delivered numerous radio and TV presentations on women's health. She is a founder of the Massachusetts Coalition of Nurse Practitioners (MCNP), a member and fellow of the American Association of Nurse Practitioners, and a member of the Association of Reproductive Health Professionals (ARHP), the National Association of Nurse Practitioners in Women's Health (NPWH), and the North American Menopause Society (NAMS). She has won several awards, including the 2012 Lifetime Achievement Award from the MCNP.

Advanced Health Assessment of Women

CLINICAL SKILLS AND PROCEDURES

Third Edition

HELEN A. CARCIO, MS, MEd, ANP-BC

R. MIMI SECOR, MS, MEd, FNP-BC, NCMP, FAANP

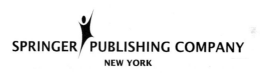

SPRINGER PUBLISHING COMPANY

NEW YORK

Springer Publishing Company, LLC
11 West 42nd Street
New York, NY 10036
www.springerpub.com

Acquisitions Editor: Elizabeth Nieginski
Composition: Integra Software Services Pvt. Ltd.

ISBN: 978-0-8261-2308-4
E-book ISBN: 978-0-8261-2309-1

16 17 18 19 / 6 5 4 3

The author and the publisher of this Work have made every effort to use sources believed to be reliable to provide information that is accurate and compatible with the standards generally accepted at the time of publication. Because medical science is continually advancing, our knowledge base continues to expand. Therefore, as new information becomes available, changes in procedures become necessary. We recommend that the reader always consult current research and specific institutional policies before performing any clinical procedure. The author and publisher shall not be liable for any special, consequential, or exemplary damages resulting, in whole or in part, from the readers' use of, or reliance on, the information contained in this book. The publisher has no responsibility for the persistence or accuracy of URLs for external or third-party Internet websites referred to in this publication and does not guarantee that any content on such websites is, or will remain, accurate or appropriate.

Library of Congress Cataloging-in-Publication Data

Carcio, Helen Nelson, author, editor.
Advanced health assessment of women : clinical skills and procedures / Helen A. Carcio, R. Mimi Secor. — Third edition. p. ; cm.
Includes bibliographical references and index.
ISBN 978-0-8261-2308-4 — ISBN 978-0-8261-2309-1 (eBook)
I. Secor, Mimi Clarke, author, editor. II. Title.
[DNLM: 1. Diagnostic Techniques, Obstetrical and Gynecological. 2. Women's Health. WP 141]
RG110
618'.0475--dc23

2014032000

Printed in the United States of America by McNaughton & Gunn.

To my sister, Dette Hunter, whose courage continues to inspire me in all aspects of my life.

—*Helen Carcio*

To my family: mom, Irene Clarke; husband, Mike; and daughter, Katherine, for their unconditional love and support.

—*R. Mimi Secor*

Contents

Unit VIII: INFERTILITY AND SUBFERTILITY ASSESSMENT

Unit IX: CONTRACEPTION

Unit X: INVESTIGATIVE PROCEDURES

Unit XI: ADVANCED SKILLS

Contributors

Ivy M. Alexander, PhD, APRN, ANP-BC, FAAN Clinical Professor and Director of Advanced Practice Programs, School of Nursing, University of Connecticut, Storrs, Connecticut

Nancy R. Berman, MSN, ANP-BC, NCMP Adult- and Menopause-Certified Nurse Practitioner, Michigan Healthcare Professionals, Southfield, Michigan

Paula Brooks, DNP, FNP-BC, RNFA Clinical Coordinator, Allied Health Care Professionals, Cape Cod Hospital, Hyannis, Massachusetts

Helen A. Carcio, MS, MEd, ANP-BC Director and Founder, Health & Continence Institute of New England, South Deerfield, Massachusetts

Kahlil A. Demonbreun, DNP, RNC-OB, WHNP-BC, ANP-BC DNP Program Faculty, Medical University of South Carolina, Charleston, South Carolina

Marcia Denine, WHNP-BC, APRN, Nurse Practitioner, Vineyard Medical Services, Vineyard Haven, Massachusetts

Jennifer Dentler Director, Women's Wellness Center, Allegan General Hospital, Allegan, Michigan

Nancy Gardner Dirubbo, FNP-C, WHNP-C, FAANP Director, Founder, Laconia Women's Health Care, Laconia, New Hampshire

Kate Green, MS, RN, CNM Clinical Assistant Professor, Nursing, University of Massachusetts–Amherst, Amherst, Massachusetts

Kathleen Haycraft, FNP/PNP-BC, DCNP, FAANP Dermatology Nurse Practitioner, Riverside Dermatology, Hannibal, Missouri

Yolanda R. Hill, MSN, FNP-BC Family Nurse Practitioner, Specialist, Occupational Health, Medicine and Occupational Health, ExxonMobil Corporation, Baton Rouge, Louisiana

Karen Kalmakis, NP, APRN-BC Assistant Professor, School of Nursing, University of Massachusetts, Amherst, Massachusetts

Cathy R. Kessenich, PhD, ARNP   Professor of Nursing, University of Tampa, Tampa, Florida

Rebecca Koeniger-Donohue, PhD, APRN-BC, WHNP-BC   Associate Professor, Nursing, Simmons College, School of Health Sciences, Boston, Massachusetts

Carol Lesser, MS, WHNP-BC   Nurse Practitioner, Boston IVF, Waltham, Massachusetts

Deborah A. Lipkin, MS, FNP-BC   Nurse Practitioner, Harvard Vanguard Medical Associates, Burlington, Massachusetts

Alison O. Marshall, FNP   Associate Professor of Practice, Director of the Family Nurse Practitioner Program, Simmons College of Nursing & Health Sciences, Boston, Massachusetts

Amy M. O'Meara, DrNP, WHNP-BC   Clinical Assistant Professor, University of Vermont, Nurse Practitioner, Planned Parenthood of Northern New England, Burlington, Vermont

Diane Todd Pace, PhD, APRN, FNP-BC, NCMP, FAANP   Clinical Associate Professor, Lowensberg School of Nursing, University of Memphis, Cordova, Tennessee

Yvette Marie Petti, PhD, APRN-BC, ANP   Associate Dean for Graduate Nursing Programs and Assistant Professor, Kirkhof College of Nursing, Grand Valley State University, Grand Rapids, Michigan

Linda Pettit, ANP   Retired Nurse Practitioner, Dover, Massachusetts

Richard Pope, PA-C, MPAS   Physician's Assistant, Department of Rheumatology, Western Connecticut Medical Group, Danbury, Connecticut

Constance A. Roche, MSN, ANP-BC   Avon Comprehensive Breast Center, Massachusetts General Hospital, Boston, Massachusetts

Frances M. Sahebzamani, PhD, ARNP, FAANP   Assistant Professor, University of South Florida, Odessa, Florida

R. Mimi Secor, MS, MEd, FNP-BC, NCMP, FAANP   Nurse Practitioner, Newton Wellesley ObGyn, Newton, Massachusetts

Susan Voss, DNP, FNP-BC, DCNP   Nurse Practitioner, Riverside Dermatology, Hannibal, Missouri

Leslie Saltzstein Wooldridge, GNP-BC, CUNP, BCB-PMD   Director, Mercy Hospital Bladder Clinic, Muskegan, Michigan

Preface

The majority of individuals who seek health care are women. As baby boomers begin to age, even more women will seek professional care. With health care reform, renewed emphasis is being placed on the knowledgeable assessment of women to provide preventative care. In today's rapidly changing health care climate, advanced practice clinicians are being viewed as a group of providers who are well qualified to care for health issues related to women. Additionally, the scope of their practice is broadening to include more advanced clinical skills and procedures. *Advanced Health Assessment of Women: Clinical Skills and Procedures, Third Edition*, brings together clear and concise factual information related to the health assessment of women.

This text provides an enhanced definition of the role and clinical skills of providers, including physician's assistants (PAs), certified nurse midwives (CNMs), and nurse practitioners (NPs). These practitioners play a vital role in managing the health of women in a variety of settings, including internal medicine, primary care, family practice, and specialty areas such as women's health care, pelvic wellness, aesthetics, and infertility.

Some of the procedures described in this manual are quite advanced and are appropriate only within certain practice settings. It must be remembered that advanced practice clinicians are under a heavy mandate to practice within the scope of legal and professional limits, as well as within their personal comfort level, when considering performing advanced techniques and procedures. Consult your state licensing board if in doubt about the legality of performing any of the procedures described. The scope of practice varies among NPs, PAs, and CNMs in relation to educational programs, practice settings, geographical location, and state laws and regulations. This text provides guidance so that each practitioner may become increasingly aware of when to practice independently, when to co-manage, when to consult, and when to refer.

Many of the assessment skills, techniques, and procedures described are fast becoming routine to the advanced practice clinician. Practitioners are educated in a variety of different ways, with differing approaches within today's conventional medical model. College curricula provide basic content for the beginning practitioner, but most curricula offer little in relation to advanced assessment and practice. This text is designed to fill that gap.

This third edition of *Advanced Health Assessment of Women: Clinical Skills and Procedures* offers an integrated and unique approach to the health care of women. It goes beyond content commonly found in texts related only to health assessment. It provides an excellent resource to link theory to clinical practice using critical thinking skills. This manual is practical and user friendly. It provides detailed descriptions, enhanced by tables and figures, to clearly describe these advanced skills. The assessment of many aspects of care related to women is outlined, with sample assessment forms integrated throughout.

An outline format was chosen because this clear and concise layout allows the information to flow in a logical sequence without one having to wade through unnecessary jargon. Where techniques are explained, a comprehensive list of equipment necessary for each technique or procedure is given as well as information on patient preparation and recommended follow-up. The entire text is enhanced with a plethora of boxes, figures, and tables. The casual format offers easy access to pertinent information.

The different techniques and procedures were selected because they are within the expanding scope of the practitioner's experience but are often not described in assessment books. This manual delineates strategies that are on the leading edge in the expanded role of the advanced practice clinician. Obviously, one cannot expect to learn the technical aspects from simply reading about them. This manual provides a foundation for, and an understanding of, the rationale behind the assessments and procedures described. It is a good idea to observe a new procedure first and then be supervised for as many times as it takes to feel comfortable performing that procedure. Always carefully read manufacturers' recommendations that accompany any instrumentation you might use in addition to the information found in this text. This manual is not meant to dictate how procedures should be performed or to supply a strict recipe for techniques and procedures. It does, however, provide a clear starting point for developing guidelines specific to each individual's clinical style and practice setting.

The text begins with a comprehensive review of the basic anatomy and physiology of women. A complete understanding of the complexities of the menstrual cycle and normal vaginal flora, examined at the cellular level, is imperative for accurate understanding and diagnoses of conditions that affect women.

The health history chapter discusses elements of a comprehensive, developmentally relevant health history with a unique approach to the physiologic, psychological, and sociocultural components involved. Advanced health history techniques are detailed in which interaction is viewed as an equal partnership between provider and patient. Critical issues related to the assessment of HIV infection are summarized. The basic techniques of the physical examination—with a focus on the gynecologic exam—are outlined, with possible clinical alterations listed for each area assessed. Evaluation of the breast includes basic techniques with a section on how to examine the augmented breast (an explanation not commonly found in traditional health assessment books).

Assessment of vulvar pain addresses the diagnoses of vulvodynia and vestibulitis. Obesity is becoming a national epidemic. This text includes a chapter that explores the assessment of obesity and body mass index (BMI).

New chapters have been added in response to suggestions from colleagues and the changing focus of health care. These topics include the assessment of skin and aesthetics, lesbian health, pelvic pain, dysfunctional uterine bleeding, and polycystic ovarian syndrome (PCOS). With the aging population, detection of skin cancer and accurate diagnosis of dermatologic conditions are essential. The new chapter on lesbian health addresses critical aspects of taking a history and special considerations that all clinicians need to be familiar with. Abnormal uterine bleeding, also known as abnormal vaginal bleeding, is a problem most clinicians will need to evaluate properly in order to diagnose and manage these patients appropriately. PCOS is increasingly common and clinicians need to know how to assess, diagnose, and manage this condition, which is associated with serious sequelae.

Pelvic health issues will become more in evidence as the population of women ages. Three new, unique chapters have been added to the investigative procedures and advanced skills sections as an adjunct to the pelvic organ prolapse and urinary incontinence chapters and include electrical stimulation of the pelvic floor, electromyography of the pelvic floor, and percutaneous tibial nerve stimulation.

Information provided in the vaginal microscopy chapter is the most comprehensive description of the interpretation and evaluation of the wet mount available in any current text. In the Pap smear, HPV chapter ("Cervical Cancer Screening"), recommendations for interpretation and follow-up of an abnormal Pap smear are outlined, reflecting the new American Society of Colposcopy and Cervical Pathology (ASCCP) guidelines for screening and follow-up. The new recommendations for HPV testing are also included.

The chapter on urinalysis offers a fresh look at an old test. Differential diagnosis of gynecologic versus urologic conditions is always challenging in women. This chapter contains an in-depth analysis of the components of urinalysis, and a step-by-step explanation of urine microscopy—a skill with which every advanced practice clinician should feel comfortable. Concerns of older women are addressed in the comprehensive new sections on menopause and urinary incontinence.

Two newly emerging techniques that are becoming an integral part of assessment of women are sonohysteroscopy and bone densitometry. The various machines used are described and interpretation of results is clearly explained.

Up-to-date information on emerging topics such as *BRCA* gene testing is provided. Content on *BRCA* gene testing will help identify those women at risk and provide the clinician with skills necessary to help a woman choose whether or not to be tested.

The infertility section has been entirely reworked and updated and presents guidelines for the assessment, evaluation, and management of the woman who is unable to conceive. Controversies and clinical dilemmas are explained. Techniques for evaluation of the infertile woman and intrauterine and donor insemination are clearly delineated.

This text contains critical information regarding the woman at risk. A nationally tested questionnaire is included to help identify the victims of violence and abuse. Management and follow-up of the rape victim are also included.

Another unique section of this text is the chapter on pessary insertion. Such descriptive information is not found in any comparable text. As baby boomers age, the incidence of genital prolapse, often accompanied by incontinence, is increasing. Today pessaries offer a viable alternative to urologic surgery. The fitting of pessaries requires patience, knowledge, and experience. Advanced-level clinicians are in a key position to assume care of this rapidly expanding population of women.

Technical skills related to insertion of various contraceptive devices are outlined. Characteristics such as the advantages and disadvantages, mechanisms of action, and contraindications of each device are necessary to educate the woman in making an informed decision regarding her contraceptive management. The technique of fitting contraceptive devices and follow-up care are outlined in detail. New information on the technique of insertion and removal of Implanon and use of the FemCap are clearly described, with figures supplied for clarification. The intrauterine contraception chapter has been expanded to include Mirena.

In the final section, the more advanced techniques are explained. Performing endometrial biopsy surgery requires skill and practice. It is also important to understand the indications for biopsy study, the implications and interpretation of the results. One chapter describes the necessary equipment required and walks the practitioner through each step. Mastering the technique of acrochordonectomy, or the removal of skin tags, will please many patients bothered by unsightly skin tags. New information on how to perform a cystometrogram is important in diagnosing the cause of urinary incontinence.

Advanced Health Assessment of Women offers a variety of clinical tools to enhance content. Feel free to use any information provided and adapt it to your organization. End-of-chapter appendices contain a special patient education series that may be used and/or adopted for use by your practice.

We hope to offer some real guidance to students and practitioners. The content reflects an extensive review of current literature, integrated with our years of clinical experience and teaching. Experts in various women's health forums have generously shared their expertise as contributors and reviewers.

Helen A. Carcio

R. Mimi Secor

Acknowledgments

Thanks to my husband Frank, and sons Marc, Ben, and CJ, who are willing to share me with a computer. It wasn't always easy but it is certainly always rewarding.

Helen A. Carcio

Thanks to Helen for all her support as we updated this textbook with new chapters involving new authors. I also want to thank my husband Mike, daughter Katherine, and my mom for their understanding and support throughout this process. It was an interesting and rewarding experience.

R. Mimi Secor

We gratefully thank Elizabeth Nieginski, Executive Editor, Nursing, and Jenna Vaccaro, Assistant Editor, for their professionalism, knowledge, insight, patience, and invaluable support through the lengthy publication process. You were both always extremely responsive to all our questions and concerns. Special thanks to Elizabeth for always being enthusiastic and extremely optimistic and for her "gentle reminders," which helped keep us on track. Her "you can do it" attitude helped spur us on.

We sincerely thank all the contributing authors for finding time in their already busy schedules to contribute to our book; for their attention to format, content, and keeping to deadlines. Thanks to Quinetta Edwards; students Trucia Casssagnol, Erica Anna Lyons, and Shoshana Violette Aronowitz; and Drs. Quinetta Edwards, Julie Adkins, and Kristine Anne Scordo for their help with research.

We both thank Springer Publishing Company for their special dedication to educating nurse practitioners and to their commitment to women's health care.

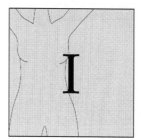

Female Reproduction

Anatomy and Physiology of Female Reproduction

Helen A. Carcio

I. **Female reproduction explained**
   A. In the female, the urinary and reproductive systems are completely separate, unlike in the male.
   B. The internal female reproductive organs are located in the lower pelvis and are safely tucked inside the bony pelvis, behind the pubic bone.
   C. External genitalia collectively include the mons pubis, the labia majora, the labia minora, the vestibule, the clitoris, and the vaginal orifice (Figure 1.1).
   D. The structures of the peritoneum are listed and compared in Table 1.1.

II. **Ovaries**
   A. Description
      1. Each ovary lies in a depression in the lateral pelvic wall, on either side of the uterus.
      2. Ovaries are small and almond shaped.
      3. The ovaries vary considerably in size among women but usually measure between 3 and 5 cm long, 1.5 and 3 cm wide, and 1 and 1.5 cm thick—about the size of a thumbnail.
      4. They are pinkish white to gray.
      5. They are not directly attached to the uterus and fallopian tubes. The ovaries lie suspended in a strong, flexible structure called the *round ligament*, which anchors them to the uterus.
      6. The uterine tubes, which consist of the oviducts and the fallopian tubes, are not directly connected to the ovaries. They open to the peritoneal cavity area near them.

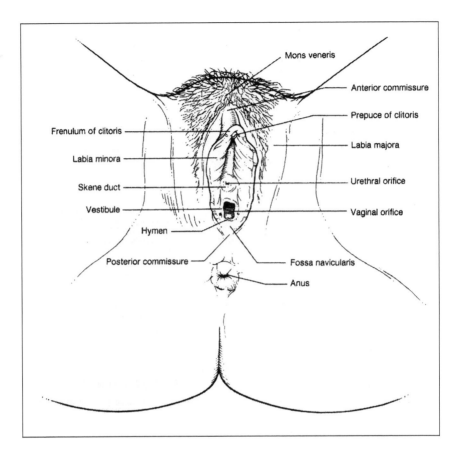

FIGURE 1.1 External female genitalia.

    B. Function
        1. The ovaries house the female sex gametes.
        2. The ovaries are counterparts to the testes in the male, in that they secrete sex hormones: estrogen, progesterone, and testosterone.
        3. The ovaries produce an ovum (egg) during ovulation in response to hormonal stimulation.

III. Fallopian tubes
    A. Description
        1. The fallopian tubes extend outward from either side of the body of the uterus and act as a connecting tunnel between the ovary and the uterus.
        2. They are approximately 13 cm (5 in), rubbery, and less than half the diameter of a pencil (.05–1.0 cm).

TABLE 1.1 Structure, Functions, and Purposes of the Organs of Female Reproduction

STRUCTURE	FUNCTION	PURPOSE
External genitalia	Sensitive to touch and external stimulation	Sexual arousal and sensation of orgasm
Vagina	Passage for intercourse Provides space for containment of sperm Excretory outlet for the uterus Becomes birth canal during the birthing process	Organ of copulation
Cervix	Fibrous, muscular band that holds bottom of uterus closed and keeps fetus inside during pregnancy	Major source of mucus production during the menstrual cycle
Uterus	Organ of menstruation	Fertilized egg implants here Maintains and protects developing fetus until birth Contracts during labor to birth the neonate
Fallopian tubes	Transport of sperm upward Transport of the egg downward	Location of fertilization of the egg Carries the egg to the uterus
Ovaries	Maturation and development of eggs Ejection of eggs Secrete hormones, including estrogen, progesterone, and testosterone	Produce eggs during ovulation

3. They have two layers—inner and outer serous layers—that surround the layers of involuntary muscle.
4. The fallopian tubes are narrow and muscular (acting as oviducts) and lined with cilia.
5. They consist of four sections.
   a. Interstitial section, which lies within the uterine wall
   b. Isthmus
      (1) The isthmus is the narrowest section closest to the uterus.
      (2) It opens into the cavity of the uterus.
      (3) It has a thick muscular wall.
   c. Ampulla
      (1) The ampulla is the longest section, about two thirds of the tube's total length.
      (2) It widens progressively to the wide distal opening in the infundibulum.

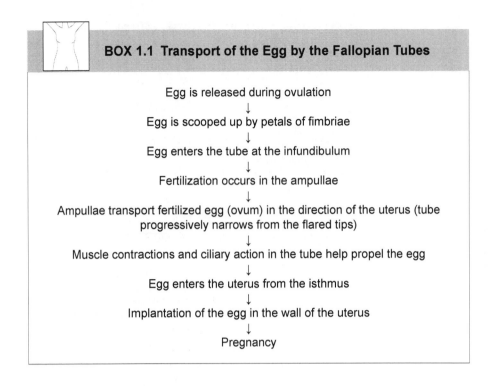

BOX 1.1 Transport of the Egg by the Fallopian Tubes

Egg is released during ovulation
↓
Egg is scooped up by petals of fimbriae
↓
Egg enters the tube at the infundibulum
↓
Fertilization occurs in the ampullae
↓
Ampullae transport fertilized egg (ovum) in the direction of the uterus (tube progressively narrows from the flared tips)
↓
Muscle contractions and ciliary action in the tube help propel the egg
↓
Egg enters the uterus from the isthmus
↓
Implantation of the egg in the wall of the uterus
↓
Pregnancy

        (3) It is thin walled.
        (4) It is the site of fertilization.
     d. Infundibulum
        (1) The infundibulum is the fimbriated end that lies in close proximity to the ovary.
        (2) Fingerlike projections at the ends of the tubes are the *fimbriae*, which sweep over the ovary, scoop up the egg, and propel it toward the inner ampullae.
B. Function
   1. Transports the sperm and the egg (Box 1.1).
     a. The inner wall of the fallopian tubes is lined with cilia, which are hairlike projections.
     b. It is believed that the beating motion of these cilia transports the fertilized egg along the tube to the uterus, where the egg is implanted.
     c. Muscle contractions in the fallopian tube assist in moving the egg along its journey, much as in intestinal peristalsis.
     d. Fallopian tubes have the unique ability to transport the egg in one direction and the sperm in the opposite direction.
   2. Collects the egg.
     a. The cilia on the fimbriae have adhesive sites that help navigate the egg into the fallopian tube.

      b. Near the time of ovulation, the fimbriae bend down in proximity to the ovaries.

      c. The swooping motion of the petals sweeps up the egg.

IV. The uterus

A. Description of the uterine corpus, or uterine body

1. The uterus is shaped like an inverted pear.
2. The uterus is hollow, thick walled, and muscular, lying between the bladder and the rectum.
3. The size and the shape of the uterus varies.
   a. Length—7.5 cm (3 in)
   b. Width—5 cm (2 in)
   c. Depth—2.5 cm (1 in)—a little smaller than a fist
4. The uterus consists of two sections, roughly divided in the middle at the isthmus.
   a. Upper portion
      (1) The corpus—the main body
      (2) The fundus—the dome-shaped portion located at the point at which the fallopian tubes enter the uterus
   b. Lower narrower portion—the cervix
5. The uterus is mobile and expands readily to accommodate a developing fetus.
6. The uterine artery is the main source of blood for the uterus.
7. The uterus is supported by the levator ani muscle and eight ligaments.
8. Major ligaments that help the uterus remain supported in midposition are the elastic broad ligaments, which act as "guide wires."
9. The position of the uterus within the pelvis varies (Figure 1.2).
   a. Anteverted/anteflexed—tilted toward the bladder
   b. Retroverted/retroflexed—tilted toward the rectum
   c. Midposition—found less frequently
   d. Positions do not affect fertility
10. Relationship of the uterine body to the cervix
    a. Anteflexed—the anterior surface bends toward the cervix
    b. Retroflexed—the posterior surface bends toward the cervix
11. Consequently, a uterus can commonly be anteverted (tilting toward the front) and anteflexed (the anterior portion bent).
12. The uterus is a freely movable organ suspended in the pelvic cavity and actual placement varies as the woman changes position.
13. The wall of the uterus consists of three layers.
    a. Perimetrium—the serous external peritoneal covering
    b. Myometrium—the middle muscular layer
    c. Endometrium—the inner layer of the cavity
       (1) The endometrium is controlled hormonally.
       (2) It is involved with menstruation or development of the placenta.

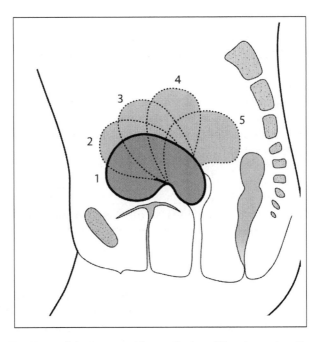

FIGURE 1.2 Positions of the uterus: (1) anteflexion; (2) anteversion, the normal position; (3) midposition; (4) retroversion; (5) retroflexion.

B. Description of the uterine cervix
   1. The uterine cervix is visible and palpable in the upper vagina and is a knob-like structure.
   2. It is smooth, shiny, and pink.
   3. It is firmer to palpation than the uterine corpus because it contains more connective tissue. (It feels like the tip of the nose.)
   4. It is covered by two types of epithelium.
      a. Squamous epithelium
         (1) The squamous epithelium is pink and shiny.
         (2) It is contiguous with the vaginal lining.
      b. Columnar epithelium
         (1) The columnar epithelium is deep red.
         (2) It is an extension of the lining of the endocervical canal.
   5. The cervical opening, the *external os*, connects the vagina to the endocervical canal, which connects to the body of the uterus.
   6. The size of the external os varies.
      a. The external os is a tiny, round opening in women who have not given birth vaginally.
      b. It is open, slitlike, and irregular in women who have had children vaginally.
      c. It becomes tight and tiny in postmenopausal women because of a decrease in estrogen levels.

C. Description of nabothian cysts
   1. The surface of the external cervix normally has endocervical glands that secrete mucus in response to hormonal stimulation.
   2. The ducts can become obstructed and cystic.
   3. The extent of obstruction varies from a few tiny cysts to large cysts covering the entire cervix.
   4. Nabothian cysts are common; however, infection may increase their number.
D. Description of endocervical canal
   1. The endocervical canal is open at both ends, connecting the external os to the internal os.
   2. The endocervical canal is about 2 to 2.5 cm (1 in).
   3. It is lined by columnar epithelium.
   4. The *ectocervix* is the cervical portion extending outward from the external cervical os.
      a. Anterior lip—the portion above the cervical os
      b. Posterior lip—the portion below the cervical os
   5. The *endocervix* is a narrow column, extending upward from the external os to the internal os of the uterine endometrium.
E. The cervical epithelium is composed of squamous and columnar epithelia.
   1. Squamous epithelium
      a. The squamous epithelium is smooth, shiny, and pink.
      b. It covers the ectocervix.
      c. It has four main layers, similar to the skin (Figure 1.3).
         (1) Basal layer—lies within the thin basement membrane. This layer has one or two cell layers.
         (2) Parabasal layer. This layer has three or four cell layers.
         (3) Intermediate layer. This layer is thicker than the parabasal and basal layers.
         (4) Superficial layer. This layer is composed of mature cells that continuously shed. It is the thickest layer.
         (5) The response to estrogen levels and presence of inflammation or infection of these four layers varies (see Chapter 23, "Methods to Detect Ovulation").
   2. Columnar epithelium
      a. The columnar epithelium is dark red and granular.
      b. It lines the endocervical canal.
      c. It secretes mucus.
   3. Squamocolumnar junction or transformation zone
      a. This junction is the boundary between the squamous and columnar epithelia.
      b. Squamous metaplasia occurs naturally as columnar epithelium is changed to squamous epithelium. (It is differentiated.)

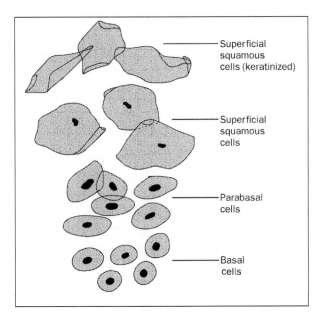

FIGURE 1.3 Layers of squamous epithelium.

   c. This area of metaplasia is the area of endocervical cells, which is critical to sample during the routine Pap smear because it is particularly susceptible to neoplastic changes.

   d. The location of this junction varies with hormonal variation.

      (1) In adolescents, the junction is visible on the external cervix.

      (2) The junction extends up the canal as estrogen levels decrease.

   e. It is termed *eversion, ectropion,* or *ectomy* if visible on the ectocervix as a granular, red, well-circumscribed area.

  F. Cervical mucus—changes in response to hormonal variations (Table 1.2)

TABLE 1.2 Comparison of Fertile and Nonfertile Cervical Mucus

OVULATORY FERTILE MUCUS	NONOVULATORY MUCUS
Clear to slightly cloudy	Opaque
Abundant	Scant
Stretchy, like raw egg white	Nonstretchy
Slippery	Rubbery
Dries without residue	Leaves white flakes when dry

V.   Vagina
   A.   Description of the vaginal canal
      1.   The vaginal canal is a fibromuscular canal about 7.5 cm (3 in).
      2.   It is located between the rectum, posteriorly, anterior to the urethra.
      3.   It is lined with squamous epithelia arranged in folds called *rugae*, extending from the cervix to the vestibule.
      4.   It extends from the vaginal opening on the outside of the body to the uterus.
      5.   The muscular coat of the vagina is much thinner than that of the uterus.
      6.   The uterine cervix enters and protrudes into the upper vagina, causing the formation of deeper rings around the cervix, called *fornices*.
      7.   The vagina can stretch and contract easily during intercourse or delivery.
      8.   It is usually pinkish red.
      9.   It does not contain any mucus-secreting glands.
         a.   It is moistened by cervical secretions.
         b.   Additional fluids percolate into the vagina from other fluid compartments during sexual arousal.
      10.   The blood supply of the vagina is carried by the vaginal branches of the uterine artery.
   B.   The function of the vagina is as a passageway.
      1.   Menstrual flow to exit the uterus
      2.   Fetus to be expelled from the uterus
      3.   Sperm to travel toward the egg
   C.   Vaginal ecology
      1.   The epithelium contains large amounts of glycogen.
      2.   Normal bacterial florae of the vagina consist of *Lactobacillus,* which metabolizes the glycogen.
      3.   Lactobacilli produce lactic acid.
      4.   Lactic acid helps maintain the vaginal pH as acidic, thus decreasing bacteria (see Chapter 31, "Vaginal Microscopy," for further explanation).
   D.   Hymen
      1.   The hymen is located at the outer opening of the vagina.
      2.   It is a folded membrane of connective tissue.
      3.   It may nearly occlude the vaginal opening in women who have never had sexual intercourse or who have never used tampons.
   E.   Bartholin glands
      1.   The Bartholin glands are two small, bean-shaped glands.
      2.   They secrete a mucousal substance that helps lubricate the vaginal canal.
      3.   They are located on either side of the vagina, deep in the labia minora.

F. Fornix
1. The fornix is a deep ring that posteriorly surrounds the cervix where it protrudes through the upper vagina.
2. It is comparatively thin walled and allows the ovaries and the uterus to be felt with palpation.
3. The fornix may act to pool semen after ejaculation, allowing a time-release effect as the sperm intermittently swim through the cervix.

VI. Pelvic support
  A. All the internal reproductive organs are supported in a sling-like fashion by ligaments that are covered by peritoneal folds.
  B. The pelvic and urogenital diaphragms provide support for the perineum.
    1. The pelvic diaphragm
      a. The pelvic diaphragm contains the levator ani and coccygeus muscle.
      b. It forms a broad sling within the pelvis that swings forward at the pelvic outlet to surround the vagina and the rectum as a form of sphincter.
      c. The pubovaginalis is the actual sphincter that acts as a sling for the vagina. It is the main muscular support of the pelvic organs.
      d. These muscles act as a diaphragm to close the lower end of the pelvic cavity.
      e. Levator ani are divided into the pubic and iliac portions.
      f. The pubic portion is a 2- to 2.5-cm band the fibers of which pass backward from the pubis to encircle the rectum with some fibers passing behind the vagina and supporting the lateral wall of the vagina.
      g. The normal resting tone of the muscles squeezes the rectum, vagina, and urethra closed by compressing them against the pubic bone.
      h. The pelvic floor muscles run like a hammock from the pubic bone in front to the tailbone in the back.
      i. The muscles and ligaments within the pelvis support the bladder, uterus, urethra, and rectum—they hold the organs in position and help them function properly.
      j. The iliac portion is a wide, flat, and sheet-like muscle that forms a shelf on which the upper pelvic organs rest.
      k. They function in combination in a swing-like fashion to maintain a constant low level of contraction for postural support of the internal organs.
    2. The urogenital diaphragm
      a. The urogenital diaphragm is the triangular area between the ischial tuberosities and the symphysis pubis.

    b. It contains urethral striated sphincter muscles, trigone fascia, and the inferior urogenital trigone fascia.

    c. It provides support for the lower urethra and the anterior wall of the vaginal canal.

VII. Uterine ligaments

A. Broad ligaments

    1. The broad ligaments are two worm-like structures extending from the lateral margin of the uterus to the pelvic walls, dividing the uterine cavity into anterior and posterior compartments.

    2. Cardinal ligament

        a. The lower portion of the cardinal ligament is composed of dense connective tissue that is firmly joined to the supravaginal portion of the cervix.

    3. The broad ligaments support the vagina and prevent uterine prolapse.

B. Round ligaments

    1. The round ligaments are fibrous cords.

    2. They attach to either side of the fundus, just below the fallopian tubes.

    3. They extend through the inguinal canal and end in the upper portion of the labia minora.

    4. They aid in holding the fundus forward.

C. Uterosacral ligaments (two)

    1. The uterosacral ligaments are cord-like structures.

    2. They extend from the posterior cervical portion of the uterus to the sacrum.

    3. They help support the cervix.

        a. The uterovesical ligament is a fold of peritoneum that passes over the fundus, extending to the bladder.

        b. The rectovaginal ligament is a fold of peritoneum that passes over the posterior surface of the uterus.

VIII. Associated pelvic organs

A. Bladder

    1. Location

        a. The bladder is located anteriorly in the pelvis, immediately posterior to the pubic symphysis.

        b. The upper surface is rounded and is covered by the peritoneum of the anterior wall of the pelvis.

        c. Posteriorly, it passes on to the uterus at the junction of the cervix and corpus.

        d. When the bladder is empty, usually the uterus rests on its superior surface.

e. The sympathetic nervous system controls detrusor relaxation and urethral and bladder neck contraction.
f. The parasympathetic system stimulates bladder contraction.
g. The somatic nervous system controls the external sphincter and the pelvic floor via the pudendal nerve.

B. Urethra
   1. Description
      a. The urethra is a small tube 2.5 to 5.0 cm long.
      b. It is 2 to 8 mm wide.
   2. The orifice lies between the labia minora, anterior to the vaginal opening and posterior to the clitoris.
   3. The urethra opens into the vaginal vestibule, about 2 cm posterior to the clitoris.
      For further information on the pelvic floor, bladder, and urethra, see Chapter 17, "Pelvic Organ Prolapse."

Bibliography

Bates, B. (2012). (written by Lynn Bickley, MD). *A guide to physical examination and history taking* (12th ed.). Philadelphia, PA: Lippincott.

Secor, M., & Fantasia, H. (2012). *Fast facts about the gynecologic exam for nurse practitioners.* New York, NY: Springer Publishing Company.

The Reproductive Cycle

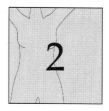

Helen A. Carcio

I. **Reproductive cycle**
   A. The female reproductive cycle is regulated through the highly co-ordinated functions of the brain, the hypothalamus, the pituitary, the ovaries, and the uterus.
   B. Each component must be in communication with the others to stimulate or suppress one of the other hormones.

II. **Hormonal influences explained**
   A. Two hormones affect the female reproductive tract. These hormones are directly concerned with gonadal function and, therefore, are classified as gonadotropic hormones.
      1. Follicle-stimulating hormone (FSH) stimulates the development of the follicles in the ovary, which leads to the ripening of the follicle, ovulation, and the secretion of estrogens.
      2. Luteinizing hormone (LH) stimulates the maturing follicle before its rupture.
      3. FSH stimulates the first part of the ovarian cycle; LH, together with FSH, influences preovulatory enlargement, ovulation, and development of the corpus luteum (Box 2.1).
   B. The ovary, under the influence of the gonadotrophic hormones, secretes two hormones: estrogen and progesterone.
      1. Basic function of estrogen
         a. Estrogen produces all the physical characteristics of a mature female.
         b. It helps prepare the endometrium of the uterus for implantation by a fertilized egg.
         c. It helps regulate the production and release of FSH and LH by the pituitary gland.
         d. It intensifies the effects of progesterone.
         e. Together with FSH, it helps promote the growth and development of the primary follicle.

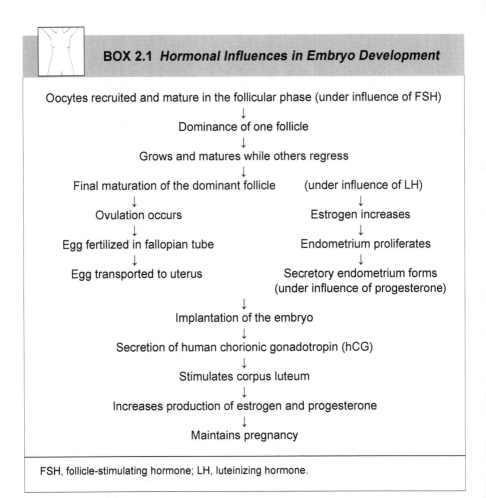

BOX 2.1 *Hormonal Influences in Embryo Development*

Oocytes recruited and mature in the follicular phase (under influence of FSH)
↓
Dominance of one follicle
↓
Grows and matures while others regress
↓
Final maturation of the dominant follicle   (under influence of LH)
↓   ↓
Ovulation occurs   Estrogen increases
↓   ↓
Egg fertilized in fallopian tube   Endometrium proliferates
↓   ↓
Egg transported to uterus   Secretory endometrium forms
                                             (under influence of progesterone)
↓
Implantation of the embryo
↓
Secretion of human chorionic gonadotropin (hCG)
↓
Stimulates corpus luteum
↓
Increases production of estrogen and progesterone
↓
Maintains pregnancy

FSH, follicle-stimulating hormone; LH, luteinizing hormone.

2. Basic function of progesterone
   a. After ovulation, progesterone prepares the uterus for pregnancy by promoting the growth of secretory endometrial cells.
   b. If pregnancy occurs, progesterone acts to maintain the placenta and inhibits uterine contraction to prevent abortion of the embryo.

III. Ovarian cycle
   A. Basics of the ovarian cycle
      1. During hormonal stimulation, the ovary undergoes many changes that result in the development and release of an ovum and in the formation of the corpus luteum.
      2. The ovarian cycle consists of the follicular phase, ovulation, and the luteal phase.

B. Follicular phase explained
1. At birth, each ovary contains about 400,000 primordial egg cells (oocytes).
2. These oocytes have a large nucleus with clear cytoplasm surrounded by theca and granuloma cells.
   a. Oocytes secrete fluid to create the ovarian blister.
   b. Theca cells are the primary source of circulating estrogens.
   c. Granuloma cells are the source of estrogens in the follicular fluid.
3. A *primordial follicle* comprises an egg cell and its surrounding cells.
   a. The production of primordial follicles stops around the time of birth of the fetus.
   b. The primordial follicles are considered permanent cells.
   c. Additional eggs are not produced throughout the woman's life cycle.
4. At the time of puberty, about 30,000 primordial follicles remain, which will either mature into eggs or disintegrate in the approximately 30 years of active ovarian activity between puberty and menopause.
5. In normally ovulating women, one egg will mature within a follicle each month, totaling between 300 and 400 eggs during the reproductive years.
C. Ovulation explained
1. As the egg matures and the fluid pressure increases, the egg and the follicle are naturally moved toward the outside of the ovary.
2. The mature egg and the follicular fluid are now called a *graafian follicle.*
3. At some point, the graafian follicle thins to the outside edge of the ovary and ruptures into the area outside of the ovary.
4. The fimbriated edges of the fallopian tube draw the egg toward the tube.
D. The luteal phase explained
1. Development of the corpus luteum
   a. After ovulation, the spot at which the egg ruptured transforms itself.
   b. The cells remaining in the follicle become filled with yellow material, and the follicle is now called the *corpus luteum.*
2. The development of the corpus albicans
   a. About 8 days after ovulation, the corpus luteum reaches full maturity.
   b. It slowly begins to evolve into a white body called the *corpus albicans.*
3. If conception and pregnancy occur, the corpus luteum increases in size and governs hormonal requirements during gestation, particularly for the first 4 months.

4. The principal hormone secreted by the corpus luteum is progesterone.
5. If conception does not occur, the progesterone secreted by the corpus luteum controls the postovulatory phase of the menstrual cycle for about 2 weeks.

IV. **The endometrial cycle**
    A. Basics of the endometrial cycle
        1. This section refers to cyclic changes in the *endometrium,* which comprises the cells lining the uterus.
        2. The endometrial cycle is broken into three phases: proliferative, secretory, and ischemic (menstruation).
        3. These cycles correspond directly to phases that are occurring in the ovary (Table 2.1).
    B. The proliferative phase explained
        1. At the end of menstruation, the endometrium is thin and considered ischemic.
        2. Within the second week of the cycle, hormonal production of estrogen increases and the endometrium becomes thicker.
        3. The cells undergo proliferative growth and become taller as the glandular cells become deeper and wider.
        4. This thickness can increase up to eight times.
        5. Glands of the endometrium become more active, secretory, and nutritive.
        6. At the same time, the follicles (i.e., theca cells) are producing more follicular fluid containing estrogen, which further primes the uterus.
        7. The proliferative phase is also called the *follicular phase* or *estrogenic phase* (to signify that the predominant hormone at this time is estrogen).
    C. The secretory phase explained
        1. The secretory phase comprises the last 2 weeks (days 14–28 after ovulation) of the cycle.
        2. After the egg is released from the follicle, the cells of the corpus luteum secrete progesterone, which governs the second half of the endometrial cycle.

TABLE 2.1 Comparison of Nomenclature for the Various Phases of the Reproductive Cycle

	PREDOMINANT HORMONE	OVARIAN CYCLE	ENDOMETRIAL CYCLE	MENSTRUAL CYCLE
Days 1–14	Estrogenic phase	Follicular phase	Proliferative	Menstrual (days 1–7)
Days 14–28	Progestational phase	Luteal phase	Secretory	Premenstrual (days 21–28)

3. Under the influence of progesterone and estrogen, the endometrial glands grow even more fluid filled and congested.
4. The blood supply of the endometrium increases, and the lining becomes filled with vacuoles and reservoirs that contain nutrient fluids.
5. The vascular arterioles become more spiral, twisted, and looped back, allowing for a nutritive layer if conception should occur.
6. Other names for this phase are *luteal* (referring to the ovary), *progestational* (referring to the dominant hormone), and *premenstrual* (see Table 2.1).

D. Menstruation explained
1. If conception does not occur, the function of the corpus luteum wanes and levels of progesterone and estrogen decrease.
2. The lining of the endometrium becomes ischemic and cell degeneration occurs.
3. As further cell degeneration occurs, the cells rupture, bursting small arterioles.
4. The deteriorated endometrium sloughs off the uterine wall and passes through the vagina.
5. Menstruation allows the endometrial wall to be rebuilt with each monthly cycle, ensuring a fresh new lining for each possible conceptus.
6. This phase is called the *ischemic phase* or *menstruation*.

V. **Hormonal regulation and feedback mechanisms (Figure 2.1)**
A. Each ovarian and endometrial cycle is regulated through the complex interaction of hypothalamic, pituitary, and ovarian hormones secreted in varying concentrations throughout the cycle.
B. To integrate the system, various feedback mechanisms organize the sequencing of hormones.
C. Within the hypothalamus, which is connected to the pituitary by a network of vessels called the *hypothalamic–hypophyseal (pituitary) portal system,* gonadotropin-releasing hormone (GNRH) is secreted.
D. GNRH moves down the portal system to control the secretion of FSH, LH, and gonadotropin from the anterior pituitary.
E. FSH is active in midcycle and controls the release of the ovum; LH is active in the luteal phase.
F. The hypothalamus is influenced by changes in neural and cerebral environments.
G. Prostaglandin also influences the cycle by influencing receptors in the hypothalamus.
H. At the start of each menstrual cycle, the pituitary secretes larger amounts of FSH, which, together with LH, promotes the maturation of several ovum follicles.
1. The emission of LH and FSH in combination promotes the secretion of estradiol, the most active estrogen and the primary estrogen of younger women.

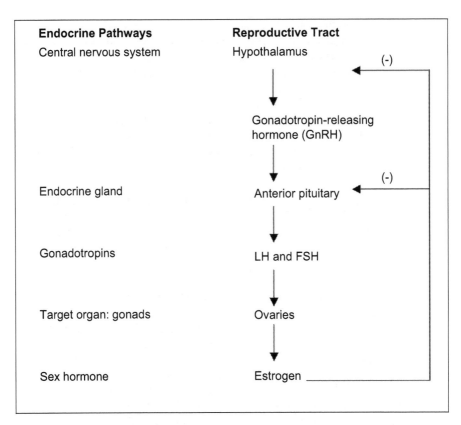

Endocrine Pathways	Reproductive Tract
Central nervous system	Hypothalamus
Endocrine gland	Anterior pituitary
Gonadotropins	LH and FSH
Target organ: gonads	Ovaries
Sex hormone	Estrogen

FIGURE 2.1 Feedback mechanism of the hypothalamic–pituitary–ovarian axis. Estrogen inhibits both the hypothalamus and the anterior pituitary.

   2. Blood levels of estradiol begin to increase, and these increasing levels of estradiol provide negative feedback on the hypothalamic–pituitary secretion of FSH.
   3. The level of FSH begins to decrease, but FSH continues to work on the follicle in combination with LH to ripen one follicle.
   I. On approximately day 12 (about 2 days before ovulation), most of the follicles that have ripened—except one—begin to degenerate or undergo atresia.
   J. The follicle that is most mature continues to grow and, in turn, estrogen activity increases markedly.
   K. Increasing amounts of estrogen secreted at this time promote secretion of GNRH (positive feedback), which causes LH and FSH to be released from the pituitary.
   L. This LH spike provides the final stimulus for maturation of the follicle, and ovulation takes place within 1 to 2 days.
   M. Changes in estrogen levels before ovulation prepare the cervical mucus to allow sperm to migrate up the reproductive tract.

N. Changes in mucus
   1. During the period immediately after menstruation, the mucus in the cervix is thick, scanty, and opaque.
   2. Around the time of ovulation, the mucus becomes much thinner, clear, and stretchable to allow the passage of sperm.
   3. *Spinnbarkeit,* or stretchability of midcycle mucus, provides a good clinical assessment of cyclic changes (see Chapter 23, "Methods to Detect Ovulation").
   4. Table 1.2 in Chapter 1, "Anatomy and Physiology of Female Reproduction," compares ovulatory with nonovulatory mucus.
O. After ovulation
   1. The ruptured follicle becomes a corpus luteum, which is supported by LH.
   2. The corpus luteum begins to secrete progesterone, and by days 19 to 21, progesterone secretion is at its maximum to prepare for implantation.
   3. Increased progesterone levels after ovulation inhibit the secretion of FSH and LH (negative feedback).
P. If implantation occurs, another hormone produced by the chorionic villi of the conceptus/trophoblast called *human chorionic gonadotropin* (the hormone assayed in pregnancy tests) converts the corpus luteum into a corpus luteum of pregnancy to maintain its function to support the developing pregnancy.
Q. If pregnancy does not occur, the corpus luteum deteriorates, progesterone levels decrease markedly, and, without hormonal support, the endometrium begins to degenerate and slough off as menstrual flow.

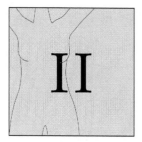

II

Health Assessment

The Health History   3

Helen A. Carcio and Paula Brooks

I. **Definition of sexual health**
   A. *Sexual health* is defined as the integration of somatic, emotional, intellectual, and social aspects of sexual beings in ways that are positively enriching and that enhance personality, communication, and love.
   B. It is multidimensional and involves sexual attitudes, behavior, practices, and activity.
   C. Its definition incorporates the whole person, including sexual thoughts, experiences, and values about being male or female. The three key elements of sexual health include
      1. A capacity to enjoy and control sexual and reproductive behavior in accordance with a personal and social ethic
      2. Freedom from fear, shame, guilt, false beliefs, and other psychological factors that inhibit sexual response and impair sexual relationships
      3. Freedom from organic disorders, diseases, and deficiencies that interfere with sexual and reproductive functions

II. **Elements of a comprehensive, developmentally relevant sexual health assessment**
   A. Interviewing to gather information about a patient's sexual history is an art requiring a grace and skill that can only come with practice.
   B. Sexuality underlies much of who and what a person is, and it is an inherent, ever-changing aspect of life from birth to death.
   C. The goal is to help a patient remember, identify, and verbalize.
   D. The sexual assessment must include a physiologic, psychological, and sociocultural evaluation, as well as elements that focus on age-related issues.

1. The physiologic component: Data should be gathered regarding the client's sexual response cycle (i.e., excitement, plateau, orgasm, and resolution) and any alterations in those phases. Also ask about
   a. Attempts to conceive
   b. Previous high-risk pregnancies
   c. Previous postpartum difficulties
   d. Contraceptive choices and any associated problems
   e. Data relating to past and present illnesses, surgeries, and medications
2. The psychological component: A woman's view of herself as female incorporates concepts of gender identity; the sense of having characteristics customarily defined as feminine, masculine, or both; and body image. Data should include
   a. The client's self-concept and body image
   b. Client's view of the self as a sexual being
   c. Level of confidence in ability to function sexually
   d. Past and current psychiatric problems or illnesses, including anxiety and depression
   e. Information about use of psychotropic medications
   f. Satisfaction with current relationship
   g. History of sexual abuse
3. The sociocultural component: A women's view of herself as female can be defined by her sociocultural upbringing and environment. Data should include
   a. Information about the client's perceptions of gender-appropriate roles for men and women in relationships and her perception of her ability to fulfill those roles competently
   b. Information about the client's religious affiliation and beliefs
   c. Information about the client's ethnic and cultural belief system
   d. The woman's sources of sexual education, when she received it, and her reactions to the information. It is always important for the health care provider to assess whether the information that the client received was correct and accurate.
E. Age-related issues
   1. Toddler and preschool child: Toddlers are able to identify themselves as "I'm a girl" or "I'm a boy," but they cannot integrate gender identity into their self-concept until they are 3 or 4 years of age, when they are able to understand that gender is a permanent condition.
      a. Children at this age are extremely curious. Assist parents in giving children the message that they and their bodies—including its sexual parts—are valuable and important.

    b. Family is the most important source of learning about sexuality issues in this age group, and the parents' attitudes and behaviors begin to shape feelings about sexuality.

    c. Provide parents with information about "normal" sexual behavior, and emphasize which developmental tasks are expected at approximate ages.

    d. Assist the parents in defining limits of appropriate and inappropriate behavior (e.g., it is not acceptable for a 3-year-old girl to discuss with a stranger on the bus the fact that she and her mother have vaginas but that her father and brother have penises).

    e. Stress the importance of teaching the child about appropriate and inappropriate touching from other people.

    f. Always assess for sexual abuse in all children in any health assessment.

2. School-age child: School-age children continue to have a high level of curiosity about sexuality, their bodies, and their environment, and, because they are aware of the pleasure stimulation gives, may actively seek sexual arousal.

    a. Masturbation and sex games are typical, and both homosexual and heterosexual encounters are commonly seen.

    b. By the time a child reaches school age, or about 8 years of age, he or she begins to understand the significance of sexuality. This is an important time for the clinician to start discussing pubertal changes with parents and to encourage parents to discuss these changes with their child.

    c. The same principles of inclusiveness and freedom from assumptions apply when taking a family history of a pediatric patient. A mother or father may be homosexual. The parent or parents may live alone, in a group house with other men or women, with the family of his or her origin, or with a partner.

    d. Children are now experiencing sexual activity at a younger age. Assess the child's understanding and activity. Begin to address these issues as you would during adolescence (see below).

    e. As in any age group, assess for sexual abuse.

3. Adolescence: Sexual awareness and changes in sexual feelings occur during adolescence.

    a. It is a time of developing a capacity for sexual intimacy, sexual curiosity, and experimentation.

    b. Adolescents are fitting their sense of sexual being into their evolving self-image and personal identity.

    c. They are learning about their bodies' sensual and sexual responses to stimulation and are developing a sense of the moral significance of sexuality. The sexual history that is gathered from adolescents is designed to

(1) Collect information

(2) Give the adolescent permission to ask questions and receive reliable information regarding issues of sexual concern.

- Reinforce privacy and confidentiality
- Communicate an aura of comfort with the client; create an atmosphere that is free of prejudice; and avoid imposing one's values.
- Assist the adolescent in feeling validated and comfortable revealing concerns and asking questions.
- Ask questions that give the message that you expect the client is changing and is aware of and curious about these changes (e.g., "How are you feeling?" "How's your body?" "Do you notice that you are getting taller?").
- Ask questions to give the message that you care about the client's feelings ("How does that make you feel?" "Do you wonder sometimes about what is happening to your body?").
- Always listen thoughtfully and carefully to the client's input, and respond positively by answering the client's questions as fully as possible while being calm, friendly, and open.

(3) Allow the health care provider to incorporate sexuality-specific education as a normal component of anticipatory guidance.

- Always give appropriate and factual information.
- Offer complete, accurate information conveyed in an open, professional manner.
- Assist the adolescent in understanding the physical, emotional, and psychological changes of puberty, and inform the client of the true risks associated with premature sexual activity.
- Ask questions to give the message that sexual changes are as expected and normal as other body changes ("Have you noticed your breasts getting any bigger?").
- Sexually transmitted diseases and vaginitis occur most frequently during the reproductive years and reach peak incidence during adolescence and young adulthood. For this reason, it is necessary for a health care provider to offer services, education, and counseling.

- Reinforce that sexual activity under the influence of alcohol or drugs can lead to unsafe sexual practices and the risk of unwanted intercourse, pregnancy, and sexually transmitted diseases.

(4) The American College of Obstetricians and Gynecologists (ACOG) recommends that the first visit to the OB/GYN for screening and preventive services begin between the ages of 13 and 15 years.

- The focus of this visit is education and does not include a pelvic examination unless indicated (see Section VI (b).

4. Early adulthood and the reproductive years (21–40 years of age): This is a critical period during which developmental tasks include achieving maturity in a sexual role and in the relationship tasks started in adolescence.

a. Many of the problems experienced by this age group in terms of sexual relationships involve poor communication between partners.

b. Major concerns in this age group include

(1) Balancing careers

(2) Raising children

(3) Nurturing and maintaining relationships

(4) Experiencing pregnancy, the postpartum period, and lactation

(5) Dealing with infertility

c. Assess use of safe sexual practices (monogamy, condom use), discuss family planning and contraceptive choices, and address fertility concerns.

d. Assist in facilitating communication between sexual partners, to teach clients about sexuality, and to clarify any misconceptions by providing information about sexual behavior, sexual activity, and sexual response.

e. Provide information about intercourse, good hygiene practices, and foreplay, and to reinforce the practice of health-promotion activities (i.e., breast self-examinations, yearly Pap smears).

5. Middle adulthood (41–65 years): This is a critical period for expanded sexual freedom and major physiologic changes.

a. The primary tasks of midlife and later years are

(1) Reappraisal, which includes a review of past and present accomplishments

(2) Reassessment of goals and life direction

(3) Redirection of energies or rededication to life's goals

b. Most women have established their careers and families by midlife. The children are often grown, and responsibilities of the mother may be decreased. More time can now be spent focusing on herself and her partner.

    c. During this period, women experience menopause (around the age of 50 years in the United States). Many fear the loss of sexual attractiveness and capacity.

    d. Health problems of either partner can be a major source of concern during these years.

III. **Advanced health history techniques**

    A. The interview: The gynecologic interview is primarily intended for gathering information. For many women, this may be the woman's sole source of preventive health care. Therefore, the purpose of this visit is fivefold.

      1. Provides information to develop problem lists, diagnoses, and plans

      2. Screens for other existing or potential health problems

      3. Provides general health maintenance and prevention of illness

      4. Establishes a relationship between the care provider and the patient

      5. Sets a tone for the entire visit and for subsequent visits

    B. Patient–practitioner interaction is an equal partnership.

      1. Each partner contributes expertise.

      2. The provider has knowledge about health and health care in general.

      3. The patient has knowledge about her history and her body.

      4. When a practitioner expresses respect for what the patient brings to the encounter, the setting and implementation of common goals become possible.

        a. Expressing respect through verbal communication: This begins with the introduction.

          (1) Always go into the waiting area to call the patient rather than having the receptionist bring the patient into the examination room. This allows the patient to meet the practitioner for the first time while the patient is fully dressed. This sets a more personal tone and promotes a feeling of equality in the patient–practitioner relationship.

          (2) Determine how each wants to be addressed. Many practitioners establish relationships with patients on a first-name basis. This is both equal and personal. However, others may find this disrespectful. Ask the patient how she wants to be addressed (e.g., first name, last name, Ms., Mrs., or Miss). Some practitioners are most comfortable being called Ms., Mrs., Miss, or Mr.; consequently, the patient should be addressed in an equivalent manner.

        b. Expressing respect through nonverbal communication, including facial expressions, eye contact, posture, and, when appropriate, touch

    (1) Smiling: When appropriate, smiling conveys warmth and caring.

    (2) Eye contact: Maintaining eye contact by frequently looking up from writing or waiting to write until the end of a conversation sends a message of interest. A practitioner who continually looks down at the chart or stares off into space establishes social distance.

    (3) Posture: Sitting up in one's seat or leaning toward the patient creates an impression of interest.

    (4) Touch: Touching may or may not be appropriate. Be aware that touch has meaning; use it to instill trust rather than distrust. In our culture, a handshake is always a respectful form of physical contact. However, other cultures find touching intrusive. Be aware of cultural norms, and use this information to guide your practice.

  c. Expressing respect through the environment: When possible, try to positively manipulate the environment.

    (1) Use round tables or couches and chairs rather than sitting behind a desk to conduct the interview. This eliminates the feeling of authority emanating from the behind-the-desk posture.

    (2) Ensure privacy by shutting the doors and pulling the curtains. If this is not possible, at least ensure "psychological privacy" by using a soft voice and avoiding any interruptions.

5. Be aware of your own sexual biases: To provide adequate sexual health care, the health care provider must

  a. Be aware of his or her own sexual biases

  b. Be comfortable with his or her sexuality

  c. Have a genuine desire to help the client

  d. Understand that personal barriers may prevent clinicians from comfortably addressing sexual issues

    (1) It is critical to address any barriers and not make assumptions about a woman's sexual behavior, feelings, or attitudes.

  e. Continually monitor personal responses to detect negative or embarrassed feelings that may easily be conveyed to the client.

6. Setting the stage

  a. Choose a private location where the client is comfortable, and assure her that the information will be held in strict confidence.

  b. Sufficient time must be given to build trust and develop a rapport before soliciting information that the client may consider highly personal or intimate.

    c. Avoid obtaining a sexual health history when the client is experiencing an acute health problem.

    d. Obtain permission to ask questions in this potentially sensitive area: "I would like to ask you some questions about your sex life. I don't mean to embarrass you and it's okay if you'd rather not answer some of them. May I begin?"

7. Begin with open-ended questions: Ask open-ended questions at the beginning of the interview and at the beginning of each of its sections.

    a. This gives the practitioner a chance to assess the language used by the patient and reveals the concerns that are most important to the patient.

    b. More pointed questions can then be asked to specify the conditions that are important for the practitioner to know about.

8. Avoid using excessive medical terminology: Language must be understood clearly by both the provider and the client.

    a. Make sure that both you and the client know the meaning of the terms used.

    b. Sometimes it may be helpful to use technical and nontechnical words in the same question: "Have you ever had hypertension or high blood pressure?"

9. Avoid euphemisms: Inclusive language should be used while taking the patient history and going through the review of systems.

    a. Follow a standard procedure, ask every patient the same questions, and make no assumptions.

    b. Avoid wording such as "slept with."

    c. Use gender-neutral terms to refer to significant others, such as "partner" or "spouse."

    d. Frame inclusive questions when asking about sexual activity, but when the questions are pertinent to the complaint or workup, make inclusive questions about the sexual activity as specific as possible.

    e. Rather than using the words "coitus" and "intercourse," or the even more vague "sexual activity" or "sexual relations," inquire about "oral sex," "anal sex," and "vaginal intercourse (or) sex."

    f. If the client does not understand, describe the behavior being asked about (e.g., "Have you ever taken a man's penis into your rectum or mouth?").

    g. Most practitioners are uncomfortable discussing sex, particularly specific sexual acts. The only way to overcome such discomfort is through routine exposure.

10. Universalizing: Universalizing should be used only in appropriate situations.

    a. Prefacing questions with phrases such as "Many people" or "Research shows that" may make the client feel more comfortable when answering sensitive questions.

    b. Do not presume a client is heterosexual because the patient discusses an opposite-sex spouse or has children.

    c. Sexual orientation and sexual behaviors encompass a broad spectrum; the astute clinician recognizes that outward appearances may not be definitive.

    d. Do not assume that a woman who identifies herself as a lesbian is having sex only with women.

    e. Avoid labels that the patient does not use. For example, people who might acknowledge same-sex sexual behavior may not identify themselves as homosexual.

11. Move from simple to complex items: Always begin the interview with least threatening material and explain to clients the purpose of the questions. This approach will help build trust and rapport.

    a. A general guideline is to begin with questions about the individual's sexual learning history, such as childhood sexual education; then proceed to personal attitudes and beliefs about sexuality; and finally, assess actual sexual behaviors.

IV. Special approaches to sexual health history

    A. A thorough sexual health history is the cornerstone of accurate diagnosis and identification of health risk factors and lays the foundation for health promotion. There are three basic types of sexual health histories:

    1. Initial or comprehensive history: A comprehensive sexual history is a detailed history that encompasses all aspects of sexual information about the individual, as well as his or her family of origin, siblings, and significant relationships.

        a. The initial or comprehensive history includes information concerning

        (1) Each phase of sexual development

        (2) Body image

        (3) Learned attitudes

        (4) Feelings relating to sexuality

        (5) Sexual debut

        (6) Sexual orientation

        (7) Range of sexual behaviors

        b. The purpose of this type of history is to create an accurate and complete account of the patient's health status.

        c. It is a lengthy process that may not be accomplished at the first visit or with a single interview.

    2. A well-interim history: This history focuses on in-depth family and lifestyle information and is used to form the basis of health maintenance and health promotion.

3. A systematic or problem-focused history: This type of history is obtained when the patient presents with a specific symptom. The focus is to gather information regarding the patient's current health problems and any confounding health factors.

   a. The systematic history focuses on the presenting symptom or assessment of specific behaviors, such as the risks for becoming pregnant or the acquisition of sexually transmitted diseases.

   b. Problem-oriented sexual histories: These histories are shorter, more direct, and specific to the immediate issue.

      (1) Indications that make it necessary to conduct the problem-focused pelvic examination:

      - Information obtained from the history, with or without symptoms
        - Maternal diethylstilbestrol (DES) exposure
        - Multiple (contemporaneous or serial) sexual partners
        - Unexplained infertility
      - New or recurrent sentinel symptoms
        - Change in character, frequency, regularity, or duration of menses
        - Midcycle, postcoital, or postmenopausal vaginal bleeding
        - Lower abdominal pain or swelling, especially when it is unilateral
        - Painful sexual intercourse (dyspareunia)
        - Vulvar or vaginal pruritus
        - Change in quantity or character of vaginal discharge
        - Urinary incontinence
        - Burning or pain on urination (dysuria), with or without diagnosed urinary tract infection
        - Lower back pain or any symptoms that bear consistent relationship to menstrual cycle
        - Unexpected onset of menarche or menopause
        - Bilateral lower limb edema (unexplained)

V. **The reproductive health history**

A. Preconception care and counseling: The goal of preconception counseling is to optimize the health of the woman and the health of her potential infant. To reach this goal, the National Institutes of Health expert panel recommends that preconception counseling begin prior to 1 year before conception of a planned pregnancy (see Chapter 7, "Assessment of the Pregnant Woman").

   1. Preconception assessment data: Includes history, physical examination results, and laboratory data

a. History

   (1) A complete medical, social, reproductive, and family history must be obtained.

   (2) Information should be specific to the client's family, medical, reproductive, and drug history, and HIV risk factors.

   (3) Nutrition and lifestyle choices should also be evaluated.

   (4) The use of a comprehensive screening tool, such as the sample prenatal genetic screen, can be useful (see Appendix 3.1).

b. Physical examination

   (1) Should include screening, evaluation and counseling, and immunizations based on age and risk factors

   (2) A complete physical examination, including a routine breast and pelvic assessment, should be performed, along with a Pap smear, cultures for gonorrhea and chlamydia, and a wet smear evaluation depending on the patient's age and sexual activity.

     • The ACOG recommends that the annual pelvic examination be performed on patients 21 years of age or older and include cervical cancer screening.

     • Data does not support the necessity of performing a pelvic examination prior to initiating oral contraceptives in an otherwise healthy, asymptomatic patient under the age of 21 years.

c. Laboratory testing

   (1) Rubella titer and antibody screen

   (2) Serology for syphilis

   (3) Complete blood count (CBC) with indices

   (4) Blood type and Rh

   (5) Random blood sugar

   (6) Urinalysis

   (7) If sickle cell disease or thalassemia is a concern, hemoglobin electrophoresis should be performed.

   (8) Screening for viral diseases, such as HIV, human papillomavirus (HPV), hepatitis, cytomegalovirus (CMV), or toxoplasmosis, should be encouraged.

   (9) For those under 21years of age, nucleic acid amplification testing on urine samples or vaginal swabs are acceptable for gonorrhea and chlamydial, yeast, trichomoniasis, and bacterial vaginosis infections.

2. Client education and counseling

a. Menstrual cycles and basal body temperature (BBT): Advise client to keep accurate record of her menstrual and ovulation cycles to help establish gestational dating (see Chapter 26, "The FemCap™").

   b. Exercise and nutrition
      (1) Vitamin and mineral supplements
      (2) Folic acid supplementation
      (3) Ideal weight before conception
      (4) Exercise program to improve cardiovascular status and
          impart a feeling of overall well-being
      (5) Balanced diet
   c. Avoidance of teratogens: Warn the client that potential
      teratogens can be related to occupation and lifestyle
      (see Appendix 3.2). These teratogens can include
      (1) Cleaning solutions
      (2) Hair coloring and perms
      (3) Photography solutions
      (4) Radiation
      (5) Chemicals used in processing food and textiles
      (6) Drugs, including prescription, over-the-counter, and
          recreational drugs
   d. Affirmation of pregnancy decision: Stress that the couple
      needs time to affirm the decision to attempt pregnancy.
   e. Readiness for parenthood: Assess the couple's social,
      financial, and psychological readiness for pregnancy and
      commitment to parenthood.
   f. Identification of unhealthy behaviors: Assist the couple in
      identifying and altering unhealthy behaviors, such as
      (1) Smoking
      (2) Alcohol consumption
      (3) Drug use—prescription, over-the-counter, and illegal
          drugs
   g. Treatment of medical conditions: Ensure that medical
      conditions that may jeopardize the pregnancy outcome are
      evaluated. Refer the couple to a specialist as needed.
   h. Identification of genetic risk (Appendix 3.1).
      (1) Indications for genetic counseling
          • Women who are pregnant or are planning pregnan-
            cies and will be 35 years of age or older at delivery
          • Couples or individuals who have had a previous
            fetus or child with a genetic disorder, birth defects, or
            mental retardation
          • Individuals who have or are suspected to have a
            genetic disorder
          • Individuals who have a parent with a genetic disorder
          • Couples or individuals with a family history of a
            genetic disorder, birth defects, mental retardation,
            learning disabilities, cancer, or other conditions
          • Families with members who have been diagnosed
            with the same mental or physical condition

- Couples or individuals with a history of pregnancy loss or miscarriages, or with unexplained infertility
- Individuals who are known carriers of a genetic disorder
- Couples or individuals of specific ethnic backgrounds known to have a higher incidence of certain disorders
- Women who were exposed during or before pregnancy to teratogenic drugs, infections, x-ray studies or radio therapy, or occupational hazards
- Couples who are first cousins or close blood relatives
- Women planning to undergo amniocentesis or chorionic villus sampling
- Women with abnormal findings at fetal ultrasonography
- Women with abnormal results on prenatal screening tests

i. Preconception classes: Where appropriate, refer the couple to community adult educational resources for preconception classes, such as

(1) March of Dimes

(2) Prenatal, pregnancy, birth, and after-childbirth classes

(3) Parent training and sibling relations classes

(4) Cardiopulmonary resuscitation (CPR) classes

(5) Couple to Couple League

(6) Pursuing Parenthood class

(7) Parent Encouragement Program, which offers classes on parenting, marriage, and families

j. Laboratory tests: Order all appropriate laboratory tests, evaluate the results, and discuss the findings and their implications with the client.

k. Appropriate vaccinations

(1) Rubella. If the client is not immune, administer the vaccine and advise the client to wait 3 months before attempting conception.

(2) Tetanus

(3) Hepatitis

l. Special dietary needs: If the client has special dietary needs (vegetarian, cultural, diabetes, overweight, underweight), refer her to a dietitian. Women are highly motivated to improve their nutritional status when planning a pregnancy.

VI. **Techniques for screening for sexual abuse**

A. Screening for sexual abuse is imperative when obtaining any health assessment (see Chapter 18, "Urinary Incontinence" and Chapter 19, "The Sexual-Assault Victim").

VII. HIV risk assessment

A. HIV is transmitted by the exchange of infected body fluids, including blood and semen. High-risk behaviors include

1. Sexual activity: Unprotected intercourse with multiple partners. Homosexual men are at greatest risk, but all sexually active people are at risk depending on the risk factors of, and number of, sexual partners.
2. Intravenous (IV) drug abuse
3. Persons who received blood products before 1985. Highest risk is for those who received blood transfusions between 1975 and March 1985.
4. Hemophiliac clients who received pooled plasma products
5. Children of HIV-infected women
6. Health care workers (e.g., those at risk for accidental needle sticks)

B. Questions to include

1. Are you a health care worker? Have you ever been stuck by a contaminated needle?
2. Do you have sex with men, women, or both?
3. How many partners have you had in the past year?
4. Have you had intercourse without a condom? When did you start using condoms?
5. Have you performed oral sex on a man or a woman without a barrier (such as a dental dam, plastic wrap, or a condom)?
6. Have you been treated for a sexually transmitted disease?
7. Do you smoke cigarettes, drink alcohol, or use other drugs?
8. Have you had unprotected sex while under the influence of alcohol or other drugs?
9. Have you had sexual partners who are at high risk for HIV (e.g., those who have a high-risk sexual history or needle-use history)?
10. Do you, or have you in the past, injected drugs?
11. Have you shared hypodermic needles, other drug equipment, or other skin-piercing or cutting instruments with another person (for injection drug use, steroid use, vitamin injection, tattooing, body piercing, or scarification)?
12. Do you use crack cocaine? If yes, have you had sex in crack houses?
13. Have you received a tattoo from an unlicensed tattoo artist or when you were not sure that the needle used had been properly sterilized?
14. Did you, or do you, receive any blood transfusions or have you undergone surgery (most important between 1975 and 1985)?

C. Components of the history when assessing an HIV-positive individual (see Appendix 3.3). The patient with HIV infection requires an initial evaluation, ongoing psychosocial support, and medical assessment. A complete history is needed, and questions should be directed to gather information specifically about HIV-related illnesses, vaccination history, history of sexually transmitted diseases, and assessment of HIV transmission category (please refer to Section IX for sample questions to ask to obtain this information). The history should include

1. Medical history, including information on cardiovascular disease; pulmonary disease; gastrointestinal disease; renal disease; neurologic disease; cancer; endocrine disease; ear, nose, and throat disease; liver disease; skin disease; chicken-pox or shingles; viral hepatitis; bacterial infections; gyneco-logic problems; exposure to tuberculosis; and psychiatric treatment (outpatient or inpatient treatment)

2. Current medications and treatments: Over-the-counter drugs, vitamins, and, especially, immunosuppressive therapy (e.g., in an asthmatic patient who intermittently requires corticosteroids)

3. Identification of when a patient's acute HIV illness occurred, which may be helpful in determining the patient's prognosis
   a. At least half of all HIV-positive patients may report a history of acute HIV infection, which presents clinically as a mild to severe mononucleosis-like illness lasting 1 to 2 weeks.
   b. The incubation period (time from exposure to onset of illness) for the acute syndromes may range from 5 days to 3 months but is usually 2 to 4 weeks.
   c. Symptoms include fever, diaphoresis, malaise, myalgia, arthralgia, pharyngitis, retro-orbital headaches, and, in some patients, lymphadenopathy or aseptic meningitis.
   d. Other less common manifestations of acute HIV infection include a history of polyneuropathy, brachial neuritis, and odynophagia with esophageal ulcers.

4. Common HIV-related illnesses: Oral candidiasis (thrush), persistent diarrhea, varicella zoster (shingles), oral hairy leu-koplakia, *Pneumocystis carinii* pneumonia, recurrent bacterial pneumonia (in 12 months), cryptococcal meningitis, toxoplas-mosis, Kaposi's sarcoma, candidal esophagitis, disseminated *Mycobacterium avium* complex, CMV infection, and tuberculosis

5. HIV-related symptoms: Fever, night sweats, changes in sleep pattern, changes in appetite, weight loss, stomach pain, vomit-ing; diarrhea, skin rashes or lesions, oral thrush or ulceration, painful swallowing, swollen lymph nodes, unusual headaches, difficulty thinking, chest pain, cough, shortness of breath, numb-ness or tingling in hands or feet, muscle weakness, changes in vision; and changes in neurologic function or mental status

6. Vaccination history: Measles, mumps, rubella (MMR), last tetanus booster, HPV, hepatitis B, and pneumococcal vaccine

    a. Tuberculosis history should include information on any known exposure to tuberculosis, date of last purified protein derivative (PPD) test, and history of positive PPD test result. If positive, was prophylaxis given? If yes, what was the duration and type?

7. Sexually transmitted diseases: Information about possible contact with syphilis, gonorrhea, genital herpes, chlamydia, condyloma (warts), HPV, gastrointestinal parasites, hepatitis B, and trichomoniasis. The history should also include

    a. Questions about where the patient has lived and traveled

    b. Questions about current sexual practices (type and number of sexual partners). Specifically, a sexual history should be taken to assess the patient's current sexual practices and to determine whether sexual partners are aware of the patient's possible HIV status and have been tested for HIV.

    c. Questions about the types of contraception used

    d. Questions about past or present IV drug use

    e. Questions about behaviors that might lead to further transmission of HIV

8. Drug use: Active IV drug users should be asked about their drug-using practices; their source of needles; whether they share needles and, if so, with whom.

9. Psychosocial history

    a. Depression is common among HIV-infected patients, and the history should include questions that focus on changes in

      (1) Mood

      (2) Libido

      (3) Sleeping patterns

      (4) Appetite

      (5) Concentration

      (6) Memory

    b. Patients should also be asked specifically about whom they have informed of their HIV status, how they have been coping with the diagnosis of HIV infection, and what types of support they have been receiving.

    c. It is important to know about the patient's family, living situation, and work environment and how these have been affected by the diagnosis of HIV infection.

10. Assessment of the patient's level of awareness about HIV infection and treatment

    a. Evaluate the patient's educational needs, and determine the form that such support might take.

    b. Assessment of patient education should include information on safer sex guidelines, use of condoms and spermicide, and safe versus unsafe practices.

    c. Drug use and abuse must be discussed and must include issues of needle sharing, the use of bleach to sterilize needles, and drug treatment options.

VIII. Sample questions and screening tools
  A. General initial history
    1. Sexual activity: When were you last sexually active? Have you had sex in the past few months?
    2. Sexual orientation: Are you intimate with males, females, or both?
    3. Number of partners: How many sexual partners do you or did you have? How long have you been with your current partner? Quantify the number and sex of sexual partners over the past few months or years.
    4. Types of sexual activity: Do you or did you have vaginal, anal, or oral sex? If anal or oral, ask Do you give it or receive it, or both?
    5. Pregnancy and contraception: Do you desire to become (make your partner) pregnant? Is it possible that you are (she is) pregnant now? What are you doing to prevent pregnancy?
    6. Sexually transmitted diseases: Do you have vaginal discharge, itching, or pain on urination? Do you have any sores or lumps? Have you or any of your partners ever been treated for a sexually transmitted disease? Which one? How long ago? Do you or any of your partners have risk factors for HIV or AIDS, such as blood transfusions, IV drug use, frequent sex with multiple partners or strangers, sex for money or drugs?
    7. Protection from sexually transmitted diseases: Do you or did you use a condom or other protection during sex or when you have had sex in the past? If no, ask Why not? Do you ever have sex without protection? How recently?
    8. Violence and abuse: Have you ever been hurt or abused by your partner? Have you ever been raped? If the answer is "yes," assess the situation.
    9. Satisfaction: Is sex satisfying for you? If no, ask Why not?
    10. Sexual concerns: Do you have any problems with or concerns about your sexual function?
  B. Comprehensive adolescent sexual history
    1. Background data: Age (birth date), parents' ages, parents' religion, parents' educational levels, parents' occupations, parents' marital status, amount of affection in relationship (parent to parent), feelings toward parent or parents
    2. Childhood sexuality: What were your parents' attitudes about sexuality when you were a child? In what way did your parents handle nudity? Who taught you about sex? From whom did you learn about sex play, pregnancy, intercourse, masturbation, homosexuality, venereal disease, birth? When do you first recall

seeing a nude person of the same sex? Of the opposite sex? How often did you play doctor–nurse or engage in other sex play with another child? Tell me about any other sexual activity or experience that had a strong effect on you.

3. Adolescent sexuality: How old were you at your first period? Onset of breast development? When did pubic hair appear? What were the characteristics of onset of menstruation (age, regularity of periods; initially, now)? What hygienic method do you/did you use (pads, tampons)? How were you prepared for menstruation? By whom? What were your feelings about early periods? Later periods? Have you had unusual bleeding?

4. Body image: How do you feel about your body? What about your breasts and genitals? How much time do you spend nude in front of a mirror?

5. Masturbation: How old were you when you began? What were others' reactions to your masturbation? What methods do you use? What are your feelings about masturbation? Do you fear that you are overdoing it?

6. Necking and petting: How old were you when you began? How often? How many partners do you currently have?

7. Intercourse: How often have you had intercourse? How many partners? How often do you initiate sex? How often are you currently having sex? How often have you had oral sex?

8. Contraceptive use: What kind of contraceptives have you used? What are you using now?

9. Homosexuality: What does it mean to you to be homosexual? How many homosexual persons have you known? How often have you had homosexual feelings? Have you and how often have you been approached? How often have you had homosexual experiences? What kinds of experiences? What were the circumstances?

10. Seduction and rape: When have you seduced someone sexually? When has someone seduced you? Have you been raped? Have you raped someone? How often have you forced someone to have sex?

11. Incest and abuse: What kinds of touching did you receive in your home? From your mother? Father? Brother? Sister? Other relatives?

12. Prostitution: What feelings do you have about prostitution? Have you ever accepted money for sex?

13. Venereal disease: How old were you when you learned about venereal disease? Have you ever had a venereal disease? Gonorrhea? Syphilis?

14. Pregnancy: Have you ever been pregnant? At what age? How was the pregnancy resolved—miscarriage, abortion, adoption, marriage, single parenthood?

15. Abortion: What are your feelings about abortion? Have you had an abortion? If yes, at what age? What were your feelings? What about your feelings now? What about your feelings immediately afterward? What about your feelings after 1 year?

C. Content areas of reproductive health history for adolescent females
   1. Menarche
      a. Age of onset
      b. Duration of flow: How many days do your periods usually last?
      c. Frequency: How often do you have your period? Do you keep track of them by using a calendar?
      d. Date of last normal menstrual period (LNMP): When was the date of your LNMP?
      e. Dysmenorrhea: During your periods, do you ever have cramps? If so, does it affect your activities or school attendance? Do you use any remedies and medications? What is the name of the drug, the dosage, and the frequency of ingestion?
   2. Sexual activity
      a. Age of sexual debut: Have you had in the past or are you currently having sex? If so, at what age did you have your first sexual experience? (Some youths may not have initiated intercourse and are seeking services before sexual debut [volitional or coerced].) Has anyone ever touched you on any part of your body where you did not want to be touched? (Issues of past sexual abuse or date rape by an acquaintance may be important areas of discussion.)
      b. Sexual orientation: Who do you find yourself most attracted to, men or women, or both? (Allows youth to respond to feelings of attraction and does not connote a behavior such as actually having intercourse with a same-sex individual.) Have you ever had sex or been sexually intimate with a person of your sex?
      c. Frequency of coitus: How often do you have sex? Once a month? Once a week? Twice a week? (Allow adolescents a range of choices.) What was the last episode of intercourse?
      d. Number of sexual partners: How many partners have you had in the past 2 months? How many in the past year? How many since you first started having sex? Have you had prior sexual contact with a sexual partner or intravenous drug user?
      e. Sexual practices: Include questions that involve a full range of sexual expression, including activities such as kissing, touching, masturbation (solo or mutual) to oral, vaginal, and anal intercourse. To counsel youth regarding safer sex practices, the clinician must be aware of the teen's entire repertoire of behaviors.
      f. Sexual pleasure: Is having intercourse or sex pleasurable for you? Are you satisfied with your sexual life the way it is now? Do you think your partner is satisfied?

3. Contraceptive use
   a. Current method of birth control used: It may be helpful to list the choice of specific methods (e.g., foam, condoms, withdrawal or "pulling out," birth control pill). Ask the teen the frequency with which she uses a method (e.g., never, sometimes, always). Ask whether she has any perceived or real side effects from using a specific method. Ask whether a condom is used with new partners.
   b. Communication skills regarding use of contraception: Are condoms or other barrier methods used as a method of fertility control or to prevent the transmission of sexually transmitted diseases?
4. Obstetric and gynecologic
   a. Number of pregnancies: List the exact number and outcome, including number of live births and spontaneous and therapeutic abortions.
   b. Recent gynecologic procedures: Dilation and curettage (D&C), recent abortion, complications after the procedure
   c. History of pelvic inflammatory disease: When did the disease occur, and where was it treated? Did you have inpatient or outpatient management?
5. Sexually transmitted diseases
   a. History of previous sexually transmitted disease: Type, date, type of treatment.
   b. Was your partner treated?
6. Drugs
   a. Onset, duration, and frequency of use: Ask about the use of cigarettes, alcohol, or illicit drugs. Ask about intravenous, inhalation, or injection drug use. Inclusion of this information is essential in the assessment of behaviors that may place the client at risk for HIV infection.
7. Partner
   a. Partner involvement: Is the adolescent female's partner involved in the visit today? Was there prior discussion regarding contraception or other topics?
   b. Male partner sexually transmitted disease assessment: Ask whether the male partner has any symptoms of infection. Include symptoms of urethritis (discharge or dysuria), any open sores, or warts on the genital region.
8. Support system
   a. Parents and friends: Who is aware of your sexual activity? Have you experienced any potential negative effects regarding disclosure of your behavior to parents or friends? Have you had any support?

D. Adolescent sexual problem history
1. Have the adolescent describe the sexual concern, problem, issue, or difficulty: How do you feel about discussing this problem? How long have you had it? When did this problem begin? What do you think caused you to have this problem? What might be contributing to this problem? What kinds of things have you done to treat or solve this problem? What health professionals have you seen? What, if any, medications have you taken or are you taking? Have you talked to a friend or relative? Have you read any books to solve this problem? What books?

Bibliography

American College of Obstetricians and Gynecologists. (2012). Well-women visit. Committee opinion no 534. *Obstetrics and Gynecology, 20,* 421–424.

Bates, B. (2012). (written by Lynn Bickley, MD). *A guide to physical examination and history taking* (12th ed.). Philadelphia, PA: Lippincott.

MacLaren, A. (1995). Primary care for women: Comprehensive sexual health assessment. *Journal of Nurse Midwifery, 40*(2), 104–119.

Secor, M., & Fantasia, H. (2012). *Fast facts about the gynecologic exam for nurse practitioners.* New York, NY: Springer Publishing Company.

APPENDIX 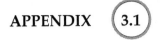 3.1

Sample Prenatal Genetic Screen

1. Will you be 35 years or older when the baby is due?   Yes ❑   No ❑

2. Have you or has the baby's father or anyone
   in either of your families ever had any of the
   following disorders?
      Down syndrome (mongolism)   Yes ❑   No ❑
      Other chromosomal abnormality   Yes ❑   No ❑
      Neural tube defect, spina bifida   Yes ❑   No ❑
      (meningomyelocele or open spine), anencephaly
      Hemophilia   Yes ❑   No ❑
      Muscular dystrophy   Yes ❑   No ❑
      Cystic fibrosis   Yes ❑   No ❑
      If yes, indicate the relationship of the affected person
      to you or to the baby's father.

3. Do you or does the baby's father have a   Yes ❑   No ❑
   birth defect:
   If yes, who has the defect and what is it?

4. In any previous marriages, have you or has the   Yes ❑   No ❑
   baby's father had a child, born dead or alive,
   with a birth defect not listed in question 2?
   If yes, what was the defect and who had it?

5. Do you or does the baby's father have any close   Yes ❑   No ❑
   relatives with mental retardation?
   If yes, indicate the relationship of the affected person
   to you or to the baby's father: Indicate the cause, if known.

6. Do you or does the baby's father or a close relative   Yes ❑   No ❑
   in either of your families have a birth defect, any
   familial disorder, or a chromosomal abnormality
   not listed above?
   If yes, indicate the condition and the relationship of the
   affected person to you or to the baby's father.

7. In any previous marriages, have you or has the   Yes ❑   No ❑
   baby's father had a stillborn child or three or more
   first-trimester spontaneous pregnancy losses?

8. Have either of you undergone a chromosomal   Yes ❑   No ❑
   study?
   If yes, indicate who and the results.

9. If you or the baby's father is of Jewish ancestry,   Yes ❑   No ❑
   have either of you been screened for Tay-Sachs
   disease?
   If yes, indicate who and the results.

10. If you or the baby's father is Black, have either of   Yes ❑   No ❑
    you been screened for sickle cell trait?
    If yes, indicate who and the results.

11. If you or the baby's father is of Italian, Greek, or   Yes ❑   No ❑
    Mediterranean background, have either of you
    been tested for beta thalassemia?
    If yes, indicate who and the results.

12. If you or the baby's father is of Philippine or South-   Yes ❑   No ❑
    east Asian ancestry, have either of you been tested
    for alpha thalassemia?
    If yes, indicate who and the results.

13. Excluding iron and vitamins, have you taken any   Yes ❑   No ❑
    medications or recreational drugs since being preg-
    nant or since your last menstrual period? (Include
    nonprescription drugs.)
    If yes, give name of medication and time taken
    during pregnancy.

APPENDIX (3.2)

Environmental Exposure History Form

1. Have you ever worked at a job or a hobby in which you came in contact with any of the following by breathing, touching, or ingesting (swallowing)? If yes, please place a check beside the name.

Acids	Ethylene dichloride	Pesticides
Alcohols (industrial)	Fiberglass	Phenol
Alkalies	Halothane	Phosgene
Ammonia	Isocyanates	Radiation
Arsenic	Ketones	Rock dust
Asbestos	Lead	Silica powder
Benzene	Manganese	Solvents
Beryllium	MDI (methy-lenediphenyl	Styrene
Cadmium	diisocyanate)	Toluene
Carbon tetrachloride	Mercury	TDI (toluene
Chlorinated naphthalenes	Methylene chloride	diisocyanate)
Chloroform	Nickel	Trichloroethylene
Chloroprene	Polybrominated	Trinitrotoluene
Chromates	biphenyls (PBBs)	Vinyl chloride
Coal dust	Polychlorinated	Welding fumes
Dichlorobenzene	biphenyls (PCBs)	x-rays
Ethylene dibromide	Perchloroethylene	Other (specify)

2. Do you live next to or near an industrial plant, commercial business, dump site, or nonresidential property?   Yes ❑   No ❑

3. Which of the following do you have in your home?   Yes ❑   No ❑
   Please circle those that apply.

Air conditioner	Electric stove (gas or oil?)
Air purifier	Wood stove
Central heating	Humidifier
Gas stove	Fireplace

4. Have you recently acquired new furniture or carpet, refinished furniture, or remodeled your home?   Yes ❑   No ❑

5. Have you weatherized your home recently?

6. Are pesticides or herbicides (bug or weed killers; flea and tick sprays, collars, powders, or shampoos) used in your home or garden, or on pets?   Yes ❑   No ❑

7. Do you (or any household member) have a hobby or craft?   Yes ❑   No ❑

8. Do you work on your car?

9. Have you ever changed your residence because of a health problem?   Yes ❑   No ❑

10. Does your drinking water come from a private well, city water supply, or grocery store?   Yes ❑   No ❑

11. Approximately what year was your home built?   Yes ❑   No ❑

If you answered yes to any of the questions, please explain.

APPENDIX (3.3)

Summary of Critical Issues in the HIV Initial History

HIV testing

When did the patient first have a positive test result for HIV?

Where was the first test conducted that resulted in positive HIV status?

What was the reason for being tested?

Does the patient have documentation of a positive enzyme-linked immuno-sorbent assay (ELISA) and Western blot test results?

Has the patient ever had a negative HIV test result?

What is the patient's usual source of health care?

What is the patient's most recent CD4 cell count (if known)?

Medical history

Cardiovascular disease

Pulmonary disease

Gastrointestinal disease

Renal disease

Neurologic disease

Cancer

Endocrine disease

Ear, nose, and throat disease

Liver disease

Obstetric and gynecologic illness

Skin disease

Chickenpox or shingles (varicella)

Psychiatric treatment

HIV-related illnesses

Oral candidiasis (thrush)

Persistent diarrhea

Varicella zoster (shingles)

Oral hairy leukoplakia

Pneumocystis carinii pneumonia

Recurrent bacterial pneumonia (in 12-month period)

Cryptococcal meningitis

Toxoplasmosis

Kaposi's sarcoma

Candidal esophagitis

Disseminated *Mycobacterium avium* complex

Cytomegalovirus (CMV) infection

Tuberculosis

Invasive cervical cancer

Other HIV-related illnesses

Vaccination history

Measles, mumps, rubella (MMR)

Last tetanus booster

Hepatitis B

Hepatitis A

Pneumococcal vaccine

Tuberculosis history

Any known exposure to *M. tuberculosis*

Date of last PPD test

History of positive PPD test result?

 If yes, was prophylaxis given?

  If yes, duration and type?

Sexually transmitted diseases

Syphilis

Gonorrhea

Genital herpes

Chlamydia (nongonococcal urethritis [NGU] or cervicitis)

Condyloma (warts)

Gastrointestinal parasites

Hepatitis B

Trichomoniasis

Pelvic inflammatory disease (PID)

Gynecologic history

Has the patient ever been pregnant?

　If yes, how many:

　　Full-term pregnancies

　　Premature births

　　Miscarriages or abortions

　　Living children

Have there been any pregnancies since the patient has learned of her HIV status?

What was the beginning date of the client's last menstrual period?

Was the last menstrual period normal?

Is the patient pregnant now?

　If yes, was a prenatal care referral made?

Does the patient use a birth control method?

　If yes, specify what type.

When was the patient's last Pap test? Was it normal?

Medication

Current medications and treatments (include over-the-counter drugs and vitamins)

Habits

Does the patient smoke or has the patient smoked in the past? (Inquire about quantity.)

Does the patient use alcohol or has the patient used alcohol in the past? (Inquire about quantity.)

Does the patient use drugs or has the patient used drugs in the past? (Specify what type and the quantity used.)

HIV transmission category

Homosexual contact

Heterosexual contact

Injection drug use

Transfusion recipients (dates and location)

Hemophilia

Unknown

Patient education

Safe-sex guidelines (condoms, spermicide); safe versus unsafe practices. Is the patient sexually active?

If yes, is the partner or partners aware of the patient's status?

Has the partner (or partners) been tested for HIV?

If so, were the results positive? (Inquire about drug use [needle sharing, bleach].)

Was treatment referral offered?

Review of systems

Has the patient had any of the following symptoms in the past 3 months?

Unexplained weight loss

Swollen lymph nodes

Night sweats

Fevers

Unusual headaches

Changes in appetite or sleep pattern

Trouble thinking

New skin rash or spots on the skin

Sores or white spots in the mouth

Pain when swallowing

Chest pain, cough, or shortness of breath

Stomach pain

Vomiting or diarrhea

Numbness or tingling in the hands or feet

Muscle weakness

Changes in vision

The Physical Examination

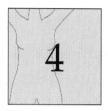

Helen A. Carcio

I. **A complete physical examination is an integral part of the health assessment of women. Components of the examination include assessment of**
   A. The thyroid gland
   B. Body habitus, including fat and hair distribution
   C. Breast examination (see Chapter 6, "Assessment of the Female Breast").
   D. Abdominal examination
   E. Pelvic examination

II. **The examination of the thyroid gland. Thyroid dysfunction can cause irregular menses, anovulation, and infertility.**
   A. Anterior approach: Examiner stands in front of the patient
      1. The woman is asked to extend her head and neck slightly.
      2. As the woman swallows, using your fingerpads, palpate below the cricoid cartilage for the isthmus of the thyroid.
      3. Ask the woman to flex her head and neck slightly forward to her right. This relaxes the sternocleidomastoid muscles, enhancing palpation.
      4. Place right examining thumb on upper portion of the left lobe, and displace the gland to anatomic right, while hooking the tips of the index and middle fingers of left hand behind right sternocleidomastoid muscle, and palpate deeply in front of the muscle with left thumb for the right lobe.
      5. Reverse and repeat procedure for the left side.
      6. The isthmus may be palpable, but the thyroid gland itself is usually not visible or palpable.
   B. Posterior approach
      1. Examiner stands behind the patient, who is seated.
      2. Instruct patient to slightly flex her chin toward her chest.
      3. Place fingerpads of both hands around the patient's neck.

    4. Palpate the isthmus by placing fingerpads in the midline of the neck, below the cricoid cartilage.

    5. Compare the right and left lobes by sliding your fingerpads laterally, below the cricoid cartilage, on either side of the tracheal rings.

    6. Ask the patient to tilt her head to the left as you displace the right lobe to the left (medially) with the right hand.

    7. Palpate the left lobe as patient swallows, using the fingerpads of the left hand.

    8. Reverse the procedure to examine the right lobe.

C. Thyroid-stimulating hormone (TSH) testing is indicated if

    1. Anomaly of the thyroid gland is palpated

    2. In the presence of associated signs or symptoms

    3. During an infertility workup, as indicated

    4. If galactorrhea is present or hyperprolactinemia is suspected (Hypothyroidism is present in 3% to 5% of women with hyperprolactinemia.)

D. Note

    1. Motion of isthmus as the woman swallows. Thyroid tissue rises with swallowing; this movement is noticeable with an enlarged gland.

    2. Compare lobes for contour, consistency, or tenderness as the patient swallows.

E. Normal findings

    1. The thyroid gland is usually not palpable.

    2. The isthmus may be felt as a band of tissue that obliterates the tracheal rings.

    3. No nodules or enlargement of the lobes should be felt.

III. **The breast examination (see Chapter 6, "Assessment of the Female Breast")**

IV. **Abdominal examination**

A. A thorough abdominal examination should precede the gynecologic examination and include assessing any palpable masses or tenderness, including inguinal lymph nodes.

B. Conducting the abdominal exam before the gynecologic examination often helps reduce some of the anxiety associated with having the gynecologic examination and may serve to "break the ice." Make sure hands are warm!

C. Position

    1. Supine, with examiner on right.

    2. Closely monitor the woman's expressions for signs of discomfort.

D. If the woman is ticklish, begin examination with her hand under the examiner's hand.

E. Inspect the abdomen for diastasis recti.
1. Is there a separation of the abdominal rectus muscles from pregnancy, multiparity, congenital weakness, or marked obesity?
    a. Ask the patient to raise her head and hold it above the pillow for 5 seconds, tensing the abdominal muscles.
    b. Note the location and length of any midline separation between the contracted muscles.
    c. Abdominal muscles should be tight together.
F. Inspect the contour and shape of the abdomen.
G. Observe for the presence of striae.
1. Striae are lines seen after normal skin has been excessively stretched.
    a. Linea alba from the stretching of the skin from pregnancy
    b. Purple lines associated with Cushing's disease
H. Palpate the lower abdomen for tenderness in the presence of pelvic pain.
I. Palpate the inguinal lymph nodes.
1. The nodes may be enlarged in the presence of herpes simplex virus.
    a. Note size, shape, mobility, consistency, temperature, and tenderness of the nodes. Refer for any hard, immobile nodes.
    b. Nodes are soft and tender in a patient with herpes.

V. **The pelvic examination explained**
A. The approach
1. The approach to the gynecologic examination must be systematic, thorough, and carried out in a calm, relaxed manner. Encourage the woman to give verbal feedback throughout the examination.
2. The pelvic examination should follow other parts of the physical examination in order to allow the woman time to become comfortable with the examiner. However, sometimes the woman is so anxious that it is best to proceed with the examination first to "get it over with."
3. Ask the patient to empty her bladder before the examination.
4. Determine whether this is her first pelvic examination. A woman undergoing a first pelvic examination is far more anxious than a woman who has undergone the examination previously. (Also remember that anxiety can increase if any previous pelvic examination was not a positive experience.)
5. Observe for signs that indicate increased anxiety as the client assumes the supine position. For example, the patient
    a. Holds or wrings hands
    b. Covers eyes or has eyes shut

      c. Places hands on shoulders
      d. Places hands over pelvis
      e. Places hands on thighs
      f. Places hands so she can hold the table
  6. Explain each aspect of the examination thoroughly before and as it is performed in order to reduce the woman's level of anxiety. Always be as gentle as possible.
      a. Explain the rationale for each aspect of the examination and provide information about what a woman might feel during the examination (e.g., "You might feel some pressure when I insert my fingers into your vagina.").
      b. Suggest coping strategies to deal with any stress the woman may be experiencing.
      c. Encourage patient to progressively relax different body parts or to try taking deep breaths and exhaling slowly at any point during the examination that she might feel tense.
      d. Teach how to use statements to herself, such as "I know this is uncomfortable but I will be fine."
      e. Reassure her that you will stop anytime she becomes uncomfortable.
  7. It is often a good idea to offer an "educational" pelvic examination by explaining about the techniques used, the sensations that the patient may feel, and the function of body parts examined.
  8. Offer the patient a mirror (a telescoping-handled type is best) so she can view her vulvar area. Such measures help patients feel more in control at a time when they may feel especially vulnerable and apprehensive.
      a. Some women are very interested in seeing their cervix, whereas others are not interested or are even "turned-off."
  9. The woman should be encouraged to give verbal feedback throughout the examination so that the examiner can be informed of any maneuvers that cause particular discomfort. This feedback will help maximize the client's cooperation and minimize anxiety regarding the examination.
  10. Explain that the whole examination should take no longer than a few minutes.
  11. Acknowledge that the woman may feel rather awkward, but she should not experience any pain unless certain conditions are present, such as herpes.
  12. The examiner may offer an alternative to the traditional pelvic examination (Table 4.1).
  13. Table 4.2 summarizes common pelvic examination problems.
B. Draping
  1. The issue of draping can be left to the woman.
  2. If draping is used, the drape should cover the patient's lower abdomen and thighs.

TABLE 4.1 Alternatives to the Traditional Pelvic Examination

ALTERNATIVE EXAMINATION	REASON
Bimanual examination without use of speculum	Only indicated for patients at low risk Perform a bimanual examination Digitally locate cervix Slide cotton swab adjacent to finger Rotate the swab over cervix several times Preliminary data support efficacy despite lack of endocervical component
Ultrasound	Virginal woman at low risk Can identify other problems, such as uterine fibroids or ovarian cysts
Sedation	Recommended for the disabled woman who cannot tolerate the examination; may use 2–8 mg/kg ketamine, 0.2–0.4 mg/kg midazolam

3. The drape should be depressed in between the knees in order to allow the patient and examiner an opportunity to see each other's faces.

4. It often helps to have the sheet draped so that the corner forms a triangle between the legs.

C. Position: The patient should be asked to assume a comfortable lithotomy position on the examination table.

1. For some women, the semisitting position is often preferable to the supine. Advantages of this position are summarized in Box 4.1.

2. Position the patient's legs in the stirrups, with buttocks slightly overhanging the end of the table.

3. The patient should be asked to keep her knees widely separated and her buttocks flat on the table. Women tend to push against their heels in the stirrups, unknowingly raising the buttocks off the table and tightening their pelvic floor muscles. Remind the patient to take the pressure off her heels.

4. The woman's hands should be across her chest or at her sides. These positions help enhance abdominal relaxation.

D. Equipment

1. A good light, either freestanding or attached to a plastic speculum

2. Vaginal speculum (metal or plastic)

3. Water-soluble lubricant (not always necessary)

4. Supplies for the Pap smear and cultures as indicated.
Note: Gloves should be worn throughout the examination and afterward when handling any equipment used. Some authorities recommend double gloving.

TABLE 4.2 Common Pelvic Examination Problems and Interventions

PELVIC EXAMINATION PROBLEM	INTERVENTIONS
Extreme anxiety	Step-by-step desensitization, relaxation techniques, deep breathing, Kegel then bear down, antianxiety meds, counseling
Inability to insert speculum due to discomfort	Use Pederson or small speculum, or use a small swab to collect samples for Pap, sexually transmitted infections (STIs), wet mount, deep breathing Consider urine testing for STIs
Inability to insert speculum due to dryness	Palpate introital tissues, or palpate cervix before speculum insertion Apply scant lubricant to tip of speculum
Inability to insert speculum due to small and/or tight introitus	Use small, Pederson speculum or nasal speculum, Kegel and bear down, or use dacron swab, encourage deep/slow breathing
Inability to visualize cervix	Palpate cervix before speculum exam, move speculum side to side (shimmy), change angle slightly, instruct patient to bear down, try larger speculum, open wider
Vaginal walls impede visualizing cervix	Apply condom over speculum (cut off tip) Use larger blade speculum such as Graves or Clinton, open wide Guttman, or "Snowman" lateral vaginal wall
Inability to view cervix because of extreme posterior position	Use large, extra-long speculum, such as "Clinton Pederson" open wide Palpate cervix before Push down on suprapubic area Instruct patient to bear down Lift hips, spread thighs, knee stirrups
Speculum comes out unless clinician holds it	Seek an assistant to hold the speculum while you collect specimens, remove speculum, then prepare tests
Patient unable to tolerate speculum in situ secondary to anxiety and/or pain	Collect samples, remove speculum, then prepare tests Remember, samples are stable on sampling tools
History of sexual abuse and extreme phobia of pelvic exams—with or without vaginismus	Co-manage with a specialized counselor Use step-by-step desensitization program May not be able to complete a pelvic exam for several visits (may take months or years)

Source: R. Mimi Secor © 2009.

BOX 4.1 *Advantages of the Sitting Position During a Pelvic Examination*

- More comfortable for the patient
- Relaxes the rectus and abdominal muscles
- Increases eye contact
- Allows the woman to hold the mirror more easily
- Enables the patient to feel less vulnerable

VI. Inspection of the external genitalia

A. Some comments

1. Examination of the external genitalia is conducted before the internal speculum and bimanual examinations.
2. The examiner should sit on a stool at the end of the table facing the client.
3. Position the light to obtain maximum illumination of the peritoneum.
4. Inspection begins by viewing the suprapubic and inguinal regions superiorly, and then progressing inferiorly to include the clitoral hood, clitoris, urethral meatus, vaginal introitus, fourchette, and posteriorly, the anal and sacral areas.
5. Visual inspection of the genitals is also conducted in a medial to lateral fashion, from the vaginal introitus laterally to the labia minora, labia majora, and upper and inner thigh regions. A thorough visual inspection also includes gentle palpation as needed to view overlapping tissues.
6. A saline-moistened cotton-tipped applicator may also be used to separate overlapping skin surfaces (and to assess for areas of tenderness) and is particularly helpful in examining the labia and introital and hymenal structures.
7. Always remember to touch the thigh gently before actually touching the genitals.
8. For physical changes related to genital atrophy, see Chapter 12, "Atrophic Vaginitis, Vulvovaginal Atrophy."
9. For assessment of pelvic organ prolapse, see Chapter 17, "Pelvic Organ Prolapse."

B. Assess the mons pubis to determine the dermatologic condition of the pubic hair and underlying skin.

1. Note general hygiene, hair distribution, and any lesions.
2. Normal findings: Clean, coarse pubic hair extending in an inverse triangle, with the base over the mons pubis. No lesions should be present.

3. Clinical alterations
   a. Dirty-appearing hair shafts from pediculosis
   b. Localized inflammation at the base of the hair shaft caused by folliculitis
   c. Scaly epidermal plaques from psoriasis
   d. Sparse hair associated with hormonal problems or advancing age
   e. Racial variations
      (1) Blacks: Shorter hair that is more tightly coiled.
      (2) Asians, Native Americans, and Alaskan Natives: Hair is generally sparser.
   f. *Phthirus pubis* (lice) or their eggs (nits). Bites seen as small red maculopapules.
C. Tanner staging
   1. Pubic hair growth begins between 8 and 14 years of age.
   2. Staging should be assessed in adolescent girls as an assessment of the maturity of the pituitary–ovarian axis. It should be performed as routinely as possible.
D. Quantify the signs of androgen excess.
   1. *Hirsutism* is defined as the presence of hair in a location where hair is not commonly found in women. Hair varies due to ethnic and racial factors.
   2. Hair morphology and distribution should be graded. The most functional and widely used instrument is the Farriman-Galloway (F-G) scale, which semiquantitatively grades hair growth in nine body areas.
   3. Cinical alterations
      a. More than 10% of adult women have hair that extends up the abdomen to the umbilicus. This distribution is usually associated with racial variations
      b. Absent or scant hair distribution may indicate endocrine dysfunction.
      c. Mild hirsutism associated with polycystic ovarian syndrome (sideburns, chin, chest, and lower abdomen).
E. Inspect the vulva for genital lesions.
   1. Note cysts, warts, chancres, ulcerations, and areas of hyperpigmentation.
   2. Normal findings: Labia majora are hair-covered epidermal surfaces; labia minora are pink, glistening mucosal surfaces. Hart's line is present.
   3. Clinical alterations.
      a. Nontender, firm nodules of sebaceous cysts
      b. Micropapillomatosis labialis
         (1) Can be differentiated from condyloma, in which multiple papillae converge toward a single base, each finger-like papillomatous projection having its own base.

      (2) Often related to chronic infections, such as trichomonas or candidiasis.
- **c.** Wartlike protrusion singly or in clusters from condyloma acuminatum or condyloma latum
- **d.** Genital warts
- **e.** Round, clear umbilicated vesicles of molluscum contagiosum
- **f.** Nontender chancre with a well-demarcated border from primary syphilis
- **g.** Chancroid
- **h.** Single or clustered, tender vesicles or ulcerations of genital herpes
- **i.** Irregular, nontender hyperpigmented lesions related to carcinoma of the vulva
- **j.** Genital mutilation associated with certain cultures
- **k.** Varicosities associated with pelvic congestion (pregnancy)

F. Inspect the vulva for discoloration and pigmentation.
- **1.** Normal findings: Pink with varying shades of white, brown, and red, depending on racial characteristics
  - **a.** Usually the same color as the skin covering the external parts of the rest of the body.
  - **b.** Color due to fine network of superficial blood vessels located just below the thick epidermal layers of the skin and the amount of melanin.
- **2.** Clinical alterations
  - **a.** Redness or erythema occurring in response to inflammation
    - **(1)** A reddened vulva with no specific lesions suggests extensive vaginal discharge that is irritating the delicate vulvar skin.
    - **(2)** Dilatation of blood vessels and edema occur in such inflammatory conditions as *Candida* infection, seborrheic dermatitis, and psoriasis.
  - **b.** Dark or pigmented lesions usually caused by increase in the amount or concentration of melanin
    - **(1)** Dark lesions require biopsy study to exclude the diagnosis of malignant melanoma.
    - **(2)** Most dark lesions are either harmless freckles or nevi.
    - **(3)** Routinely monitor nevi because of their potential to develop into melanoma.
  - **c.** White lesions are related to
    - **(1)** Decreased vascularity
    - **(2)** Depigmentation (decrease in melanocytes in the basal layer)
    - **(3)** Changes in the keratin in the presence of moisture. (The presence of water turns the keratin white, as if a hand or foot was soaked in water for 10 to 20 minutes.)
    - **(4)** Common conditions that cause white lesions are lichen sclerosus and squamous hyperplasia.

G. Examine the external genitalia for any bruises that might indicate sexual assault.
H. Examine the clitoris.
  1. Note the size.
  2. Normal findings: Round, pink erectile tissue under the fourchette. Approximately 2 cm (0.75 in) in length and 0.5 cm in width.
  3. Clinical alterations
    a. Enlargement in masculinizing conditions, excess testosterone secretions, and use of testosterone-containing medications
    b. Atrophy to the point of disappearance with lichen sclerosis
I. Inspect the urethral orifice.
  1. Note erythema or purulent discharge.
  2. Normal findings: Pink tissue without discharge
  3. Clinical alterations
    a. Caruncle associated with estrogen deprivation is seen as a small red protrusion through the orifice. It resembles a polyp.
    b. Prolapse of the urethral mucosa, which forms a swollen red ring around the urinary meatus. This condition is often associated with menopause.
    c. Leaking of urine associated with stress incontinence.
J. Examine the vaginal orifice.
  1. Note presence of discharge, hymen, and bulging of vaginal tissue or cervix through the orifice.
  2. Normal findings: Small amount of white to clear discharge; intact hymen or hymenal remnant surrounding the orifice; no bulging.
  3. Clinical alterations.
    a. Discharge secondary to vaginitis or cervicitis
      (1) Perform wet mount evaluation on any discharge present (see Chapter 31, "Vaginal Microscopy").
    b. Thick, pink membrane overlying the vaginal orifice from an imperforate hymen
    c. Anterior bulging of vaginal tissue through the orifice from a cystocele
      (1) A cystocele is the prolapse of the bladder against the anterior vaginal wall.
      (2) It is generally related to the weakening of vaginal and pelvic support due to childbirth.
      (3) It is aggravated by obesity.
    d. Posterior bulging of the vaginal tissue from a rectocele
      (1) A rectocele is the prolapse of the rectum against the posterior vaginal wall. It is generally related as above.
  4. It is sometimes useful to draw a diagram of any anomalies.

K. Inspect perineum and anus.
  1. Posterior skin of the perineum between the vaginal introitus and the anus should appear smooth.
  2. If woman had an episiotomy, a scar may be visible.
  3. Note any skin tags, fissures, or hemorrhoids in anal area.

VII. Palpation of the external genitalia
  A. Some comments
    1. Avoid startling the patient by telling her when she will be touched and where.
    2. Palpation of the external genitalia is conducted using a gentle approach and, if tenderness is elicited, a cotton-tipped applicator may be used to assess more specifically the location and severity.
    3. Placing the finger beneath the urethra along the anterior vaginal wall may help identify the presence of a urethral diverticulum or express any material that might be present in the Skene's glands.
    4. During palpation of the introitus, obese and parous patients may also be asked to perform a Kegel contraction followed by a Valsalva maneuver to assess tone and laxity of the pelvic musculature and to detect any degree of cystocele or rectocele.
    5. Avoid excessive "fingering" of the genitalia, which otherwise might be interpreted as sexual.
  B. Assess Bartholin's glands and Skene's glands.
    1. Technique: Insert index finger into the vagina with thumb remaining outside on the posterior portion of the labia majora. Press thumb and index finger together at the 5 o'clock and 7 o'clock positions of the lateral labia minora.
    2. Note any swelling, masses, discharge, or tenderness.
    3. Normal findings: Skene's and Bartholin's glands are normally not palpable. The surface should be homogenous, nontender, and without discharge.
    4. Clinical alteration: Varying degrees of enlarged gland from a Bartholin's cyst. Marked warmth and tenderness may indicate an abscess.
    5. If discharge is present, a gonorrheal culture (GC) should be performed because gonorrhea may cause a Bartholin's abscess.
  C. Assess paraurethral gland and urethra.
    1. The technique: Insert the gloved hand slowly into the vagina, palm upward. Exerting upward pressure, remove finger, milking the urethra.
    2. Note discharge from the urethra or paraurethral glands, or any tenderness.
    3. Normal findings: Negative discharge
    4. Clinical alteration: Purulent discharge related to gonococcal or chlamydial urethritis.

   D. Evaluate vaginal wall support.
   1. Technique: Spread the vaginal orifice with thumb and forefinger, and ask patient to bear down. Assess any degree of prolapse. You may also ask woman to cough.
   2. Note any anterior or posterior bulging of the vaginal wall. Some leakage of urine from the urinary meatus may also be noted during this maneuver.
   3. Normal finding: No protrusion through the vaginal orifice.
   4. Clinical alterations
      a. Anterior bulging of vaginal tissue in varying degrees through the introitus indicating a cystocele or cystourethrocele.
      b. Posterior bulging. A rectocele will balloon upward toward the introitus during the Valsalva maneuver.
      c. Cervix visible at the opening, which may indicate a uterine prolapse.
   E. Assess pelvic muscle tone (see Chapter 17, "Pelvic Organ Prolapse").
   1. The pelvic floor muscles are attached to the pubic bone in front and the tail bone in back. Their character and strength are easily accessed during the vaginal digital examination (see Figure 4.1).
      a. Place one finger 2 cm inside the woman's vagina. Palpate the pelvic floor muscle at 5 o'clock. Ask her to tighten her pelvic floor muscle by contracting her rectal muscles. Repeat maneuver in the 7 o'clock position.
      b. Compare strength.
   2. Examiner should feel upward pressure on the fingers.
   3. Normal findings: Maintains tension for 5 seconds.
   4. Clinical alteration. Impaired strength due to
      a. Vaginal deliveries (traumatic or multiple)
      b. Older age, particularly with decreased estrogen levels in women not receiving hormone replacement
      c. Neurologic impairment such as multiple sclerosis
   5. Impaired tone may cause urinary or fecal incontinence.

VIII. The bimanual examination
   A. Special considerations
   1. Any pelvic mass detected during the bimanual examination should be described in terms of its position, motility, consistency, and size in centimeters.
   2. It is very important for the patient to relax completely because voluntary guarding of the abdominal musculature will prevent effective palpation of any pelvic organs.
   3. Controversy exists regarding which portion of the pelvic examination should be performed next. Many clinicians believe that the bimanual examination should precede the speculum examination. There are many advantages (Box 4.2).

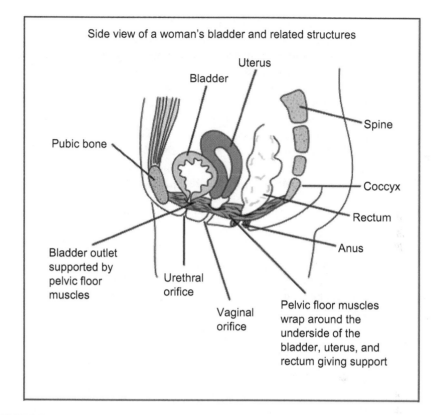

Side view of a woman's bladder and related structures

Uterus

Bladder

Spine

Pubic bone

Coccyx

Rectum

Anus

Bladder outlet
supported by
pelvic floor
muscles

Urethral
orifice

Vaginal
orifice

Pelvic floor muscles
wrap around the
underside of the
bladder, uterus, and
rectum giving support

FIGURE 4.1 Note how the urethral and vaginal orifices and rectum pass through the strap of the pelvic muscles.

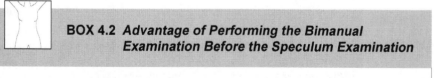

BOX 4.2 *Advantage of Performing the Bimanual Examination Before the Speculum Examination*

- Able to use woman's own vaginal secretions for lubrication
- Facilitates insertion of the speculum
- Eliminates use of messy gels
- Clues the examiner to palpated anomalies that require further inspection
- Perceived by the patient as less invasive
- Helps the inexperienced clinician determine the position of the cervix in order to make insertion of the speculum and location of the cervix easier

a. This technique helps facilitate the insertion of the speculum, because the woman's own vaginal secretions can be used as a lubricant, thus eliminating the use of messy gels.

b. Water applied to the gloved hand may be used in place of a lubricant.

      c. Once any anomalies are palpated, they can be thoroughly inspected during the speculum examination. Most lesions within the deep folds of the vagina are better palpated than visually inspected.

      d. When the bimanual examination is performed before the speculum examination, the clinician can better determine the position of the cervix, which makes the speculum insertion easier for both the patient and the clinician.

      e. Gentle palpation may be perceived as less invasive to the woman than inserting the speculum first.

      f. A disadvantage of this technique is the possibility of mixing cervical and vaginal flora together, altering the accuracy of any subsequent vaginal microscopic analysis.

    4. The bimanual examination involves using both hands, with one inside the vagina and the other hand palpating the pelvic structure through the abdominal wall.

    5. It is very important that the patient be relaxed during the bimanual examination because guarding and tightening of the abdominal muscles will greatly alter the examiner's ability to palpate the underlying structures beneath the rigid musculature.

    6. A metal speculum can be warmed by keeping it on a heating pad or running it under warm water.

    7. Some clinicians touch the blades of the speculum to the inside of the client's thigh before insertion to let the client know what it feels like and to be sure that the temperature is comfortable.

    8. A virginal orifice easily admits a single examining finger. Modify the technique so as to use the index finger only. Should the orifice be too small, a single finger in the rectum can be used for a fairly accurate bimanual examination. Be sensitive to the invasiveness of the procedure.

    9. Box 4.3 lists the advantages and disadvantages of using a plastic speculum.

  B. Technique

    1. Stand between stirrups.

    2. Insert the index and middle fingers of your gloved hand, exerting firm pressure primarily downward. (The thumb should be abducted, with the ring and little finger flexed into the palm.)

  C. Palpation of the cervix: The cervix should be palpated by sweeping the fingers around the protruding knob in the area of the fornices. Move knob back and forth.

    1. The cervix should normally be able to be moved without discomfort.

    2. Note depth and angle of the cervix.

      a. Should the cervix be markedly tilted to the right or left, or fixed, endometriosis or adhesions (or both) should be suspected.

BOX 4.3 *Advantages and Disadvantages of the Plastic (Disposable) Speculum*

Advantages of the Plastic Speculum

● Provides an unobstructed view of the vaginal walls through its clear blades
● Eliminates the need to warm the speculum
● Reduces patient anxiety because clear plastic is generally less "threatening" to patients than metal
● More comfortable due to the rounded edges of the speculum blades
● Can attach to a light source
● If attached: Enhances illumination of the cervix and vaginal walls; reduces risk of contamination of lamp from adjusting an external light source

Disadvantages of the Plastic Speculum

● Accumulation of medical waste that needs to be disposed of
● The speculum can break—it should not be used with obese or restless patients
● A click occurs during the opening and closing of the blades that may startle the patient

   3. Note size, shape, and consistency (like the tip of the nose).
   4. Note any palpable lumps.
   5. Clinical alterations
      a. Presence of cervical motion tenderness (CMT), which is indicative of pelvic inflammatory disease
      b. A fixed cervix due to endometriosis or a tumor displacing it
      c. Small lumps associated with nabothian cysts
      d. Prominent anterior lips from maternal use of diethylstilbestrol (DES)
      e. An anterior-pointing cervix suggests a retroverted uterus
      f. A posterior-pointing cervix suggests an anteverted uterus
      g. Projection of the cervix into the vagina more than 3 cm (1.2 in) may indicate a pelvic or ovarian mass.
   D. The vagina should be carefully palpated for tenderness, lesions, masses, or foreign bodies (e.g., forgotten tampons).
   E. Palpation of the uterus.
      1. Some comments
         a. The uterus is sometimes difficult to palpate effectively.
         b. It may not be palpable in an obese woman or in one whose abdominal muscles are tense and rigid.
         c. If the uterus is not palpable in a thin, relaxed woman, it may be absent, or tipped posteriorly (retroverted).

2. The technique
   a. Place the abdominal hand on the abdomen, midway between the umbilicus and the symphysis pubis.
   b. Insert the first and second fingers of the other hand into the vagina, with the palmar surface facing anteriorly.
   c. Apply firm pressure on the posterior surface of the cervix to ballot the uterus into the lower abdomen, raise the cervix upward against the abdominal palpating hand, and try to grasp the uterus between the two hands. Assess the uterus with the abdominal hand (Figure 4.2).
3. Note anteflexed, retroflexed, anteverted, or retroverted position
   a. The uterus is normally anteverted and slightly anteflexed.
   b. If it is retroverted and immobile, suspect endometriosis.
   c. A retroverted uterus is not palpable during a bimanual examination (Figure 4.3).
4. Consistency, size, and shape
   a. Mobility
      (1) It should be normally mobile in the anteroposterior plane.
      (2) It has limited mobility in the transverse plane because it is held by the cardinal ligaments.

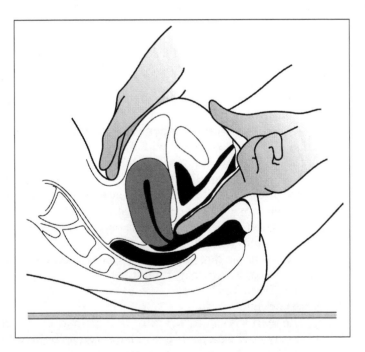

FIGURE 4.2 Bimanual palpation of an anteverted uterus.
Source: Gray (1980).

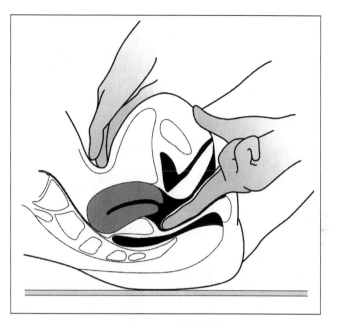

FIGURE 4.3 Bimanual palpation of a retroverted uterus. The examiner is unable to palpate the body of the uterus between the vaginal and abdominal examining fingers. *Source:* Gray (1980).

   (3) Immobility in the anteroposterior plane suggests scar tissue due to previous pelvic inflammatory disease, endometriosis, or surgery.
  b. Tenderness
  c. Palpable masses
  d. Normal findings: Smooth, firm surface; mobile, without tenderness of masses
  e. Clinical alterations
   (1) Soft enlargement from an intrauterine pregnancy.
   (2) Tenderness of the uterus suggesting possible infection, endometriosis, or pregnancy.
   (3) An irregular, firm uterus is related to the various shapes and positions of fibroids (Figure 4.4).
   (4) An immobile, tilted uterus is associated with endometriosis or an abdominal mass.

IX. Palpation of the ovaries and fallopian tubes
 A. Some comments
  1. The ovaries are small (the size of a thumbnail) and difficult to assess, particularly in the presence of extra adipose tissue or muscle rigidity. In endometriosis, the ovaries may be located behind the uterus, making them difficult to assess.

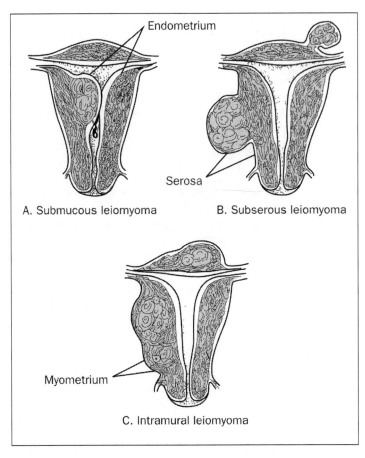

FIGURE 4.4 Appearance of uterine fibroids: (A) submucous leiomyoma, (B) subserous leiomyoma, (C) intramural leiomyoma.

2. The ovaries should not be palpable in postmenopausal women; if they are palpated, they should be considered abnormal and should be investigated.
3. Advise the patient that there may be a fleeting sensation of discomfort when the ovaries are palpated.
4. The fallopian tubes are normally not palpable. If they are enlarged, the examiner should suspect salpingitis or an ectopic pregnancy.

B. The technique
1. The ovaries are evaluated by first locating the vaginal fingers to either the right or left sides of the lateral fornix.
2. Move the abdominal hand to the lower abdominal quadrant on the same side as the internal hand.
3. Apply firm and steady pressure, beginning medially to the anterior iliac crest. Sweep your abdominal hand inward toward the vaginal hand and down to the mons pubis.
4. Repeat the procedure on the opposite side.

    C. Note
      1. Size, tenderness, and masses
      2. Location
      3. Thickening or enlargement
    D. Normal findings
      1. Ovaries may normally be tender.
      2. The fallopian tubes should be nonpalpable and nontender.
    E. Abnormal findings
      1. Enlarged, cystic ovaries are related to polycystic ovarian syndrome.
      2. Enlarged ovary owing to an ovarian cyst or ovarian cancer. If the condition is suspected, a pelvic ultrasound should be ordered to confirm the diagnosis.
      3. Palpable tubes. The tube may feel like fibrous bands, suggesting previous salpingitis or endometriosis.

X. **Rectovaginal examination**
    A. Instruct client to bear down when the finger is inserted into the rectum; then relax and continue to inhale and exhale slowly. The exam is usually uncomfortable and is considered invasive.
    B. Technique
      1. After applying a new glove, insert one lubricated, gloved finger rectally and one gloved finger vaginally, palpating the rectovaginal septum.
      2. Insert the fingers as far in as possible.
      3. With the other hand on the abdomen, push the uterus as posteriorly as possible.
      4. Palpate the posterior surface of the uterus and the rectal wall with the internal fingers.
      5. Note any masses, tenderness, hemorrhoids, or the presence of a retroverted uterus.
    C. Guaiac assessment for occult blood
      1. Take stool adhered to the examining glove and wipe on the appropriate section of the test paper.
      2. Place one to two drops of developing solution over sample.
      3. Wait 30 seconds.
      4. A positive response is the appearance of a blue or dark green color.
    D. Flexible sigmoidoscopy screening
      1. Colon cancer is the second most common cause of death from malignant disease in the United States.
      2. When individuals become symptomatic, most tumors have spread beyond the bowel.
      3. Early screening for asymptomatic colorectal cancer is important.
      4. Suggest screening of average-risk women from 50 years of age every 3 to 5 years.

5. High-risk women include those with advancing age, a diet high in fat, or a family history of colon cancer.
6. Recommend screening of high-risk women from 40 years of age every 2 years.
7. Education is critical.

XI. **The speculum examination**
   A. Some comments
      1. The diameter and tone of the introitus influences the size and type of the speculum that is selected.
      2. Select a speculum size that will be comfortable for the patient while allowing optimal viewing of the cervix.
      3. If a metal speculum is used, it should be warmed or lubricated with tap water.
      4. Commercial lubricants may interfere with the Pap smear, cultures, and vaginal microscopy tests.
      5. The patient should be told that the speculum will be inserted. Showing the patient the speculum before it is inserted often lessens anxiety during the procedure. (However, it may increase anxiety in others.)
   B. Choice of speculum. Either a plastic or metal speculum may be used.
      1. Plastic speculums can be purchased with an attached light. This feature greatly enhances visualization because it allows direct illumination of the vaginal vault.
   C. Technique
      1. Using your nondominant hand, spread the labia with index and middle fingers while applying downward pressure at the lower margin.
      2. This helps avoid pinching or dragging the labia into the introitus as the speculum is inserted.
         a. Some examiners suggest a woman bear down at this point as it eases insertion of the speculum, and consequently increases the patient's comfort.
      3. Hold the speculum at an angle during insertion. This places the long blades parallel to the longitudinal slit of the vaginal opening.
      4. The speculum is next gently directed downward toward the sacrum, while putting downward pressure against the peritoneum until it is fully inserted.
      5. Gradually open the blades, and bring the speculum back to the horizontal position as the cervix comes into view. This technique reduces the risk of irritating the sensitive urethral tissues.
         a. If the visible vaginal wall is rugated, the speculum is probably anterior to the cervix; if the visible wall is smooth, it is probably placed posterior to the cervix.

6. Be careful not to pinch the labia or pull on any pubic hair.
7. Sometimes, a side-to-side movement of the blades will help you visualize the cervix.
8. Small adjustments in speculum angle may also be helpful.
9. The bimanual examination, if previously performed, will help you know where to direct the speculum and locate the cervix.
10. The blades may be held open by either tightening the screw of a metal speculum (be careful not to catch any pubic hair) or by clicking the plastic blades into an open position.
    a. There is no need to secure the blades wide open. It is sometimes more comfortable for the patient if the blades are held partially open for the short time during which the vagina and cervix are inspected.
11. The vaginal canal is inspected as the speculum is removed. This is enhanced with a lighted plastic speculum.

D. Inspection of the vagina
1. Note the quantity, quality, color, and odor of any vaginal discharge.
   a. A vaginal pH, whiff test, and a wet mount are recommended for all women who are concerned regarding their fertility and for complaints of a change in vaginal discharge in order to confirm the presence of normal vaginal flora, and to detect any vaginal infections or estrogen deficiencies (see Chapter 31, "Vaginal Microscopy").
   b. Abnormal flora can interfere with the movement of sperm that is deposited in the vagina.
   c. Research suggests that bacterial vaginosis (BV) and streptococcus may be linked to preterm labor and many gynecologic problems.
   d. It is now recognized that lactobacilli-dominant flora is important for all women of reproductive age, including those who are attempting pregnancy. A culture for gonorrhea or chlamydia may be indicated if the wet mount shows an abundance of polymorphonuclear white blood cells.
2. The vaginal mucosa should be examined as the speculum is slowly rotated and withdrawn from the vagina. This is facilitated by use of a clear plastic speculum. Special attention should be given to any lesions that were palpated earlier.
3. Note any abnormal alterations.
   a. Presence of rugae (mucosal folds): Rugae indicate a good estrogen effect. In a woman with low estrogen levels, the mucosa will be thin, atrophic, and without rugae.
   b. A spatula or cotton-tipped applicator is used to collect a lateral vaginal wall sample to assess pH, perform a whiff test, and prepare the wet mount.

    c. Cervical mucus may alter the pH and wet mount reading, so it should be avoided, if possible.

E. Visualization of the cervix. If discharge obscures the view, gently remove it by using a large cotton swab or rectal probe. Culture any unusual discharge. Pay special attention to any anomalies previously palpated. Note

  1. Size and shape of the cervical os

    a. Normal findings and clinical alterations

      (1) Slit associated with vaginal delivery

      (2) Lacerations from a tear during a precipitous delivery

      (3) An oval os is found in nulliparous women

      (4) A tiny os, which may be partially obliterated, may be found in menopausal women who are not taking hormone replacement therapy.

  2. Characteristics of the cervix, such as friability or lesions

    a. A friable cervix may be related to a cervical infection, such as chlamydia or vaginitis.

    b. Lesions of Bartholin's cysts appear smooth, round, small, yellow, and raised.

    c. A wartlike excoriation is associated with cervical cancer. (Cervical cancer is usually not visible in the early stages.)

  3. Cervical surface

    a. A cervical erosion is a denuded area of squamous epithelium with a clearly defined but slightly irregular border.

    b. Varying amounts of squamous epithelium are visible on the ectocervix, depending on the patient's age and hormonal status.

    c. Conditions affecting the cervix are listed in Table 4.3.

  4. Cervical mucus. Evaluate for quality and quantity, including clarity, opacity, and mucus. Perform a wet mount, if indicated (see Chapter 10, "Assessment of Menopausal Status").

  5. Signs of DES exposure (Box 4.4)

  6. Color of the cervix: It is normally pink but may have a bluish hue in early pregnancy or increased vascularity.

  7. Schiller's test

    a. If suspicious lesions are noted, paint the cervical surface with Lugol's solution. Normal tissue will take up the stain. Abnormal tissue will appear whitish pink.

    b. Use of this test has been replaced by colposcopy.

    c. The disadvantage is that it is nonspecific; normal areas, such as a cervical erosion, may not pick up the stain.

XII. On completion of the pelvic exam

  A. The woman should be given verbal reassurance and offered tissues with which to wipe herself. A pad should be given if any bleeding is present.

TABLE 4.3 Conditions Affecting the Cervix

CONDITION	SYMPTOMS IDENTIFIED DURING ASSESSMENT
Nulliparous cervix	Os is small and either round or oval Covered by smooth epithelium
Parous cervix	Slit-like appearance
Cervical polyp	Small berry-like protrusions Usually arise from the endocervical canal becoming visible when they protrude through the cervical os
Nabothian cyst	Vary in size, can be single or multiple Appear as translucent nodules on the cervical surface Often caused by chronic cervicitis
Ectropion	An extension of the endocervical columnar epithelium onto the ectocervix Often seen with increased estrogen production, such as pregnancy or use of birth control pills
Erosion	Friable tissue surrounding os from an infected ectropion Might be first evidenced by bleeding with a Pap smear

BOX 4.4 *Signs of Diethylstilbestrol (DES) Exposure*

Cockscomb: Prominent anterior portion of the cervix
Collar: Flat rim or hood surrounding the posterior cervix, covered with columnar epithelium
Pseudopolyp: Lypoid appearance of cervix resulting from circumferential groove, thickening of stroma of anterior or posterior endocervical canal
Hypoplastic cervix: Cervix less than 1.5 cm in diameter
Other: Columnar epithelium that covers most of the cervix; may extend to the vaginal wall

B. Provide the woman privacy to dress; then return to complete the visit. Allow ample time to address any questions arising from the examination.

C. At this point, information obtained from the comprehensive health history is combined with findings related to the physical examination.

D. The resulting assessment will help guide the course of the evaluation process.

> **BOX 4.5** *Charting a Normal Pelvic Examination (Sample)*
>
> **External genitalia:** Normal distribution of pubic hair. No lesions or growth. No deformities or discoloration. No masses or discharge from the Bartholin's glands or urethra.
> **Vagina:** Pink; rugated without bulging; clear mucus discharge without odor; good muscle tone.
> **Cervix:** Pink, intact, no lesions; no cervical motion tenderness.
> **Uterus:** Anterior; firm without enlargement, tenderness, or masses; motile.
> **Adenexae:** Ovaries palpated without tenderness of masses.
> **Rectovaginal:** No fissures, masses, or fistulas.

E. All factors should be clearly reviewed with the woman.
F. Review timing of the results of any testing done.
G. Document findings clearly and accurately (Box 4.5).
H. Arrange for any follow-up or additional testing.

Bibliography

American College of Obstetricians and Gynecologists. (2012). Well-women visit. Committee opinion no. 534. *Obstetrics and Gynecology, 20*, 421–424.

Bates, B. (2012). (written by Lynn Bickley MD). *A guide to physical examination and history taking* (12th ed.). Philadelphia, PA: Lippincott.

Bates, C. K., Carroll, N., & Potter, J. (2010) The challenging pelvic examination. *The Journal of General Internal Medicine, 26*(6), 651–657.

Harmanli, O., & Shier, M. (2010). Using lubricant for speculum insertion. *Obstetrics and Gynecology, 116*, 415–417.

Richman, S. M., & Drickamer, M.A. (2007). Gynecologic care of elderly women. *Journal of the American Medical Directors Association, 8*(4), 219–223.

Secor, M., & Fantasia, H. (2012). *Fast facts about the gynecologic exam for nurse practitioners.* New York, NY: Springer Publishing Company.

Assessment of the Skin

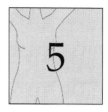

Kathleen Haycraft and Susan Voss

I. Dermatology assessment: Review of basic cutaneous anatomy
    (Figure 5.1)
    A. The epidermis and the dermis rest on the subcutaneous layer. These
        layers form the integumentary system.
    B. Epidermis is the outer layer of the skin.
        1. It is composed of the following layers
            a. Sratum germinatum (above the dermis)
            b. Stratum spinosum
            c. Stratum granulosum
            d. Stratum corneum (top layer of the skin)
        2. The epidermis has four types of cells
            a. Keratinocytes (produce keratin) create the hornified outer
                layer of the skin.
            b. Melanocytes (have dendritic connections to keratinocytes)
                are responsible for the production of melanin (protection
                from ultraviolet rays).
            c. Langerhans cells are derived from the bone marrow and are
                present in the first three layers of the epidermis. They play
                an important role in the immune system of the skin.
            d. Merkel cells are neuroendocrine cells.
    C. Dermis
        1. The papillary dermis is directly below the epidermis. It consists
            of capillaries, fibers, and collagen.
        2. The thicker reticular dermis consists of dense connective tissue,
            larger blood vessels, and elastic and collagen bundles.
        3. Fibroblasts are the predominant cell type of the dermis. The
            cells produce collagen and elastic fibers.
        4. Collagen represents the majority of the dermis. Elastic fibers
            represent approximately 1% but have a significant role in coun-
            tering deforming forces.

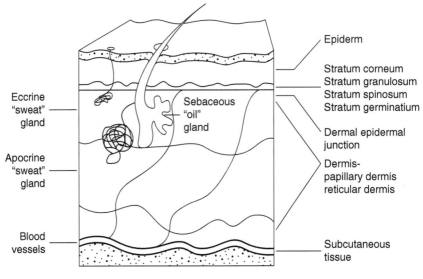

FIGURE 5.1 Skin anatomy.

D. The dermal–epidermal junction is an undulating membrane that connects the dermis to the epidermis. This layer flattens with aging. This is a focal point of attack in diseases like bullous pemphigus.

E. Epidermal appendages include hair follicles, nails, sweat (eccrine) glands, sebaceous glands, apocrine glands, and mammary glands.

F. Vascular supply
    1. The cutaneous vessels play a critical role in thermal regulation.

II. Cutaneous assessment: The color of the skin can add valuable clues to the patient's state of health. To examine the skin, you must listen to the patient's history and current concerns; you must look at all of the skin; you must touch the skin as you examine it; and you must smell for any unusual odors.

A. Pigment changes (see Table 5.1)

B. Temperature and turgor
    1. Very cool skin can be seen with exposure to cold or shock.
    2. Skin that is excessively warm may be associated with high fever and/or infection.
    3. Good skin turgor is the ability of the skin to resume its normal shape after being tented with the thumb and forefinger for

TABLE 5.1 Dermatologic Assessment

COLOR	ASSOCIATED WITH
Yellow to orange	Liver, renal, or hypercarotenemia
Blue	Cyanosis (low oxygen) or argyria (excess silver)
Red or erythema	Red man syndrome (allopurinol, rapid intravenous [IV] fluoroquinolone) or erythroderma (exfoliative dermatitis, which can be fatal and may require hospitalization) Excess flushing from embarrassment, fever, or infection
Absence of pigment	Vitiligo, Addison's disease, uremia, anemia: In a lesion it may represent a morpheaform basal cell cancer.
Hyperpigmentation	Medications (minocycline, amiodarone, and many others), postinflammation: In a lesion it may represent melanoma or a pigmented basal cell cancer.

about 10 seconds. If the skin does not rapidly resume its shape, poor skin turgor is present and dehydration may exist (this may occur with aging skin).

C. Scars
1. Location
2. Tenderness
3. Cause
4. Hypertrophic (large scar at site) or keloids (large scar that extends beyond the original scar site)

D. Presence of dryness (frequently associated with aging) or oiliness (seen with acne)

E. Odor may range from the smell of infection, renal failure, liver failure, intestinal obstruction, diabetic fruitiness, and a wide range of smells.

F. Oral assessment
1. Teeth and gum assessment is important to the complete assessment.
2. Assess the gums for signs of gingivitis, which include bleeding and inflammation of the gums. Patients with symptoms of gingivitis should be referred to a dentist. Gingival hypertrophy is a side effect of many medications, and either gum disorder requires a dental referral.

3. Cavities and excessive plaque should be referred to a dentist.
4. Lesions of the gums, tongue, palate, or buccal mucosa should be referred to a dentist or an ear, nose, and throat (ENT) specialist for prompt evaluation.
5. A thick-ridged hard palate is a normal finding and is referred to as a *torus palatine.*
6. Oral health has strong implications for overall health. Every opportunity should be taken to stress the overall health benefits of brushing of the teeth and regular flossing.

G. Fingernails/toenails: The nails may add to the assessment of systemic and localized illness (see Table 5.2).

H. Hair
   1. Loss of hair is referred to as *alopecia.*
   2. Examination of the scalp is an important part of hair assessment.
      a. Any unusual scalp lesions should be referred for possible biopsy.

TABLE 5.2 Nail Changes Associated With Systemic Diseases

NAIL CHARACTERISTIC	ASSOCIATED CONDITION
Clubbing of fingernails	Chronic lung/heart conditions
Spoon nails (koilonychia)	Anemia and kidney disease
Melanoma of the nails	Seen as a dark spot or line usually at the proximal nail
Rippled nails	Thyroid, diabetes, and circulation disorders
Nail pitting	Psoriasis, lichen planar pilaris, alopecia areata, and other cutaneous disorders
Yellow nail syndrome	Lymphedema and respiratory conditions
Terry's nails (opaque nails with dark tips)	Diabetes, congestive heart failure, liver disease, and malnutrition
Beau's lines	Injury or illnesses where the cuticle growth has been interrupted (e.g., fever, severe illness, malnutrition, or other serious illnesses)
Onycholysis	Psoriasis, lichen planar pilaris, psoriasis, thyroid disease, drug reactions, and a wide range of other illnesses
Lyndsay's nails (half & half nails)	Renal disease
Leukonychia	Trauma
Thickened white or yellow nails	Fungal/mold infections of the nails

Note: The interdigital areas of the toes and soles of the feet need to be examined for erythema, scale, and/or maceration associated with yeast, fungal, mold, or mixed-web infections.

    b. Note whether the scalp is erythematous, boggy, or tender.

    c. Question the patient whether the scalp is itchy.

    d. Erythema and scalp edema are associated with infectious and inflammatory disorders and require referral to dermatology.

    e. Scalp pruritus is frequently associated with contact dermatitis and/or excessive hair washing. Sulfite/sulfate-free shampoos can be helpful.

    f. Persistent pruritus should be referred for evaluation.

3. Loss of hair due to prolonged relaxation is referred to as *telogen effluvium* and is common postpartum, with low iron levels, and with use of some medications.

4. Loss of hair due to anagen effluvium is rapid and frequently due to medications, such as chemotherapeutic agents.

5. Androgenic effluvium is due to changes in hormonal balance. The hair follicle itself thins and the hair pattern loss is greater at the front than the back.

6. Alopecia areata is hair loss due to immune activity in which the hair follicle is destroyed by the immune system.

    a. It is seen with other autoimmune system disorders.

    b. When promptly treated, alopecia aereata may be halted.

    c. It is usually first noted as "spot baldness."

    d. When it occurs all over the body (axilla, genitalia, eyebrows, eyelashes, and so forth), it is known as *alopecia universalis.*

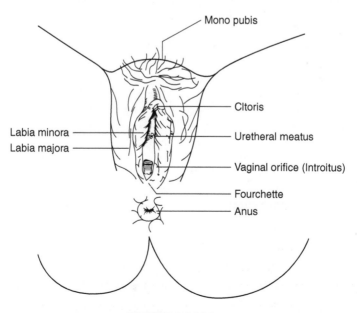

FIGURE 5.2 Vulva.

      7. Scarring alopecias occur with lupus, dissecting cellulitis, lichen planar pilaris, and folliculitis decalvans, to name a few.
   a. Most scarring alopecias are associated with an erythematous tender scalp.
   b. Must be promptly identified and referred immediately to prevent permanent hair loss.
I. Rashes or pruritus
   1. How long has it been present?
   2. Is it associated with pain?
   3. Is it associated with any recent activities or changes in environment?
   4. What has been used or provides relief or worsening of symptoms?
J. Petechiae or ecchymosis should prompt questioning of any trauma, recent or current symptoms of infection, and any other associated bleeding. Bleeding skin lesions should prompt evaluation for immediate biopsy.
K. Hyperhidrosis or hypohidrosis
   1. Excessive sweating can be associated with carcinoma, thyroid disorders, hormonal changes, and infectious disease.
   2. Hyperhidrosis is generally a benign condition but is associated with significant social embarrassment.
   3. Hypohidrosis is associated with increased risk of heat stroke/exhaustion.
L. Fitzpatrick scale to assess skin color (see Table 5.3)
M. Vulvar assessment (Figure 5.2): Melanoma, human papillomavirus (HPV)–related vulvar intraepithelial neoplasia (VIN), lichen sclerosis, and other dermatologic conditions and precancers may be noted during the genital exam.
   1. The mons pubis is the rounded mass of skin with underlying fatty tissue over the pubic bone.
      a. Note the hair growth, as sparse hair may be associated with hypoactive endocrine gland activity and heavy hair growth may be associated with hyperactive endocrine gland activity.

TABLE 5.3 Fitzpatrick Scale

SKIN TYPE	COLOR	FEATURES
I	White/freckled	Always burn, never tans
II	White	Burns easily, tans poorly
III	Olive	Mild burn, gradually tans
IV	Light brown	Burns minimally, tans easily
V	Dark brown	Rarely burns, tans easily
VI	Black	Never burns, always tans

    b. Examine for the presence of unusual looking lesions on the mons pubis. This is of particular importance in women who use sun-tanning beds or who tan without wearing a bathing suit.
2. Labia majora are the two prominent cutaneous folds that extend from the mons pubis to the perineum. Elongated labia majora are called *labia majora elongata* and are a normal variant.
3. Labia minora are the two inner mucosal/cutaneous folds that form the vaginal orifice. The labia minora may also be enlarged and are also referred to as *labia minora elongata*.
4. The introitus is the vaginal orifice. The introitus is examined for the presence of prolapse.
5. The clitoris is a small mound of erectile tissue found above the urethral meatus and under the clitoral hood near the anterior junction of the labia minora.
    a. It is involved in sexual arousal and orgasm.
    b. Persistent genital arousal disorder is occasionally associated with clitoral priapism. This may be an adverse effect of antidepressants.
    c. Enlargement of the clitoris may be an effect of excessive androgen production.
6. The fourchette is the area where the labia minora meet posteriorly. It is an area that is involved if episiotomy is needed during delivery.
7. For more information on the vulvar examination, see Chapter 4, "The Physical Examination."

III. Dermatologic issues related to pregnancy
  A. Changes in the skin: Three factors involved in the development of changes of the skin during pregnancy are increased hormones, compression from the expanding uterus, and intravascular volume expansion.
    1. Estrogen increases melanocytic activity, resulting in increased pigmentation, cutaneous vasodilatation, keratin growth, increased permeability, and increased angiogenesis.
    2. Progesterone also enhances melanocytic activity and reduces the lysis of collagen.
    3. Hormones produced by the pituitary gland (gonadotropins, adrenocorticotrophic hormones, and melanocytic hormones) all have effects on the skin.
    4. The sources of these hormones are the endocrine glands as well as the placenta.
  B. Pigment changes
    1. Melasma and chloasma ("mask of pregnancy") occur in 70% of pregnant women, usually in the third month of pregnancy and regresses postpartum.
    2. Melasma is worsened by sunlight and is more pronounced in patients with higher Fitzpatrick skin types (types I–VI, see Table 5.3).

3. Avoid the standard treatments during pregnancy (hydroquinone, retinoic acid, and fluocinolon).
4. Broad-spectrum sunscreens and sun avoidance are the mainstays of prevention and treatment.
5. Additional areas of increased pigment changes include the areola, anogential, axilla, and inner thighs.
6. Linea nigra is found in 75% of pregnant females. This is a darkened line from the umbilicus (occasionally substernal) to the symphisis pubis.
7. Freckles, nevi, and scars may become more pigmented during pregnancy. They may expand as the patient expands; however, rapidly expanding lesions are a hallmark of malignancy and need to be carefully evaluated.

C. Vascular changes
1. Vasomotor instability may result in excessive facial flushing. The majority resolve in the postpartum period.
2. Spider telangectasias occur in 60% of pregnant women.
   a. Erythematous macules or papules with central redness surrounded by radiating capillaries
   b. Frequently develop in the first trimester and frequently resolve after delivery. They occur on the upper part of the body (drained by the superior vena cava). They do not require treatment. If numerous lesions appear suddenly, concern for hepatic disease is raised.
3. Acral (hands/feet) erythema is common in the first trimester and usually resolves in the postpartum phase.
4. Vascular proliferation is evidenced by hyperplasia and erythema of the gingiva.
   a. Pyogenic granulomas (pregnancy epulus/epulus gravidarum) appear as fleshy erythematous growths.
   b. Can occur anywhere but are often found in the oral cavity.
   c. Fragile and tend to bleed
   d. Spontaneous regression is observed in the postpartum period.

D. Structural changes
1. Striae gravidarum are of great concern and occur in 60% to 90% of pregnant White women.
   a. Less common in other ethnic groups
   b. Risk factors include maternal weight gain, high neonatal birth weight, and younger age.
   c. No proven preventive measures
   d. Laser and retinoid creams may be of some help but should be limited to postpartum.
2. Acrochordons (skin tags) are common during the second half of pregnancy and frequently shrink after delivery. If they persist, they may be treated after delivery by electrocautery or snip removal.

E. Adnexal changes
  1. Hair decreases in the telogen phase resulting in thickening of the hair.
     a. Increased hair can also occur in undesirable hirsutism of the face, trunk, and extremities.
     b. Usually reversed postpartum
     c. Excessive hair loss (shedding) can occur in the postpartum phase.
     d. Generally resolves in 6 to 15 months
  2. Nails grow faster during pregnancy and may become more brittle.
  3. Hormonal influence on sebaceous glands may result in acne.
     a. More common in the last trimester
     b. All "cyclin" antibiotics should be avoided as well as many retinoids.
     c. Topical benzoyl peroxide and macrolide antibiotics may be used.
  4. After the sixth week of pregnancy, the sebaceous glands of the areola enlarge.
     a. Appear as elevated dark tan papules that regress after delivery
     b. Occurs in about 50% of women
  5. Eccrine (sweat) glands increase progressively during pregnancy. Milia appear as small papules that appear clear.
  6. Fox-Fordyce (purplish macules/papules in the labia) usually reduce during pregnancy, as does hidradenitis suppurativa (chronic marble- or pea-sized lumps in the axilla and groin that are painful and drain).
F. Specific dermatologic issues related to pregnancy
  1. Atopic eczema of pregnancy (AEP) is the most frequent dermatosis of pregnancy.
     a. It develops as an itchy rash on the flexural surfaces.
     b. Prurigo features (nodules formation) may occur with eczema of pregnancy.
     c. Soap and water may aggravate the disorder, and mild soaps and limited bathing followed by emollients are the mainstays of treatment.
  2. Polymorphic eruption of pregnancy (PEP) is nonspecific eczema-like patches and papules.
     a. Are not associated with elevated immune globulin (AEP has increased immune globulin)
     b. Usually presents in the last trimester of pregnancy. The incidence is less than 1% and is more frequent in the first pregnancy.
     c. Spontaneous remission usually occurs after delivery.

d. If the pruritus is severe, antihistamines and topical/oral steroids may be needed. The risk/benefit of treatment needs to be evaluated.

3. Pemphigoid gestationis (previously known as herpes gestationis) is associated with the development of tense bulla (blisters) usually in the second or third trimester in multiparous women.
   a. Pruritus usually precedes the development of the blisters.
   b. Pruritus usually develops in the periumbilical area and extends to the abdomen.
   c. Tense bullae develop on the trunk and limbs and usually spare the face.
   d. Treatment with oral or ultra-potent topical steroids may be indicated. The risk/benefit of treatment needs to be evaluated.

4. Intrahepatic cholestasis of pregnancy usually presents in the third trimester as intense nocturnal pruritus.
   a. If skin lesions are present, they occur due to scratching. The symptoms resolve postpartum and the disorder is likely to reoccur in future pregnancies.
   b. This disorder is significant as it is associated with higher incidence of neonatal mortality and morbidity.
   c. Liver enzyme and bile salt levels need to be monitored and the disorder is treated with cholestyramine and/or ursodeoxycholic acid.

IV. **Dermatologic issues related to contraception**
A. Acne is a chronic inflammation of the sebaceous glands of the face, chest, and/or back. Stress the need for chronic treatment and gentle cleansing of the acne areas. Despite popular traditions, the skin should not be inflamed or irritated by rough abrasives or harsh astringents. The lesions of acne include papules, pustules, comedos, cysts, and nodules. The types of lesions as well as the number of lesions determine the severity of acne.
B. Pathology of acne (see Table 5.4)
C. Treatment focuses on reduction of sebum (benzoyl peroxide, salicylic acid, and retinoids), antibiotics (topical or oral) to reduce *P. acnes*, and opening of the pores with retinoids (the mainstay of acne treatment). Birth control pills are an effective acne treatment.
   1. Acne is generally improved by estrogen and may be affected by progesterone.
   2. Avoid birth control pills that contain androgenic progestin. Generally, a higher estrogen dose improves acne (30-35 mcg).
   3. Acne is affected by contraception choices.
      a. Birth control pills are an effective treatment for acne.
      b. Implanon, intrauterine devices (IUDs), or Depo-Provera injections deprive the acne-prone patient from the benefits of estrogen potentially precipitating or worsening acne.

TABLE 5.4 The Two Paths of Acne Pathology

PATH 1: HORMONE DRIVEN	PATH 2: INCREASED CELL PRODUCTION
Many hormones (DHEA-S, progesterone, testosterone, insulin-like growth factor) influence the sebaceous gland to increase sebum production	Hyperkeratinization
The sebum is rich in triglycerides	Causes plugging of the sebaceous gland
Triglycerides provide abundant food that promotes the proliferation of *Propionibacterium acnes* (*P. acnes*)	Probably genetically driven
P. acnes stimulates the toll-like receptors (TLR) along the sebaceous unit resulting in inflammation	Results in the development of comedones; when the pore is closed, they become papules or pustules, and when the pore is open, they are commonly known as "blackheads" (oxidized sebum/cells)

     c. Assessing the patient for acne history is a vital component of contraception counseling and selection of contraceptive methods.

  D. Erythema nodosum is an inflammatory condition of the fat cells under the dermis.

    1. Presents as erythematous tender nodules or lumps over the shins

    2. May be preceded by a mild fever, fatigue, and arthralgias

    3. Usually resolves within 6 weeks

    4. May be triggered by a wide variety of infectious processes, autoimmune disorders, carcinoma, pregnancy, and medications including birth control pills

    5. Treatment is focused at removing the etiologic agent. Elevation of the legs and compressive stockings may provide symptomatic relief.

V. **General dermatology**

  A. Rosacea is a common dermatologic condition in women's health.

    1. Rosacea is an inflammatory cutaneous condition of the face.

    2. Its pathology involves the presence of a demodex mite with associated inflammation and increased vascularity.

    3. It presents as a central erythema of the face with associated papules and thickening of the skin.

    4. Rosacea has four types (see Table 5.5)

TABLE 5.5 Rosacea Types

Erythrotelengectatic	Erythema of the central face Treatment includes intense pulsed-light therapy or bromocriptine
Ocular	Onsets frequently with erythematotelangiectatic rosacea (ETR) Best treated with oral "cyclins" and/or sulfa ophthalmic drops
Papular/pustular	Erythema associated with these lesions Treatment includes metronidazole, azelaic acid, and oral "cyclins"
Granulomatous	Thickening of the skin Best treated with oral "cyclins," laser, and/or isotretinoin

    B. Skin cancers/carcinoma
        1. Cutaneous carcinoma is the most common cancer.
        2. During the well-women exam, a practitioner has abundant opportunity to examine the skin and identify skin cancer in the early stages, leading to appropriate treatment and reduction in mortality and morbidity.
        3. Types of skin cancer (see Table 5.6)
        4. Risk factors for cutaneous carcinoma (see Table 5.7)

VI. Cosmesis and photo-aging
    A. Cutaneous aging
        1. Aging is associated with a number of changes in the skin, including
            a. Reduction in sebaceous glands resulting in xerosis (dry skin), more irritated skin, and resultant pruritus
            b. Collagen fibers thicken and dominate over elastin fibers resulting in rhytides (wrinkles).
            c. Skin thins and paper-like skin that is prone to injury occurs and angiomas develop.
            d. Blood vessels become more fragile resulting in easy bruising.
            e. Collagen production is reduced.
            f. Subcutaneous fat is reduced resulting in hollowing.
            g. Pigment formation is dysfunctional, resulting in "blotchiness."
            h. Keratinocyte repressor genes fail in areas resulting in seborrheic keratosis.
        2. The above are intrinsic factors associated with aging (genetic and chronologic).
        3. Extrinsic factors associated with aging (smoking and ultraviolet rays) may result in increased rhytides, lentigo (pigmentation), and telangectasias (spider vessels).

TABLE 5.6 Common Skin Cancer Types

TYPE OF CANCER	ID FEATURES/TREATMENT
Basal cell cancer (BCC) 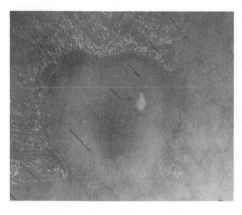	*Most common* skin cancer Rarely occurs in the Black race 85% occur on the head and neck Usually presents as bleeding or scabbed lesions or a pimple that does not heal or recurs *Rarely deadly* If untreated it can penetrate and infiltrate the surrounding tissues Nodular BCC usually presents as a pearly white or pink dome-shaped papule Superficial BCC presents as a patch or erythematous skin that extends peripherally and develops telangiectatic vessels Morpheaform BCC presents as a white patch of sclerotic skin and is frequently missed until advanced There are patients who have multiple BCCs that are genetically linked; this is Gorlin syndrome
Squamous cell cancer (SCC) 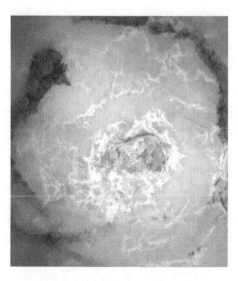	*Second most common* form of skin cancer *Presents on sun-exposed skin* Most common sites are face and back of the hands SCC usually present as an erythematous, scaly, papule They may grow rapidly or slowly Although it rarely causes death, the immune-suppressed patient is at much greater risk of death from metastasis and death from SCC If the SCC is found on the mucosa or tongue, it has a much higher risk for metastasis It may occur in burns (Marjorin's ulcer) Human papilloma virus (HPV) has been associated with SCC in the anogenital area

(continued)

TABLE 5.6 Common Skin Cancer Types *(continued)*

TYPE OF CANCER	ID FEATURES/TREATMENT
Melanoma 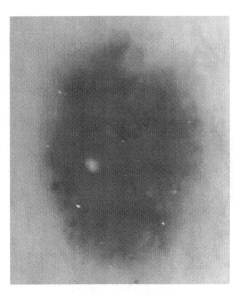	*Third most common* type of skin cancer Previously referred to as the most deadly skin cancer; however, Merkel cell cancer is much rarer and much more deadly Early detection is important Treatment, prognosis, and 5-year survival are determined by tumor thickness and lymph node involvement Lesions may appear anywhere on the body It does not have to be in a sun-exposed area Lesion may be noted in the scalp, mouth, vulvar area, under nails, and on the feet, including between the toes Although not totally precise, the *ABCDEs of melanoma* detection have helped increase melanoma detection by lay/nonmedical individuals These are danger signs that may indicate the need to biopsy and/or refer. A–Asymmetry. When viewing the lesion in half, both vertically and horizontally, the two halves do not match. B–Border irregularity. The borders of the lesion may be uneven, scalloped, or notched. C–Color variation. The lesion may have two or more colors. D–Diameter enlargement. The lesion may be larger than 6 mm or ¼ inch. This is roughly the size of a pencil eraser. E–Evolving. The lesion may be evolving or changing from its original presentation. An experienced practitioner should only excise melanoma. Suspicious lesions should not be monitored but referred promptly to an experienced dermatology practitioner.

TABLE 5.7 Risk Factors for Cutaneous Carcinoma

Family history
Sun exposure
Fair skin
Tanning beds
History of actinic keratosis
History of sunburns
Immune suppression

Melanoma-specific risk factors:
   All of the above
   Multiple melanocytic nevi especially dysplastic nevi
   Past history of melanoma
   Family history of melanoma (*BRAF* gene)
   Higher altitude or closer to the equator

4. Ultraviolet rays are very harmful to the skin.
   a. UVA waves penetrate deep in the dermis. They are associated with premature aging, skin cancer, and autoimmune disease. UVA waves can penetrate glass and clothing.
   b. UVB waves penetrate the epidermis and result in tanning and sunburns. They are strongly associated with skin cancer.
   c. UVC waves are reflected by the ozone layer and have an oncogenic effect where ozone layers are depleted.
B. Cosmetic approach to reducing/preventing photo-aging
   1. To reduce photo-aging, use broad-spectrum sunscreen daily, avoid the midday sun, and wear broad-rimmed hats and sunglasses. A recent study in Australia showed that daily application of sunscreen from head to toe reduced cutaneous aging.
   2. Antioxidants reverse the daily damage from ultraviolet (UV) exposure. Many antioxidants are available and include green tea, vitamin E, vitamin C, coffee berry, blueberry, caffeine, alpha-lipoic acid, hydroquinone, kojic acid, tocopheryl, polyphenols, and a wide variety of others.
   3. Retinoids will reduce small rhytides (wrinkles), pigmentation, and inflammation; they reduce aging.
      a. Retinols are available over the counter, whereas the more powerful retinoids are available by prescription.
      b. Retinoids are much more potent.
      c. Retinols do convert to retinoids but at a much lower concentration.
   4. DNA and stem cell serums are available on the market and promote claims to reverse DNA damage to the skin. The data is inconclusive at this time.

5. Dermabrasion is an ablative technique that uses a wire brush or diamond wheel, causing the upper layer of the skin to be injured.
   a. As the wound heals, the technique results in new skin formation.
   b. It is used with acne scarring, uneven skin tones, tattoos, and striae. This is not to be confused with microdermabrasion, which is performed with brushes and is not done in the office setting.
6. Laser and light therapy can reduce skin laxity, increase collagen, and improve pigment issues. By reducing the appearance of wrinkles, age spots, and pigment changes, they are powerful tools in the armament of cosmetic therapy.
7. There is a wide variety of chemical peels that add to the arsenal of treatment for acne scarring, melasma, hyperpigmentation, acne, and rhytides. Adverse effects from peels include scarring, changes in pigmentation, and infection. Only experienced providers should use them.

C. Fillers and neuromodulators
   1. Botulinum toxin type A (Botox, Dyport, and Xeomin) is a neuromodulator that modulates the neuromuscular synapse by binding to the receptor site on the motor nerve terminal. This inhibits acetylcholine from activating the motor neuron.
      a. These products are very safe.
      b. Side effects are dependent on the site injected and the injector's expertise.
      c. A new topical gel administered in the provider's office is available.
      d. Areas for injection include the glabella, forehead, periocular rims, brow lift, gummy smile reduction, depressor angularis orbicularis (DAO), mentalis (chin), and nasal sidewall. The only Food and Drug Administration (FDA)–approved sites are the periocular rims (crows feet) and the glabella.
   2. Fillers
      a. Hyaluronic acid fillers are used around the lips, nasolabial folds, around the mouth, and cheeks.
      b. Calcium hydroxyl apatite is used on the cheeks, nasolabial folds, temples, and *not on the lips.*
      c. Polylactic acid fillers are used for general volume and *not on the lips.*
      d. Fillers should never be injected into the glabella, as that may be associated with blindness.

D. Fat reduction: Careful client selection is critical to patient satisfaction with the procedures. Patients may have areas of fat that have been shown to be resistant to diet and exercise. It is not an effective treatment for obesity.

    1. Cryolipolysis: This technique is a form of "controlled frostbite." It is useful for the abdomen, flanks, back, chin, and thighs. It is uncomfortable but not painful. One to two procedures per desired site will be needed. Minimal complications occur. The most common are bruising, paresthesias, and rarely postprocedure neuropathic pain.

    2. Laser: The laser is used three times a week over a 2-week period to achieve its effects. It has few side effects after the procedure but is somewhat painful during the procedure. Side effects include bruising and the risk of burning with scarring. It can be used in the same places as cryolipolysis.

E. Nonsurgical facelift: Ultrasound is administered with a convex system that allows the energy to be focused and create thermal coagulation points. When the energy is focused on the superficial musculo-aponeurotic system (SMAS; thin muscles below the skin), it creates increased collagen formation, reduction in laxity, and tightens the skin. It is used on the forehead, lower face, and neck. Bruising, burns, and numbness may be side effects (see Table 5.8).

TABLE 5.8 Aesthetics

PROCEDURE	INDICATIONS	ADVERSE EFFECTS	COST*
Neurotoxin	Reduction of dynamic wrinkles	Headache, bruising, paralysis of undesired areas, asymmetry	$200–$700 depending on the site and the type of agent used
Filler	To restore volume in the temples, chin, cheeks, nasolabial, and lips	Blindness, necrosis, injection into areas that it is not intended for with undesirable consequences. Due to its high side-effect profile, collagen is rarely used. Fat transfer is a viable filler option.	$500–$3,000 depending on the type of filler used and the number of syringes

(continued)

TABLE 5.8 Aesthetics *(continued)*

PROCEDURE	INDICATIONS	ADVERSE EFFECTS	COST*
Fat-reduction techniques	To reduce focal fat areas Not as effective in older people or those also lack skin elasticity	Laser bruising, burning with scarring Ultrasound postprocedure neuropathy	$650–$1,200 depending on procedure type and location
Nonsurgical facelift	Better results if younger, less sun exposure, and not a smoker	Bruising, swelling, paresthesia Pain may require medication	$1,500–3,000
Facelift	To reduce rhytides and promote a smoother face	All those associated with a surgical procedure	$10,975

Notes: The most important accomplishment after skill excellence is the ability to set realistic expectations. *All costs were obtained from www.realself.com. This site is excellent for determining costs, expectations, and making referrals.

    F. Varicose veins
        1. Varicose veins occur due to prolonged standing (occupational hazard), pregnancy, trauma, genetic factors, and obesity.
        2. They are veins that are close to the surface of the skin and appear most frequently on the legs.
        3. Nonsurgical treatments include weight loss, dietary sodium reduction, exercise, compression stockings, and avoiding long periods of standing and/or sitting.
        4. Small veins may be injected with sclerotherapy or treated with laser (by an experienced clinician). Larger veins may be treated by laser-guided sclerotherapy, radiofrequency, or surgery.
        5. Sclerotherapy may be performed by hypertonic sclerotherapy or foam sclerotherapy. Both require compression stockings and avoidance of prolonged standing or sitting for up to 2 weeks (some providers may limit to a few days) after the procedure. Complications include skin ulceration, thromboembolism, and allergic reactions.
    See Box 5.1 for clinical pearls.

BOX 5.1 *Clinical Pearls*

- Cutaneous carcinoma is the most common cancer.
- A pimple that comes and goes (or persists in the same spot) is frequently a basal cell cancer.
- A lesion that bleeds easily, regardless of size, is suspicious for skin cancer.
- A patch of skin that comes and goes or persists in the same area may be a superficial basal cell cancer or squamous cell cancer in situ.
- A rapidly growing lesion or one that is changing in color should be referred for biopsy.
- When examining the skin for abnormal lesions, look for the "ugly duckling," the "pretty duckling," or "what doesn't belong with the others." In other words, look for the lesion that does not appear similar to the others.
- Melanoma skin cancer can occur in areas of the body that have never been exposed to the sun.
- A Bartholin's cyst that persists despite treatment should be biopsied for carcinoma.
- Persistent genital warts that are not responsive to treatment should be biopsied for squamous cell carcinoma.
- Persistent lichen sclerosis that has not been responsive to treatment should be biopsied for vulvar carcinoma.

Bibliography

Bates, B. (2012). (written by Lynn Bickley MD). *A guide to physical examination and history taking* (12th ed.). Philadelphia, PA: Lippincott.

Bolognia, J. L., Jarizzo J. L., & Schaffer, J. V. (2012). *Dermatology* (3rd ed.). China: Saunders/Elsevier.

James, W. D., Elston, D. M., Berger, T. G., & Andrews, G. C. (2011). *Andrews' diseases of the skin: Clinical dermatology* (11th ed.). London, UK: Saunders/Elsevier.

Habif, T. P. (2010). *Clinical dermatology: A color guide to diagnosis and therapy* (5th ed.). Maryland Heights, MO: Mosby/Elsevier.

Hughes, M. C. B., Williams, G. M., Baker, P., & Green, A. (2013). Sunscreen and prevention of aging: A randomized trial. *Annals of Internal Medicine, 158*(11), 1–28.

Soutou, B., Regnier, S., Nassar, D., Parant, O., Khosrotehrani, K., & Aractingi, S. (2013). Dermatological manifestations associated with pregnancy. *Medscape*. Retrieved December 5, 2013, from www.medscape.org/viewarticle/706769_6

Assessment of the Female Breast

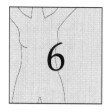

6

Jennifer Dentler and Helen A. Carcio

I. **Basics related to examination of the female breast**
   A. The examiner must possess a thorough understanding of the normal anatomy and physiology of breast structure to identify any anomalies.
   B. Physical examination of the breast by clinicians and self-examination are important for breast cancer detection. Breast cancer is not preventable; it is the early detection of breast cancer that is key to the patient's survival.
   C. The examination of the breast includes inspection and palpation of the breasts and palpation of the lymph nodes that drain the breast.
   D. Proper positioning of the patient and good lighting are key factors to inspection and palpation of the breast.
   E. It is important for the examiner to acknowledge the societal association of the breast with sexuality; this makes the assessment of the breast an emotionally uncomfortable examination for many female clients.
   F. Assessment of breast symmetry is essential; the client must have both breasts uncovered for comparison.
   G. Ideally, the breast examination should not take place immediately before a woman's menstrual period, when the breast may be normally tender and engorged.
   H. The breast examination provides the examiner with an excellent opportunity to demonstrate breast self-examination (BSE) and to reinforce teaching.
   I. Approximately 5% of women in the United States have breast implants.
      1. There are limitations in detecting breast cancer in women with implants.
      2. Proper positioning techniques can be used to overcome these limitations.

II. **Important statistics**
   A. Statistics related to breast cancer are reliable and are particularly important to review with the patient. The incidence of breast cancer in women continues to increase.
   B. Based on American Cancer Society (ACS) current incidence rates, 12.4% of women born in the United States will develop breast cancer at some time in their lives. This translates to one woman in eight being affected, with most of the risk occurring after the age of 50 years.
   C. The strongest risk factor for breast cancer is age. Almost 8 out of every 10 new breast cancer cases and almost 9 of every 10 breast cancer deaths are in women 50 years old and older.
   D. Breast cancer is the second most common cancer among women, following skin cancer. Cancer is the second greatest cause of death among women, following heart disease.
   E. Although it is rare, young women under age 45 can and do develop breast cancer. In the United States, about 10% of all breast cancer occurs in women under age 45.
      1. In the United States, 24,000 women under age 45 are expected to be diagnosed with breast cancer this year (including situ breast cancer), and more than 3,000 will die.
      2. Breast cancer is the leading cause of cancer deaths in women under age 40.
      3. The 5-year relative survival rate in the United States is slightly lower among women diagnosed with breast cancer before age 40 (82%) compared to women diagnosed at ages 40 and older (89%).
   F. The ACS estimates that in 2013 there were approximately 232,340 new cases of invasive breast cancer and approximately 39,620 women died of breast cancer.
   G. Breast cancer is far more curable when the tumor is detected early.
      1. The goal of screening exams for early breast cancer detection is to find cancers before they start to cause symptoms. Screening refers to tests and exams used to find a disease, such as cancer, in people who do not have symptoms.
      2. Breast cancers that are found because they are causing symptoms tend to be larger and are more likely to have already spread beyond the breast. In contrast, breast cancers found during screening exams are more likely to be smaller and still confined to the breast. The size of a breast cancer and how far it has spread are some of the most important factors in predicting the prognosis of a woman with this disease.
      3. Table 6.1 comes from the National Cancer Institute's SEER database. It shows survival rates and emphasizes the importance of early detection.

TABLE 6.1 Breast Cancer Survival Rates

STAGE	5-YEAR SURVIVAL RATE (%)
0	100
I	100
II	93
III	72
IV	22

H. *The breast cancer death rate is decreasing.* A new report from the ACS finds that death rates from breast cancer in the United States have dropped 34% since 1990. But the rate at which new breast cancers are diagnosed increased slightly among African American women from 2006 to 2010, bringing those rates closer to those of White women, who still have the highest diagnosis rates among women ages 40 and older.

III. **Anatomy and physiology of the breast**
   A. Breast tissue
      1. Each breast contains 12 to 20 major ducts that intertwine, with each duct opening at the nipple. Most breast cancers originate in these ducts.
      2. The breasts extend from the second or third rib to the sixth or seventh rib, and from the sternal edge to the anterior axillary line.
      3. Breasts consist of glandular tissue, fibrous tissue, ducts, fat, blood vessels, nerves, and lymph nodes (Figure 6.1).
         a. Glandular tissue is contained in the lobes.
         b. Fibrous tissue is the supporting tissue that lies between the glandular tissue.
      4. Each lobe is subdivided into 50 to 75 lobules, which drain into separate excretory ducts, which in turn drain into the nipple.
      5. These lobules in the peripheral breast tissue emerge at the nipple (the hub) like the spokes of a wheel.
      6. The lobules produce milk, and the ducts carry the milk to the areola.
      7. Each duct dilates as it enters the base of the areola to form a milk sinus, which serves as a reservoir for milk during lactation.
      8. Inframammary ridge: The ridge of fat on the lower portion of the breast is called the inframammary ridge. The breast tissue here is often more dense than the surrounding tissue. Muscle: There is very little muscle in the breast except for a small amount in the areola and the nipple, which causes the nipple to contract, facilitating the emptying of the milk sinuses.

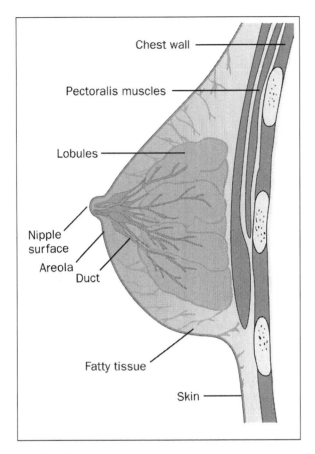

FIGURE 6.1 Anatomy of the breast.

9. The areola and nipple
   a. Dermal papillae contain sebaceous glands. The skin of the areola contains occasional hair follicles.
   b. Sebaceous glands on the areolar surface are the Montgomery tubercles.
10. Tail of Spence: More than half the ducts are present in the upper, outer breast quadrant (divide the breast into four parts, with the nipple at the center).
    a. Breast tissue feels firmer in those areas.
    b. Breast cancer is more common here (many cancers arise from ductal tissue).
11. Lymph nodes drain the area in and around the breast (Figure 6.2).
12. The breast undergoes changes during pregnancy and lactation.

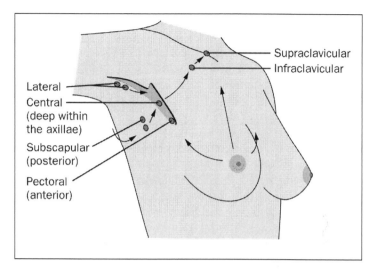

FIGURE 6.2 Arrows indicate direction of lymph flow.

BOX 6.1 *Reasons Why a Woman Might Not Perform Breast Self-Examination (BSE)*

- She may be afraid of finding a lump that is cancerous, which can actually be immobilizing.
- She may not have the confidence that she can perform the BSE efficiently, so why bother.
- She may not really believe that performing BSE will ever result in detecting a cancerous lump.
- She may simply forget to perform it regularly.

IV. **Breast self-examination: BSE is an option for women starting in their 20s. Women should be told about the benefits and limitations of BSE. Women should report any breast changes to their health professional right away.**
   A. BSE explained
      1. Few women practice BSE regularly. This is due to many different factors (Box 6.1).
      2. Recent research suggests that BSE plays a small role in the detection of breast cancer.
      3. Women are more likely to practice BSE if they know what to look for. Health education is vital.
      4. Women should report
         a. New lumps or thickness of breast or underarm (axilla)
         b. Nipple tenderness or discharge or physical change (persistent soreness)

      c. Skin irritation such as a pucker, dimple, new crease, or fold

      d. Warm, red, swollen breasts with skin resembling the skin of an orange (peau d'orange)

   5. Inform the woman that any firm lump that remains unchanged with cyclic variations is suspect and warrants a visit to her health care provider.

   6. In women who are disabled, primary caregivers or chaperones should be trained to perform BSE.

   7. Performing BSE provides the woman with a great opportunity to assume an active role in her own health care.

   8. BSE is an important screening tool for breast cancer because most breast lumps are discovered by the woman herself.

   9. Performing BSE is vital to discovering interval cancers, which are lumps that grow large enough to become palpable between annual clinical breast exams (CBEs).

  10. Point out that BSE should never act as a substitute for either CBE or mammography.

  11. A woman is more likely to detect breast cancer earlier if she practices routine BSE.

B. The technique

   1. The BSE is relatively easy to perform; however, because the area to be palpated is large, women often believe that the technique is complicated.

   2. Women must simply be informed that there is the overlying skin on the top, with the palpable ribs underneath. They must feel for the presence of any lumps or masses in between these structures.

   3. If a woman learns how to identify and even count her ribs, she will develop a sensitivity to feel for any lumps or changes in breast tissue.

   4. Educate the woman in the following:

      a. Keep the middle three fingers on the skin when palpating, varying the pressure as you palpate in dime-sized areas.

      b. Do not use the tips of your fingers, but use the pads because they have more sensitive pressure receptors.

      c. Use a systematic pattern: Either circles or strips (the vertical up-and-down pattern) seem to be the easiest to use.

      d. Be sure to cover the entire breast, beginning in the middle of the armpit, where there are many ducts.

      e. Move up and down in vertical strips (a finger's width) between the collarbone and the bra line, and progress across the breast to the middle of the hard bone of the sternum.

      f. Ask the woman whether she can count her ribs beneath the breast tissue.

BOX 6.2 *Risk Factors Associated With Breast Cancer*

Advancing age
Older than 40 years
Family history
First-degree relative: Mother, sister, daughter. Mother or sister has disease.
Relative was premenopausal at time of diagnosis. Personal history of breast
cancer or ovarian cancer.
Previous breast biopsy or benign breast disease
Atypical hyperplasia; lobular neoplasia; reproductive issues
Estrogen exposure
First pregnancy at 30 years of age or older. Early menarche (before age 12).
Late menopause (after age 55). Infertility or nulliparity. Never breastfed.
Hormonal treatments
Estrogen replacement therapy (controversial)
Recent use (within 5 years)
Long-term use
Oral contraceptive use (probably does not increase risk)
Dietary factors
Obesity (older than age 50)
High-fat diet
Alcohol use (more than two glasses per day)
Lifestyle factors
Pesticide exposure; smoking; lack of exercise
Personal or family history of colon cancer
Radiation therapy to the chest

---

    g. The average examination, depending on breast size and density, should take up to 10 minutes per breast. If it does not take the patient that long, she needs to reevaluate her technique.

    h. The examination can be performed in the shower, in the bathtub, lying in bed, or standing upright in front of the mirror.

V. **A patient history relevant to the examination of the female breast must be gathered to assess for any risk factors (Box 6.2).**

    A. Age: The older a woman is, the more the risk for breast cancer increases.

    B. Menstruation: The fewer ovulatory cycles a woman has, the lower the risk for breast cancer, as well as ovarian cancer. It is important to assess

        1. Age of menarche

        2. Date of last menstrual period

        3. Age at menopause

        4. Number of years taking oral contraceptives or estrogen replacement agents

C. Family history of breast cancer (see Chapter 34, "Genetic Testing for Heredintary Breast and Ovarian Cancer")
   1. About 5% to 10% of breast cancer cases are thought to be hereditary, meaning that they result directly from gene defects (called mutations) inherited from a parent.
D. Childbearing: Nulliparous woman and those who gave birth to a first live-born child at age 30 years or older have a somewhat increased risk for breast cancer. Ask the client about
   1. Number of children
   2. Age when children were born
   3. Breastfeeding pattern (decreases risk somewhat)
E. BSE
   1. Evaluate when and how performed, as well as how often
   2. Evaluate any findings by the client
   3. Assess level of comfort
F. Discharge from nipple: Inquire about
   1. Onset, duration, amount, color, odor, consistency, and frequency
   2. Whether it's bilateral, spontaneous, or provoked (e.g., by exercise or sexual activity); the examiner should be concerned if the discharge is spontaneous, unilateral, and persistent
   3. Use of medications that may increase prolactin levels, such as birth control pills, steroids, or antidepressants
G. Breast pain or lumps: Inquire about
   1. Onset, duration, quantity, quality, location (one or both breasts), radiation of pain, relation to menstrual cycle, and history of previous episodes
   2. Presence of predisposing factors, such as menstruation, lactation, pregnancy, or history of fibrocystic disease
   3. Presence of associated signs and symptoms, such as dimpling of the skin or discharge from the nipple
H. Breast implants: Inquire about
   1. Year surgery was performed
   2. Presence of any discomfort or tenderness in area of the implant
   3. Acute or gradual onset of pain that may be related to a ruptured implant
   4. Occurrence of any trauma in the area of the implant
I. Medications: Past or present use
   1. Use of oral contraceptives
      a. Duration
      b. Type
      c. Presence of complications or side effects
      d. Reasons for discontinuing
   2. Use of estrogen replacement therapy: Risk for breast cancer may be increased if estrogen replacement therapy is used for more than 10 years. Inquire about past or present use.
      a. Duration

      b. Type

      c. Reason for discontinuing

      d. Concomitant use of progesterone

J. Social habits pertinent to risk factors for breast cancer

    1. High-fat diet

    2. Alcohol intake (Question whether patient consumes more than two drinks per day.)

    3. Smoking history (can be cofactor in the development of breast cancer)

K. Personal history

    1. Personal history of cancer of the breast or other reproductive cancer

    2. Pelvic surgery, including oophorectomy

    3. Family history of breast cancer

L. *BRCA* testing (see Chapter 34, "Genetic Testing for Hereditary Breast and Ovarian Cancer"). Ask about

    1. Rationale for testing

    2. Results

    3. If results were positive, was any special monitoring necessary?

VI. Inspection of the breasts

  A. Position

    1. The client should be seated, with arms at her side; she should be disrobed from the waist up.

    2. Begin inspection 3 feet from the client to fully inspect both breasts.

  B. Compare the breasts.

    1. Note size, symmetry, hair pattern, location, and contour.

    2. Normal findings

      a. Breasts should be equal bilaterally; a slight asymmetry is common in adolescents.

      b. Breasts extend from the third to the sixth ribs, with the nipple and areola over the fourth or fifth rib; convex contour; sparse hair surrounds areola. (There may be racial variations.)

      c. Size of breasts varies with overall body weight, and genetic and hormonal influences.

      d. Flatter breasts are seen in geriatric clients (less fat).

    3. Clinical alterations

      a. Marked asymmetry resulting from cysts, inflammation, or tumor

  C. Assess the breast skin

    1. Note color, texture, venous pattern, temperature, and the presence of edema, dimpling or retraction, and lesions.

    2. Normal findings: Warm, smooth skin; silver striae; lighter color than exposed areas of skin

3. Clinical alterations
   a. Edema and dimpling are often suggestive of breast cancer.
   b. Inflammation is often caused by mastitis, breast abscess, or inflammatory breast carcinoma.
   c. Retraction results from a benign or malignant tumor.
   d. Dilated superficial veins result from a benign or malignant tumor of the areolar area.
   e. The breasts are engorged in pregnancy and lactation, with dilated superficial veins.
D. Inspect the areolae and the nipples.
   1. Note size, shape, texture, pigmentation of the breast, direction, pigmentation of the nipples; also, note the presence of any discharge or supernumerary nipples.
   2. Normal findings
      a. Symmetrically round or oval areolae
      b. Pigmentation should be pink to dark brown, with roughened Montgomery's tubercles; nipples should be erect and the same color as areolae.
   3. Clinical alterations
      a. Inversion (new onset) is often associated with breast cancer.
      b. Excoriation is often associated with Paget's disease.
      c. Areola is darkened during pregnancy.
E. Observe for milk lines
   1. Origin: Breast tissue arises out of the ectoderm, extending along the lines from the axilla to the groin.
   2. Accessory or supernumerary mammary glands and nipples are sometimes found along these embryotic lines. Women may have thought that they were moles or fleshy warts.
   3. Supernumerary nipples are often found 5 cm to 6 cm below the normal nipples.
F. Observe breasts when the client is in the following positions
   1. Sitting with both arms raised over head
   2. Sitting with both arms pressed firmly on hips, flexing pectoral muscles
   3. Sitting, leaning forward with arms outstretched, allowing breasts to hang freely
   4. Supine with arm above head, on the side being examined. This stretching of the pectoral muscles pulls on breast tissue and exaggerates any dimpling or pucker or retraction.

VII. **Palpation of the breast**
   A. Basics
      1. In a very large breast, it is unlikely that anything but the most obvious lesions will be discovered.

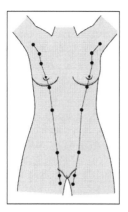

FIGURE 6.3 Milk lines. Possible sites of accessory breast tissue or supernumerary nipples, both of which may become more prominent during pregnancy and the puerperium.

2. The presence of adipose tissue affects the nodularity, density, and fullness of the breast.
   a. In a woman who has recently lost a considerable amount of weight, the breasts are lumpy because the cushion of fatty tissue is absent. The breasts may feel similar to tapioca pudding.
   b. Women who are overweight have fuller breasts.
3. Three to 5 days before menstruation, the breasts become engorged, increasing in size. The CBE should not be performed during this time.
4. Wash hands with warm water before examination.
5. Placing a small pillow under the side to be examined flattens the breast tissue and distributes it evenly across the chest wall to facilitate the detection of masses or accessory breast tissue or supernumerary nipples, both of which may become more prominent during pregnancy and the puerperium.
6. If a woman reports a problem with one or both of her breasts, examine the unaffected side first to provide a baseline for comparison.
7. Palpation may be performed with one or two hands.
8. Lower the woman's arm to relax the pectoral muscles to best examine deep in the muscles in the area of the tail of Spence.
9. Sensory component of fingertips
   a. Uses sensitive pressure receptors in the fingertips
   b. With training, fingertips can detect most 3.0 mm tumors.
   c. The structure must be denser than the surrounding tissue.

      10. Use powder if the patient's skin is moist with perspiration.

B. Palpate the four quadrants of the breast.

    1. Instructions to client: Observe how your breast is being examined so that you can use this technique at home. Describe any tenderness.

    2. Technique

        a. The examiner should lubricate his or her fingers with lotion or soap and warm water or powder.

        b. Gently palpate the breast with the pads of the four fingers.

        c. Starting at the 12 o'clock position on the upper aspect of the breast, rotate fingerpads in imaginary concentric circles or lines, toward the center of the breast, the areola, and the nipple.

        d. Do not lift fingers from the breast when moving from one section to another.

        e. In large-breasted women, use bimanual palpation, compressing the breast between hands.

        f. Next, palpate the breast with the client supine, with her arm above her head on the side being examined.

        g. Repeat for the other breast.

        h. Chart any anomalies. A diagram works best.

    3. Note temperature; size (in centimeters), location, delimitation (borders of the mass), mobility, degree of fixation, and consistency (hardness) of any masses; and breast tenderness

    4. If a mass is present, assess for the retraction phenomenon

        a. Elevate and mold the breast around the mass. Observe for any dimpling.

    5. Normal findings

        a. The breast should be warm, smooth, and elastic.

        b. No masses or discharge should be present; the breast is coarser and more nodular in a geriatric client.

        c. Generalized, uniform nodularity (may be increased in second half of cycle in a woman taking progesterone supplements)

        d. Increased density and nodularity in the area of the inframammary ridge (firm, crescent-shaped ridge of compressed tissue along the lower edge of the breast)

    6. Clinical alterations (see Table 6.2, which compares different types of lumps)

        a. Nontender, mobile, smooth, well-delineated nodules associated with fibroadenoma

        b. Nontender, immobile, or fixed nodule suggestive of breast cancer

TABLE 6.2 Comparison of Different Types of Breast Lumps

CHARACTERISTIC	FIBROCYSTIC	FIBROADENOMA	CANCER
Age	25 to 55 years (rare after menopause)	Puberty to menopause (peak 20–29 years)	Older than 30 years of age Incidence increases with age
Number	Usually multiple, may be single	Usually single	Usually single; two primary lesions may occur in the same breast
Shape	Smooth, round, may be multilobular	Smooth, lobular, round	Irregular
Delimitation	Well circumscribed	Well circumscribed	Poorly delineated from surrounding tissues
Mobility	Mobile	Mobile	Limited mobility; fixed to surrounding skin or underlying tissue
Pain	Present, cyclic (second half of menstrual cycle)	Usually not painful	Usually nontender
Axillary involvement	None	None	May be present with regional metastasis to axillary lymph nodes
Nipple discharge	Absent	Absent	Often present

    c. Tender, multiple nodes in one or both breasts associated with chronic mastitis

VIII. Palpate the nipple and the areola
    A. Technique
        1. Gently compress nipple between index finger and thumb.
        2. Repeat for other nipple.
    B. Note
        1. The amount, color, and odor of any fluid that is ejected from the nipple
        2. Shape and consistency of nipple
    C. Evaluation of the discharge (see Table 6.3, which compares the various types of nipple discharge)

TABLE 6.3 Comparison of Types of Nipple Discharge

TYPES OF NIPPLE DISCHARGE	DESCRIPTION	COMMENTS
Milky white, thin	White, thin	Lactation
Serous, thin, clear, and yellowish	Thin, clear (like the white of an egg) or yellowish	Suggests intraductal papilloma
Serosanguineous, thin	Thin, clear, and pink	Suggests fibrocystic changes or cancer
Bloody	Thick, opaque, and red	Suggests fibrocystic changes or cancer
Watery	Thin, clear, and colorless (rare)	Suggests cancer
Purulent	Thick, opaque, greenish or yellowish	Suggests infection

Note: Pap test should be performed on any nipple discharge.

1. A guaiac test may be necessary to test for blood in the discharge.
2. Cytologic examination of breast discharge
   a. Compress the nipple, and express the discharge onto a slide.
   b. Spray with fixative, as with Pap smear.
   c. A Pap test may reveal abnormal cells.
3. If bilateral nipple discharge is present, suspect galactorrhea. Measure prolactin levels to check for a pituitary tumor.

D. Normal findings: No discharge, except during lactation; nipple is erect

E. Clinical alterations
   1. Unilateral, serous (egg white), or serosanguineous discharge is suggestive of intraductal papillomas.
   2. Clear, yellowish fluid is associated with chronic mastitis.
   3. Sanguineous or dark red discharge is associated with Paget's disease.
   4. Galactorrhea is associated with the use of tranquilizers, marijuana, and high estrogen levels.

IX. **Palpate lymph nodes**

A. Technique
   1. Using the same rotating motion, gently palpate the supraclavicular and infraclavicular areas.
   2. Face the patient, abduct her right arm with your right hand, and place your left hand against the chest wall, high into the axilla.

3. Rotate your hand, cup the examining fingers, and reach high into the axilla using gentle pressure to palpate the subscapular, central, pectoral, and lateral axillary nodes as the hand slides down the axilla.
4. Support the woman's arm with the opposite hand. This approach relaxes the pectoralis muscle and permits careful evaluation of the axilla.
5. Repeat for the opposite axilla. Repeat with the client supine with her arm over her head.

B. Note location (which quadrant), size (in centimeters), shape, consistency, mobility, and tenderness of any nodes palpated. A diagram is helpful.
C. Normal findings: None
D. Clinical alterations
   1. Nontender, hard enlarged lymph nodes are indicative of metastatic breast cancer.
   2. Lymphadenitis: Freely mobile 3 to 5 mm, associated with an infection of the client's hand or arm
E. Refer any abnormal findings for further evaluation.

X. **Physical examination of an augmented breast**
A. Physical examination includes evaluation of both the natural breast tissue and the implant. The breast must also be examined for possible complications related to the implants.
B. In both the upright and supine positions
   1. Assessment procedure performed when the woman is upright with arms at her side
      a. Instruct the woman to elevate her arms over her head and then to place her hands on her hips and lean forward, flexing the pectoralis muscle when asked.
      b. Palpation of the natural breast tissue with the patient upright is often easier if she leans slightly forward.
      c. The breast tissue should be gently pinched or pulled away from the implants.
   2. Assessment procedure when the woman is in the supine position
      a. The patient's arm should not be elevated above the head, but rather relaxed at her side to relax the pectoral muscles, making the implants more mobile and compressible.
      b. Contraction of the pectoralis muscle contracts the implant into a ball.
      c. Push the implant away from each wedge of tissue as it is examined.
         (1) Some implants are soft and easily displaced.
      d. Palpate the axillary and supraclavicular area for lymph nodes as described previously.
      e. Evaluate the implant for compressibility and mobility.

   C. Note the following elements of the implant:
     1. Contour
       a. Flatness
       b. Bulges
       c. Indentations
     2. Abnormal skin changes
       a. Thickening
       b. Lesions
       c. Nipple abnormality
     3. Compare the size of the breasts, observing the location of the augmentation scar.
     4. Determine whether the implants are visible.
     5. Observe for signs of capsular contraction or abnormal shape of implants.
     6. Assess the integrity of the implant by evaluating any capsular scarring or contraction.
       a. A ruptured implant may not be evident clinically.
       b. May feel firm or hard from silicone granuloma formation

XI. Chart
   A. Carefully document physical examination findings.
     1. A diagram is helpful because it graphically documents any suspected anomalies.
     2. Divide the breast into four quadrants by drawing two imaginary lines through the nipple at right angles to each other. Tail of Spence is an extension of the upper outer quadrant.
   B. Record: Breasts symmetric; normal contour; no dimpling, retraction, or erythema; nipples erect, no discharge; areola pink; firm, smooth, elastic breasts; no masses or palpable lymph nodes

XII. Mammogram
   A. Mammography explained
     1. Radiographic examination of the breast
     2. Only reliable means of detecting breast cancer before palpation
   B. Mammography can pick up soft tissue densities not yet palpable, as well as calcifications that are too small to feel. BSE and CBE are complementary to mammography, and each test is performed to detect a mass missed by the other two.
   C. Indications
     1. To obtain a baseline mammogram in women 40 years of age, or earlier if clinically indicated
     2. To evaluate a lump or mass found during palpation of the breast by either the woman or the clinician
     3. To screen a woman for breast cancer, particularly those at risk for development of breast cancer

4. To evaluate the breast for any abnormalities before initiating estrogen replacement therapy
D. Advantages
   1. Easy to perform
   2. The sensitivity of mammography is the percentage of breast cancers detected in a given population when breast cancer is present. According to the National Cancer Institute overall sensitivity is approximately 79% but is lower in younger women and in those with dense breast tissue.
   3. Ninety percent specific for benign disease (percentage of benign disease detected by test as benign). The specificity of mammography is the likelihood of the test being normal when cancer is absent, whereas the false-positive rate is the likelihood of the test being abnormal when cancer is absent. If specificity is low, many false-positive examinations result in unnecessary follow-up examinations and procedures.
   4. Positive predictive value for cancers is 95%
   5. Relatively inexpensive
E. Disadvantages
   1. Requires special equipment and trained personnel
   2. Low sensitivity in women younger than 50 years of age because of the fat content of breasts
   3. Uncomfortable for the woman
F. Role of ultrasound
   1. Used to distinguish between solid and cystic masses
      a. If the mass is cystic, refer for possible aspiration.
      b. If solid, refer for needle localization biopsy.
G. Screening parameters as recommended by the ACS.
   1. Mammography
      a. Baseline mammography by 40 years of age
         (1) May start earlier if there is a strong family history of breast cancer, positive *BRCA* test results, fibrocystic disease (makes palpation more difficult), or breast augmentation
      b. Mammography should be performed every year after 40 years of age.
         (1) The ACS believes that age alone should not be the reason to stop having regular mammograms.
         (2) Women with serious health problems or short life expectancies should discuss with their doctors whether to continue to have mammograms or not.
      c. Women who are at high risk for breast cancer based on certain factors should get an MRI and a mammogram every year. This includes women who
         (1) Have a lifetime risk of breast cancer of about 20% to 25% or greater, according to risk-assessment tools available

        (2) Have a known *BRCA1* or *BRCA2* gene mutation

        (3) Have a first-degree relative (parent, brother, sister, or child) with a *BRCA1* or *BRCA2* gene mutation, and have had genetic testing themselves

        (4) Had radiation therapy to the chest when they were between the ages of 10 and 30 years

  H. U.S. Preventive Services Task Force (USPSTF) recommendations

    1. Routine screening of average-risk women should begin at age 50, instead of age 40.

      a. Routine screening should end at age 74.

      b. Women should get screening mammograms every 2 years instead of every year.

      c. BSEs have little value, based on findings from several large studies.

    2. Digital mammaography

      a. Similar to traditional mammography but the system uses a digital receptor and computer

    3. CBE

      a. Every 3 years between the ages of 20 and 40 years (many clinicians start earlier)

      b. Every year for women older than 40 years of age

 I. Note: The Centers for Disease Control and Prevention (CDC) states that having a CBE or a BSE has not been found to decrease risk of dying from breast cancer. At this time, the best way to find breast cancer is with a mammogram. If you choose to have CBEs and to perform BSEs, be sure you also get mammograms regularly.

 J. Special findings

    1. Microcalcifications

      a. Tiny specks of calcium in the breast

      b. Often found in areas of rapidly dividing cells

      c. Appear benign

      d. Subsequent mammography in 3 to 6 months

      e. If the microcalcifications are clustered or in small groupings, refer the patient for needle localization biopsy or removal.

    2. Macrocalcification

      a. Calcium deposits are frequently associated with degenerative changes in the breast

      b. Due to aging, old injuries, or inflammation

      c. Usually benign

      d. First appearance; subsequent mammography in 6 months

      e. Stable—mammography should be performed every year

XIII. Breast cancer risk-assessment tool

  A. For an excellent tool for screening women for breast cancer on a yearly basis go to http://www.cancer.gov/bcrisktool

Bibliography

American Cancer Society. (2013). *Cancer facts and figures 2013*. Atlanta, GA: American Cancer Society.

Bates, B. (2012). (written by Lynn Bickley MD). *A guide to physical examination and history taking* (12th ed.). Philadelphia, PA: Lippincott.

Boyd, N. F., Guo, H., Martin, L. J., Sun, L., Stone, J., Fishell, E., et al. (2007). Mammographic density and the risk and detection of breast cancer. *New England Journal of Medicine, 356*(3), 227–236.

Centers for Disease Control and Prevention. (2013). *Breast cancer statistics*. Retrieved January 14, 2014, from http://www.cdc.gov/cancer/breast/statistics

Goldman, S. (1994). Evaluating breast masses. *Contemporary OB/GYN-NP, 1*(4), 76–94.

Mann, L. (1995). Physical examination of the augmented breast: Description of a displacement technique. *Obstetrics & Gynecology, 85*(2), 178–185.

National Cancer Institute. (2013). *Breast cancer screening concepts*. Retrieved January 14, 2014, from http://www.cancer.gov/cancertopics/pdq/screening/breast/health-professional/page4

Pennypacker, H. A. (1994). Achieving competence in clinical breast examination. *Nurse Practitioner Forum, 4*(2), 45–56.

Somkin, C. P. (1993). Improving the effectiveness of breast self-examination in the early detection of breast cancer: A selective review of the literature. *Nurse Practitioner Forum, 4*(2), 345–348.

Thompson, K. (2006). Evaluation and management of common breast complaints. *Female Patient, 31*, 28–38.

U.S. Preventative Services Task Force. (2009). *Screening for breast cancer*. Retrieved December 22, 2013, from http://www.uspreventiveservicestaskforce.org/uspstf/uspsbrca.htm

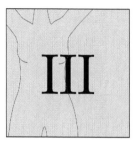

III

Evaluation of Special Populations

Assessment of the Pregnant Woman

7

Kate Green

I. **Initial prenatal evaluation.** The initial evaluation of a pregnant woman should include a thorough review of the patient's medical history and a careful physical examination. This visit is a good opportunity to screen for potential complications of pregnancy and to begin to establish a trusting relationship with the pregnant woman.

II. **Documentation of pregnancy.** Many practices require documentation in the chart of a positive pregnancy test result to verify the woman's pregnancy before the onset of the comprehensive initial prenatal evaluation. Urine and serum pregnancy tests are based on levels of human chorionic gonadotropin (hCG), which is secreted into the maternal bloodstream and then excreted through the maternal urine.

    A. Urine pregnancy tests
1. Accurate 95% to 99% of the time, depending on time used and correct use.
2. Sensitive within 7 days after implantation.
3. Possible for pregnancy to be detected before first missed period; however, this is not a certainty.
4. The test is inexpensive, private, and easy to obtain over the counter.
5. Use first morning void when possible because concentrated urine improves the pregnancy detection rate (nearly equal to that of serum).
6. The test is specific for beta subunit of hCG, eliminating cross-reactivity with other hormones.

    B. Serum qualitative or quantitative tests do not indicate pregnancy until levels rise above baseline values (may vary by laboratory, but usually around 25–30 mIU/dL).
1. hCG is detectable in serum as early as 7 to 9 days after ovulation or just after implantation.

    2. During the first 3 to 4 weeks after implantation, serum hCG level doubles every 2 days.

    3. The level should be 50 to 250 mIU/dL at the time of the first missed menstrual period.

    4. The level peaks at 60 to 70 days after fertilization, and then decreases during the first half of pregnancy, after which it remains relatively constant throughout the remainder of the second half of pregnancy.

    5. Qualitative test results are read as positive or negative (false-positive results are rare).

    6. Quantitative beta-hCG is a radioisotope test performed on a blood sample to quantify levels of hCG. It is most useful when

        a. Serial testing is desired to monitor suspected ectopic pregnancy, molar pregnancy, or spontaneous abortion.

        b. Variable results from other tests are present.

    7. Must specify qualitative or quantitative test when ordering serum hCG.

  C. Progesterone levels

    1. These levels remain constant through the first 9 to 10 weeks of pregnancy, unlike hCG.

    2. Nonviable pregnancies have much lower levels than normal pregnancies.

    3. Highly predictive of pregnancy outcome

    4. Not routinely performed

  D. Signs and symptoms of pregnancy: The diagnosis of pregnancy is based on the following

    1. Presumptive signs (Table 7.1 lists signs and symptoms)

    2. Probable signs

    3. Positive signs

III. **Estimated date of confinement (EDC)**

  A. Obtain date of start of last menstrual period (LMP)

    1. Evaluate patient's surety on the date because EDC is based on the LMP.

    2. Conception usually occurs approximately 2 weeks after the LMP in a 28-day cycle.

  B. Review of menstrual cycles

    1. Frequency of menses: If the woman does not have a regular 28-day cycle, adjust EDC accordingly.

    2. Duration of flow

    3. Question whether LMP was normal for the patient; if flow was exceptionally light or spotting only, the condition could be the result of syncytiotrophoblastic cells implanting in the endometrial lining at about the time the next menstrual cycle would have been expected. This process will cause a change in the EDC.

TABLE 7.1 Signs and Symptoms of Pregnancy

SIGNS	DESCRIPTION
PRESUMPTIVE	
Cessation of menses	Uterine lining does not shed. May have some spotting around the time of implantation.
Nausea, vomiting, "morning sickness"	Onset at 2 to 12 weeks gestation; usually subsides 6 to 8 weeks later. Most severe on awakening.
Frequent urination	Bladder irritability from enlarging fetus pressing on bladder, causing reduced capacity.
Breast tenderness	Onset at 2 to 3 weeks gestation; may be present throughout pregnancy. Soreness and tingling of breasts from hormonal stimulation.
Perception of fetal movement, or "quickening"	16 to 18 weeks gestation; should be present until delivery. Sensation of "fluttering" or motion in abdomen perceived by the mother.
Fatigue	Common early in pregnancy; usually resolves by 20 weeks gestation.
Skin changes	Abdominal striae and increased pigmentation from hormonal changes.
PROBABLE	
Enlargement of the abdomen	Palpated abdominally above symphysis pubis at 12 weeks gesatation.
Hegar's sign	6 weeks gestation; palpable softening of lower uterine segment
Goodell's sign	8 weeks gestation; softening of the cervix (changes from consistency of the tip of the nose to that of lips)
Chadwick's sign	6 to 8 weeks gestation; blue-violet hue from congestion seen on the vulva, vagina, and cervix (particularly the vaginal opening).
Braxton Hicks contractions	May be felt as early as end of first trimester. Irregular, painless, intermittent uterine contractions.
Pregnancy test	Positive 7 to 10 days after conception

(continued)

TABLE 7.1 Signs and Symptoms of Pregnancy *(continued)*

SIGNS	DESCRIPTION
POSITIVE	
Fetal heart	Ultrasound Fetal heart motion by 4 to 8 weeks gestation after conception Doppler Fetal heart sounds by 10 to 12 weeks after conception
Movement	19 weeks gestation; mother may feel movement weeks earlier but it must be verified by examiner
Visualization of the fetus	Ultrasound; visualize fetus at 5 to 6 weeks gestation Rarely used to diagnose pregnancy, more frequently used to establish estimated date of confinement

    C. Accurate dating is imperative to allow for prenatal testing to be carried out at the appropriate time intervals.
        1. Nägele's rule: Estimated by adding 7 days to the first day of the LMP; then subtract 3 months from that date to estimate the EDC.
        2. Obstetric wheels are available for calculation of EDC from many companies.
        3. Clarification of terms
           a. Pregnancy: 40 weeks (10 lunar months), or 280 days from LMP
           b. Fetal calculation: 38 weeks or 266 days from conception
    D. Pregnancy tests are probable signs of pregnancy. Only auscultation of fetal heart tone, sonographic evidence, and fetal motion (according to some authorities) are positive signs of pregnancy.

IV. **Current identifying data: These items provide general information that is current and allow the woman to answer relatively uncomplicated questions comfortably, establishing a pattern for the rest of the interview. These items should include**
    A. Current name
    B. Date of birth to screen for age-related complications
        1. If the woman is older than 35 years of age, genetic counseling should be offered.
        2. Review the risk for chromosomal abnormalities relative to maternal age (Table 7.2).
    C. Current employment: Screen for occupational hazards to the health of the mother and the developing fetus

TABLE 7.2 Risk for Chromosomal Abnormality (at Birth) at Various Maternal Ages*

MATERNAL AGE	RISK FOR DOWN SYNDROME	TOTAL RISK FOR CHROMOSOMAL ABNORMALITIES
20	1:1667	1:526
21	1:1667	1:526
22	1:1429	1:500
23	1:1429	1:500
24	1:1250	1:476
25	1:1250	1:476
26	1:1176	1:476
27	1:1111	1:455
28	1:1053	1:435
29	1:1000	1:417
30	1:952	1:385
31	1:909	1:385
32	1:769	1:322
33	1:602	1:286
34	1:485	1:238
35	1:378	1:192
36	1:289	1:156
37	1:224	1:127
38	1:173	1:102
39	1:136	1:83
40	1:106	1:66
41	1:82	1:53
42	1:63	1:42
43	1:49	1:33
44	1:38	1:26
45	1:30	1:21
46	1:23	1:16
47	1:18	1:13
48	1:14	1:10
49	1:11	1:8

*Because sample size for some intervals is relatively small, 95% confidence limits are sometimes relatively large. Nonetheless, these figures are suitable for genetic counseling.

    D. Partner's name, if involved with patient, or support person's name

    E. Partner's employment

    F. Household members

    G. Race: Screen for race- and ethnicity-related disorders (see genetic assessment questionnaire, Appendix 3.1)

        1. Ethnic populations and carrier status

           a. Black, some Hispanic, and Southeast Asian women may be at risk for sickle cell disease.

           b. Ashkenazi Jewish, French Canadian, Cajun, and Pennsylvania Dutch women may be at risk for Tay-Sachs disease.

           c. Mediterranean, North African, Middle Eastern, and Asian women may be at risk for beta-thalassemia.

           d. Asian women may be at risk for alpha-thalassemia.

    H. Religion, if any: Screen for any religious restrictions on care or nutrition or practices specific to childbearing

    I. Educational level

V. **Evaluate reactions to pregnancy: Pregnancy is the reason the woman has sought care, and it is the most important issue to her. It is wise to discuss early in the visit what her expectations are in relation to her pregnancy and to establish what care she is expecting. Additionally, the reactions of her partner and family should be explored.**

    A. Feelings about pregnancy: whether it was planned or unplanned

    B. Plans for the pregnancy, including

        1. To keep the baby

        2. To put the baby up for adoption

        3. To terminate the pregnancy

    C. Whether friends and family have been informed and their reactions

    D. Partner's response

VI. **Current physical symptoms: Include severity, when occurred, treatment or relief measures tried and their effectiveness. Table 7.3 summarizes common complaints of pregnancy and their explanation.**

    A. Nausea and vomiting (i.e., "morning sickness")

        1. Most common problem associated with pregnancy. Common in first trimester (70%–85% of pregnant women); infrequently noted later

        2. Unknown cause: Possible reaction to high levels of hCG

        3. Frequent and consistent vomiting, dehydration, weight loss, electrolyte imbalance, poor appetite or food intake, or ketonuria may indicate hyperemesis gravidarum (0.5%–2% of all pregnancies) *↳ severe type of nausea*

    B. Breast tenderness (mastalgia)

        1. Related to increased levels of estrogen, progesterone, and chorionic somatomammotropin

        2. Often, the first presumptive sign of pregnancy

TABLE 7.3 Common Complaints During Pregnancy and Their Explanation

COMMON COMPLAINT	TIME IN PREGNANCY	EXPLANATION AND EFFECTS ON WOMAN'S BODY
No menses (amenorrhea)	Throughout	Continued high levels of estrogen, progesterone, and human chorionic gonadotropin after fertilization of the ovum allow the uterine endometrium to build up and support the developing pregnancy rather than to slough as menses.
Nausea with or without vomiting	First trimester	Possible causes include hormonal changes of pregnancy leading to slowed peristalsis throughout the gastrointestinal tract, changes in taste and smell, the growing uterus, or emotional factors. Women may have a modest (2–5 lb) weight loss in the first trimester.
Breast tenderness, tingling	First trimester	The hormones of pregnancy stimulate the growth of breast tissue. As the breasts enlarge throughout pregnancy, women may experience upper backache from their increased weight. There is also increased blood flow throughout the breasts, increasing pressure on the tissue.
Urinary frequency (nondisease)	First and third trimesters	There is increased blood volume and increased filtration rate in the kidneys with increased urine production. Due to less space for the bladder from pressure from the growing uterus (first trimester) or from the descent of the fetal head (third trimester), the woman needs to empty her bladder more frequently.
Fatigue	First trimester	Mechanisms not clearly understood, but multifactorial, including increased cardiac output.
Heartburn and constipation	Throughout	Relaxation of the lower esophageal sphincter allows stomach contents to back up into the lower esophagus. The decreased gastrointestinal motility caused by pregnancy hormones slows peristalsis and causes constipation. Constipation may cause or aggravate existing hemorrhoids.

(continued)

TABLE 7.3 Common Complaints During Pregnancy and Their Explanation *(continued)*

COMMON COMPLAINT	TIME IN PREGNANCY	EXPLANATION AND EFFECTS ON WOMAN'S BODY
Leukorrhea	Throughout	Increased secretions from the cervix and the vaginal epithelium due to the hormones and vasocongestion of pregnancy result in an asymptomatic milky white vaginal discharge.
Weight loss	First trimester	If a women experiences nausea and vomiting, she may not be eating normally in early pregnancy (see Nausea previously described).
Backache (nondisease)	Throughout, may increase third trimester	Hormonally induced relaxation of joints and ligaments and the minor lordosis required to balance the growing uterus sometimes result in a lower backache. Pathologic causes must be ruled out.

    C. Abdominal pain or cramping
        1. Commonly benign and associated with round ligament pain
        2. If present, should check for symptoms of impending miscarriage, such as bleeding, or for gastrointestinal disorders
    D. Vaginal discharge or bleeding
        1. Discharge may be normal or may indicate genital tract infection
        2. Spotting may be normal and may indicate implantation of the blastocyst, resulting from invasive chorionic villi activity in the uterine lining. Spotting may occur at approximately the time a woman would have been expecting her menses if she were not pregnant.
        3. Heavy bleeding in pregnancy is abnormal and must be evaluated further. Consider
            a. Obtaining a sonogram
            b. Obtaining quantitative hCG level for later comparison
            c. Refer for follow-up
    E. Urinary frequency
        1. Frequency may be normal due to uterine position in relation to maternal bladder in the first and third trimesters.
        2. If urination is accompanied by dysuria, it may indicate a urinary tract infection.
    F. Headache: Must monitor for preeclampsia if persistent
    G. Nosebleeds: If they are mild, they are considered normal
    H. Fatigue
        1. Very common in first trimester, related to increased cardiac output.
        2. Patients need reassurance that fatigue will lessen as the pregnancy progresses.

I. Heartburn
   1. More common in late pregnancy
   2. Related to increased pressure in abdomen and softening of pyloric sphincter
J. Back pain
   1. Common
   2. Should discuss relief measures, such as good support bra, warm soaks, erect posture, and massage if no disease is noted during examination
K. Quickening, if present (patient's first awareness of fetal movement)
   1. Assists in dating pregnancy
   2. Quickening is usually not felt until approximately 16 to 20 weeks gestation
L. Skin changes may normally include
   1. Darkening of the areola
   2. Linea nigra
   3. Chloasma – Darkening of face. Brown patches appear on the face
   4. Breast and abdominal striae from stretching of skin
M. Ptyalism (excessive salivation)
   1. Reassure the patient that the problem is common and harmless
   2. Attempts at treatment largely unsuccessful, although may try remedies for nausea
N. Absence of menses
O. Constipation
   1. Common
   2. Probably related to steroid-induced suppression of bowel motility and compression of the intestine from the enlarging uterus
   3. Aggravates hemorrhoids

VII. **History since conception provides screening for agents that may increase risks for anomalies or miscarriage and risks for pregnancy outcomes for the pregnant woman and her baby.**
   A. Radiation exposure, including x-ray studies (even dental) without use of a shield (usually routinely used on women of childbearing age)
   B. Viral exposure
      1. Includes rubella exposure (German measles. Distinctive red rash)
         a. Rubella infection in pregnancy has a high rate of causing fetal malformations in early pregnancy; the risk decreases as the pregnancy progresses. Up to 50% risk if infected in the first month of pregnancy, 20% in the second month of pregnancy, 7% in the third month, and 1% to 2% in the fourth and fifth months of pregnancy.
      2. Other "childhood illnesses" the woman has been exposed to since conception
         a. Infection in pregnancy may cause varying complications or be entirely benign.

C. Fever
   1. Include how high and when occurred
   2. May provide a clue to first-trimester exposure to diseases that may affect pregnancy such as rubella or Fifth's disease (human parvovirus B-19)
D. Medications used since conception
   1. Inquire about use of
      a. Over-the-counter medications
      b. Home remedies and herbal preparations
      c. Prescribed medications
      d. Progesterone in infertility patients
      e. Vitamins, folic acid, or mineral supplements; particularly calcium and iron
   2. Drugs are rated as categories A, B, C, D, and X (Box 7.1)
   3. Medications should be checked in a drug reference if the examiner is unsure of classification or effect on pregnancy
E. Recalled or documented pre-gravid weight and weight gain since onset of pregnancy
   1. Overweight and obesity may be related to pregnancy complications of hypertension, diabetes, fetal macrosomia, and to delivery complications.

VIII. **Medical history: Include diseases that could affect the woman's health or fetal well-being during pregnancy.**
   A. Diabetes: Correlates with an increased risk for multiple maternal and fetal complications, such as preterm labor, infectious illnesses, hydramnios and hypertension (maternal), and congenital anomalies, fetal macrosomia, intrauterine fetal death, delayed fetal pulmonary maturation, and metabolic abnormalities
      1. Diabetes in pregnancy of any type necessitates close control and consultation.
      2. Screening recommended for all pregnant women during initial history. Further screening recommended between 24 and 28 weeks gestation, with initial laboratory work for diabetes with 1 hour, 50-g glucola test. Testing should be done earlier if indicated by history of gestational diabetes or high-risk factors, such as morbid obesity.
      3. Three types of diabetes to be considered in pregnancy
         a. Type 1: Insulin dependent: Should assess age at onset and amount and type of insulin used; refer the patient for insulin management and nutritional counseling
         b. Type 2: Noninsulin dependent: Refer for plan for monitoring serum glucose levels and to nutritionist for dietary counseling, and possible use of oral hypoglycemics or insulin for strict control of glucose levels

---

BOX 7.1 *Drugs During Pregnancy: Food and Drug Administration Risk Categories*

- *Category A*
Controlled studies in women do not demonstrate a risk to the fetus in the first trimester (and there is no evidence of risk in later trimesters), and the possibility of fetal harm appears to be remote.
- *Category B*
Either animal reproduction studies have not shown a fetal risk and there are no controlled studies in pregnant women, or animal reproduction studies have shown an adverse effect (other than a decrease in fertility) that was not confirmed in controlled studies in women in the first trimester (and there is no evidence of a risk in later trimesters).
- *Category C*
Either studies in animals have revealed adverse effects on the fetus (teratogenic, embryocidal, or other effect) and there are no controlled studies in women, or studies in women and animals are not available. Drugs in this category should be given only if the potential benefit justifies the potential risk to the fetus.
- *Category D*
There is positive evidence of human fetal risk, but the benefits from use in pregnant women may be acceptable despite the risk. The drug may be needed in a life-threatening situation or for a serious disease when safer drugs cannot be used or are ineffective.
- *Category X*
Studies in animals or human beings have shown fetal abnormalities, there is evidence of fetal risk based on human experience, or both, and the risk of the use of the drug in pregnant women clearly outweighs any possible benefit. The drug is contraindicated in women who are or may become pregnant.

Based on information from Yaffe (1990) and the Food and Drug Administration labeling and prescription drug advertising (1979).

---

  c. Gestational diabetes: Diabetes during pregnancy. Refer for dietary counseling and glucose monitoring, and possible oral hypoglycemics or insulin for strict control of glucose levels
 B. Hypertension: Consult as needed
  1. Chronic: Assess for method of control or use of antihypertensive medication
  2. Pregnancy related: Must monitor and refer due to increased risk to current pregnancy
 C. Cardiac disease
  1. Assess need for prophylaxis in labor if patient has mitral valve prolapse
  2. Consultation necessary for other cardiac diseases

D. Liver disease
   1. Assess risk factors for hepatitis and screen with blood testing as needed. Infants may require treatment with immunoglobulins soon after delivery if hepatitis is present.
E. Renal disease
F. Gallbladder disease: Can be exacerbated in pregnancy
   1. Counsel for low-fat diet, and refer as needed
G. Stomach or bowel disease
   1. If abdominal surgery was performed, note type of surgery and location of any scarring
   2. Consult specialist because the condition could cause deleterious effects during the antepartum or intrapartum period
H. Pulmonary disease
   1. If asthma is present, assess which medications or inhalers the patient currently uses.
   2. Assess current and recent status of asthma (mild, intermittent, severe).
   3. If pulmonary disease is present, evaluate early with consultation because of the possibility of the need for anesthesia in labor.
I. Congenital anomalies and genetic diseases: Must screen for risk to patient and fetus during pregnancy and labor.
J. Cancer
   1. If cancer of the cervix treated with cone biopsy, the patient is at increased risk for preterm labor.
K. Genitourinary tract disease
L. Varicosities and phlebitis: May worsen during prenancy
M. Anemia
   1. Inquire about sickle cell disease and sickle cell trait as well as thalassemia.
   2. Screen with initial laboratory work if status is unclear.
N. Infectious diseases
   1. Hepatitis: Assess for type and current status
   2. Tuberculosis
   3. Human immunodeficiency virus (HIV) infection
      a. Inquire about history of high-risk sexual behavior or intravenous (IV) drug use.
      b. Rate of transmission of HIV with retrovirals is approximately 2%.
O. Autoimmune disorders
   1. Increased rate of miscarriage in women with systemic lupus erythematosus (SLE)
P. Neurologic disorders or any neurologic defects
Q. Psychiatric disorders
   1. Screen for risk factors for postpartum depression
R. Multifetal gestation
S. Allergies: Document reaction

IX. Obstetric and gynecologic history
  A. Gynecologic
    1. Abnormal uterine bleeding
    2. History of sexually transmitted diseases (STDs) in self and partner
      a. Treatment of STDs; include human papillomavirus (HPV), herpes simplex virus (HSV), HIV, chlamydia, gonorrhea, *Trichomonas*, bacterial vaginosis, and syphilis
      b. Note test of cures, if done
      c. Any long-term sequelae
    3. Contraception
      a. Types ever used
      b. Most recently used method
      c. When contraception was most recently used
      d. If patient became pregnant while actively using contraception, the examiner may need to discuss effects of contraceptive type on pregnancy
    4. Gynecologic surgery: List date and reason
  B. Infertility treatments performed
    1. Include current or continuing infertility treatments
    2. Use of ovulation induction
    3. Previous attempts at pregnancy
      a. Intrauterine insemination (IUI)
      b. Assisted reproductive technologies (ART)
  C. Past pregnancy history
    1. Written as
      a. Gravida: Number of total pregnancies
      b. Para: Number of specific type of deliveries a woman has had (Box 7.2)
    2. Include
      a. Abortions
      b. Miscarriages, ectopic, and molar pregnancies
      c. Preterm deliveries
      d. Number of living children and their current health
      e. Multifetal gestations
      f. Complications with pregnancy, labor, or delivery
      g. Cesarean section deliveries

X. Surgical history
  A. Include past surgeries, types of anesthesia received, feelings about or physiologic reaction to any anesthesia received, and any complications.
    1. List all surgical procedures. Include
      a. Abdominal or pelvic surgeries that could affect pregnancy or delivery

---

BOX 7.2 *Terminology of Pregnancy*

Gravida: Refers to the number of times a woman has been pregnant, regardless of the outcome of the pregnancy or the number of babies born from the pregnancy.

Parity: Technically means the number of pregnancies that ended with the birth of a viable fetus. In practice, used as a system of digits describing the outcome of pregnancies.

First digit: Number of term babies (36 weeks gestation or 2,500 g) delivered
Second digit: Number of preterm babies delivered (28–36 weeks gestation or 1,000 to 2,499 g)
Third digit: Number of pregnancies ending in spontaneous or elective abortion
Fourth digit: Number of currently living children

Example: If a woman is currently pregnant and has one living child born at term, she is listed as G2 P1001.

---

      b. Scarring
      c. Complications
  B. Other hospitalizations
  C. Types of anesthesia ever received and any reactions
  D. Blood transfusions
  E. Accidents that caused injuries that may affect the woman's ability to labor or deliver

XI. **General health and nutrition**
  A. Exercise (Box 7.3 lists recommendations)
    1. Discuss amount and type currently practiced
    2. Use opportunity to discuss and recommend moderate, regular exercise during pregnancy
  B. Diet
    1. Inquire about current special diet requirements.
      a. Lactose, gluten, or other intolerances
      b. Vegetarian
      c. Food allergies
    2. Check for calcium intake, and recommend supplementation as needed.
      a. Sources vary; however, 1,000 to 1,500 mg daily calcium intake is usually recommended.
      b. Adequate calcium can prevent calf cramps later in pregnancy.
    3. Encourage appropriate weight gain considering woman's age, prepregnancy weight, and health status.

> **BOX 7.3** *Recommendations Relating to Exercise During Pregnancy*
>
> - Exercise of any kind should not be fatiguing and should be combined with periods of rest.
> - Consult with provider about current or new exercise program.
> - Avoid high-risk and high-impact sports and activities.
> - Decrease intensity of exercise as pregnancy progresses.
> - Regular, moderate exercise most days of the week is recommended.
> - Wear supportive bra and shoes.
> - Drink liquids before and after exercise to avoid dehydration.
> - Avoid vigorous exercise in hot weather to prevent hyperthermia.
> - Stop activity and consult provider if symptoms occur (palpitations, shortness of breath, dizziness, abdominal pain, bleeding, numbness and tingling, no fetal movement).
> - Avoid sitting or standing for long periods.

      a. Evaluate prepregnancy weight using standardized measure (e.g., body mass index [BMI], ideal body weight [IBW]). Although opinions vary, normal-weight woman should gain 25 to 35 pounds during the course of the pregnancy; less if overweight and more if underweight at the onset of pregnancy.

      b. The average additional caloric consumption to a normal diet during pregnancy is approximately 300 calories per day.

   4. Folate

      a. The Centers for Disease Control and Prevention (CDC) recommends .4 mg of folic acid per day for prevention of neural tube defects.

      b. All women of reproductive age should take folic acid daily to decrease the risk of neural tube defects and anencephaly in planned or unplanned pregnancies.

   5. Iron: Evaluate hemoglobin and hematocrit levels. If iron-deficiency anemia is present, woman should supplement with 30 to 120 g a day. (Not routinely recommended at onset of pregnancy.)

XII. Social history

  A. Substance abuse: Note past use and current use, including amount and frequency

    1. Use of any of the following substances is not recommended during pregnancy: Cigarettes, alcohol, or illicit drugs.

2. If patient is using cigarettes, alcohol, or illicit drugs, she should be informed of the potential effects on her fetus.
3. She should be advised to stop her use of the substance or substances, and be encouraged to accept a referral to an appropriate treatment or counseling center.
4. Some states have requirements regarding reporting to state agencies if there is a history of known substance abuse.
5. Inquire about
   a. Smoking: Include amount smoked in a typical day
      (1) Associated with low birth weight, stillbirth, and sudden infant death
   b. Alcohol use: Include type, amount, and pattern of use
      (1) Safety level unknown, no use of alcohol is recommended during pregnancy.
      (2) Associated with low birth weight, stillbirth, and fetal alcohol syndrome.
      (3) Fetal alcohol syndrome is a leading cause of mental retardation.
   c. Illicit drugs: Include type, amount, and pattern of use.
B. Physical abuse (see Chapter 19, "The Sexual-Assault Victim")
   1. Current or past
   2. Counseling done in past
   3. Encourage patient to assess her current safety and refer her to counseling or local agencies as needed. Abuse may intensify during pregnancy.
C. Sexual abuse
   1. Current or past
   2. Counseling done in past
   3. Encourage patient to assess her current safety and refer her to counseling or local agencies as needed. Abuse may intensify during pregnancy.
D. Financial stressors
   1. Does patient have insurance coverage or private means to pay for pregnancy? If not, refer to social worker, financial aid worker, Medicaid, or local funding organizations as needed.
   2. Does she have housing and adequate food during and after pregnancy? If not, refer to Women, Infants and Children (WIC), social services, or local agencies as needed.
E. Social support system
   1. Family or friends whom the patient can rely on during her pregnancy and after delivery
F. Patient's plans for pregnancy and postpartum recovery
   1. Does she plan to attend prenatal classes?

2. What contraception is she planning at the end of her pregnancy; if she plans sterilization, does she meet criteria within state or institution?
3. Does she plan to breastfeed or bottle-feed her baby?

XIII. Family history

A. Used for screening for potential physical and emotional complications of pregnancy and familial patterns of health or illness. Document relationship to patient and type of condition, if known.
   1. Diabetes
   2. Hypertension or gestational hypertension
   3. Heart disease
   4. Renal disease
   5. Cancer, including primary site, if known
   6. Anemia
   7. Other blood disorders
   8. Infectious diseases: Screen for patient exposure or immunization
   9. Neurologic disorders
   10. Psychiatric disorders
   11. Congenital anomalies
   12. Genetic diseases
   13. Multifetal gestations or births

XIV. Physical examination

A. A complete physical examination should be performed, including breast, abdominal, and pelvic examinations.
B. Explain to the patient specifically what you will be doing and what she may expect to feel just before and during the examination.
C. Baseline vital signs, blood pressure, height, and weight: These items will act as baseline measurements for the duration of the pregnancy.
D. Breast examination (see Chapter 6, "Assessment of the Female Breast"). In addition to routine observation and palpation, the examination should include a check of the nipples' ability to evert with a gentle squeeze of the areola, to predict eversion of nipples during breastfeeding.
E. The abdominal examination should include
   1. Notation of any abdominal scarring
   2. Fundal height in centimeters from the symphysis pubis to the top of the fundus, if the fundus is palpable (Figure 7.1)
   3. Estimation of size and position

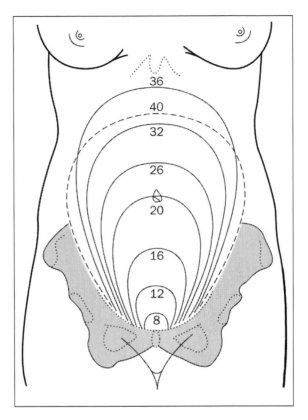

FIGURE 7.1 Uterine fundal height.

4. Assessment of fetal heart tones; can be auscultated using Doppler ultrasonography
   a. It is possible to assess fetal heart tones by 10 weeks gestation with Doppler.
5. Assess for gradual uterine and abdominal enlargement

F. Pelvic examination (see Chapter 4, "The Physical Examination"). In addition to a routine pelvic examination, evaluate
   1. Chadwick's sign
      a. A bluish color of the cervix caused by increased vascularity in pregnancy
      b. May also be apparent in the vagina and vulva
      c. Evident at approximately 6 to 8 weeks gestation
   2. Goodell's sign
      a. Mild softening of the cervix from the nonpregnant state
      b. May be evident at approximately 7 to 8 weeks gestation
   3. Hegar's sign
      a. Softening and compressibility of the lower uterine segment

4. Cervical position, length, and any dilation: Dilation or effacement (thinning of the cervical length) is abnormal until late in the third trimester.
5. Uterine size should be estimated by use of bimanual examination, and congruence with LMP should be considered in estimating the current gestational age.
   a. If incongruence of size and dates is noted, ultrasonography should be considered to establish dating, fetal viability, and probable health status
6. Adnexa should be palpated for pain or enlargement to screen for ectopic pregnancy.
   a. Ectopic pregnancy occurs when the fertilized ovum is implanted outside the uterus, usually in the fallopian tube.
   b. Symptoms initially are those of a normal pregnancy. Further symptoms may be vague or pronounced. They may include
      (1) Lower quadrant abdominal pain
      (2) Spotting
      (3) Syncopal symptoms (related to blood loss)
      (4) Adnexal tenderness
      (5) Uterus may be normally enlarged
      (6) Neck or shoulder pain with rupture
   c. Obtain pelvic ultrasound and consider quantitative serum hCG to confirm diagnosis.
   d. Obtain consultation if ectopic pregnancy is suspected.
   e. Treatment may be medical (methotrexate) or surgical.
   f. Risk factors are usually related to conditions that affect the lumen of the fallopian tubes or uterine cavity (Box 7.4).
7. The bony pelvis should be evaluated during bimanual examination, including
   a. Diagonal conjugate
   b. Sacral shape
   c. Prominence of the ischial spines
   d. Sacrosciatic notch
   e. Coccyx mobility
   f. Angle of the pubic arch
   g. Diameter of the ischial tuberosities

XV. **Laboratory tests: Routine testing is performed to identify more clearly pregnancies at risk and to provide an opportunity to prevent problems. It should include all of the following items:**
   A. Blood type and Rh factor
      1. If patient is Rh negative and partner is Rh positive, Rh incompatibility may result. The patient should be advised that she will probably receive RhoGAM during the pregnancy.
      2. If the patient's blood type is O and her partner's is A, B, or AB, there may be ABO incompatibility.

> **BOX 7.4 *Risk Factors for Ectopic Pregnancy***
>
> - Prior tubal pregnancy
> - Tubal surgery such as reversal of tubal ligation
> - Pelvic inflammatory disease in which the tubes become scarred
> - Endometriosis
> - Intrauterine device

B. Antibody screen of serum
   1. Antibodies are formed from major or minor blood group antigens.
   2. If the test yields positive results, the antibody should be identified and a titer should be performed.
   3. Screening should be repeated at 28 weeks gestation in Rh-negative women.
C. Complete blood count (CBC) with differential smear
   1. Hemoglobin and hematocrit
      a. Blood volume increases 30% to 50% during pregnancy, with plasma volume increasing more than red blood cell (RBC) volume.
      b. A decrease in hemoglobin and hematocrit levels is normal during pregnancy.
      c. Mild anemia during pregnancy is defined as less than 11 g/dL hemoglobin; severe anemia is defined as less than 9 g/dL.
      d. Anemia during pregnancy is usually iron-deficiency anemia; however, other types may coexist.
      e. Iron-deficiency anemia should be treated using iron supplements; severe anemia should be evaluated further, with referral as needed.
   2. A platelet count should be performed to detect thrombocytopenia.
   3. Leukocytes: To screen for leukemia and infection. Pregnancy values may normally reach 17,000 leucocytes. RBCs and indices are used to diagnose various types of anemia.
   4. The differential is used to identify types of leukocytes, erythrocytes, cell abnormalities, and platelets.
D. Rubella titer to indicate immune status for rubella
E. Serology
   1. The Venereal Disease Research Laboratory (VDRL) test is usually used as a screening test for syphilis; if the test result is positive, a fluorescent treponemal antibody (FTA) test is performed to confirm diagnosis.

   2. Parenteral penicillin is the only recommended treatment for syphilis during pregnancy. Dosage is dependent on stage of infection and complicating factors.
F. Hepatitis B surface antigen (HBsAg)
   1. If the test result is positive, the infant will need immuno-prophylaxis at delivery.
   2. Vaccination is acceptable during pregnancy.
G. HIV screening
   1. Recommend testing for all pregnant women as early as possible in pregnancy.
   2. Treatment for HIV can substantially lower transmission to infants of infected women from 15% to 20% to less than 2%. All pregnant women with HIV should be referred for treatment during pregnancy.
   3. Breastfeeding is not recommended in HIV-positive women because of the risk of transmission through breast milk.
H. Urinalysis to screen for asymptomatic kidney or bladder disease (see Chapter 35, "Urinalysis")
   1. The presence of bacteria, leukocytes, and erythrocytes may indicate infection.
   2. The presence of casts or RBCs may indicate pyelonephritis.
   3. Glucose level may be normal in relation to increased glomerular filtration rate, or it may indicate carbohydrate intolerance. If the second test result is positive, testing for carbohydrate intolerance should be performed.
   4. Protein: Value greater than 1+ is abnormal and may be related to
      a. Urinary tract infection
      b. Pregnancy-induced hypertension
      c. Kidney disease
I. Other screening to be considered for patients at risk
   1. Sickle cell preparation or hemoglobin electrophoresis for sickle cell trait, thalassemia, or other hemoglobinopathy
   2. Tay-Sachs screening for couples at risk
   3. Toxoplasmosis screening should be performed if the woman is exposed to cat feces or undercooked meat.
      a. Women should be warned not to change cat litter or work in the garden without gloves during pregnancy because of risk of toxoplasmosis.
   4. Cytomegalovirus screening with known exposure
   5. Tuberculosis testing (purified protein derivative [PPD])
   6. Thyroid screening if symptoms are present or as indicated
J. Cervical or vaginal tests to consider
   1. Pap smear
      a. All pregnant patients should receive a Pap smear within the year before the pregnancy ends.
         (1) Screens for cervical cancer and HPV

        (2) DNA testing should be ordered with Pap smear for high-risk HPV strains.

2. Chlamydia culture
   a. Chlamydial infection necessitates treatment during pregnancy.
   b. Culture should be repeated after treatment and 3 months after treatment for confirmation of cure.
   c. If the results are positive, treat per current CDC guidelines.
      (1) Current recommendation for treatment is azithromycin 1 g orally in a single dose or amoxicillin 500 mg orally three times a day for 7 days.

3. Gonorrhea culture
   a. Positive culture must be treated.
      (1) Current recommendation for treatment is ceftriaxone 250 mg in a single intramuscular dose *with* azithromycin 1 g orally in a single dose or doxycycline 100 mg orally twice daily for 7 days.
      (2) No repeat culture needed if patient is asymptomatic following treatment.

4. Bacterial vaginosis: If patient is symptomatic and there is a positive wet mount, treat the condition; treatment may lower incidence of preterm labor.
   a. Treatment: Metronidazole 500 mg orally twice a day for 7 days

5. HSV
   a. Women should be questioned regarding history of HSV and, if positive history, for prodromal symptoms and symptoms of outbreaks.
   b. Testing is necessary only to confirm the diagnosis of active herpes.
   c. Vaginal delivery is preferred if the woman has no prodromal symptoms and no lesions are visible at the onset of labor. If active lesions are present, caesarian section is the preferred mode of delivery.
   d. Risk to neonate varies by type of HSV and whether outbreak is initial infection or recurrence.
   e. Women should avoid any sexual contact with partners with known or suspected herpes during the third trimester.
   f. Acycolovir may be recommended to women with history of HSV to decrease risk of outbreaks at term with associated caesarian delivery

6. Group B streptococcus infection
   a. Screening recommended for all pregnant women at 35 to 37 weeks gestation.
   b. Treatment of choice is IV penicillin administered during labor. Susceptibility testing should be done on specimens from patients with known penicillin allergy.

  7. *Trichomonas*
    a. Wet mount or culture
    b. Treatment of choice is 2 g metronidazole in a single oral dose.
  8. *Candida* infection
    a. Infections tend to be more frequent during pregnancy.
    b. Short course of topical azole is the recommended treatment during pregnancy.
K. Other antenatal screening
  1. Use of ultrasonography
    a. May be performed for dating if unknown LMP or if there is a size/date discrepancy
    b. Routine screening: Frequently done at 19 weeks gestation
    c. To look for particular anomalies or complications of pregnancy
      (1) Multiple gestations
      (2) Molar pregnancy
      (3) Fetal anomalies
      (4) Maternal anomalies
      (5) Placenta previa
  2. Amniocentesis should be performed at approximately 17 weeks gestation when indicated.
  3. Chorionic villus sampling at approximately 10 weeks gestation is offered when indicated in women older than 35 years for screening for chromosomal abnormalities.
  4. The maternal serum alpha-fetoprotein (AFP) screen is offered at approximately 19 weeks gestation as a screen to detect
    a. Neural tube defects
    b. Down syndrome
    c. Various other defects
  5. Cell free fetal DNA (cffDNA) is a serum test that may be offered at approximately 9 weeks gestation for women who may be at high risk of having fetuses with trisomy 13, 18, or 21.
    a. Approved by the American College of Obstetricians and Gynecologists (ACOG) in 2012 as an initial screen only for those at high risk
    b. Significant ethical and legal concerns; cffDNA screening should be offered cautiously
L. Table 7.4 summarizes common laboratory tests, indicating changes with pregnancy and timing of the test.

XVI. Planning at initial visit

A. Most patients in the United States expect to be prescribed vitamins regardless of nutritional status. Prenatal vitamins are available over the counter or by prescription.
B. Laboratory tests should be ordered, and testing necessary in first or early second trimesters should be discussed and arranged.

TABLE 7.4 Common Laboratory Values in Pregnancy

TEST	NORMAL RANGE (NONPREGNANT)	CHANGE IN PREGNANCY	TIMING
SERUM CHEMISTRIES			
Albumin	3.5–4.8 g/dL	↓ 1 g/dL	Most by 20 weeks, then gradual
Calcium (total)	9–10.3 mg/dL	↓ 10%	Gradual decrease
Chloride	95–105 mEq/L	No significant change	Gradual increase
Creatinine (female)	0.6–1.1 mg/dL	↓ 0.3 mg/dL	Most by 20 weeks
Fibrinogen	1.5–3.6 g/L	↑ 1–2 g/L	Progressive
Glucose, fasting (plasma)	65–105 mg/dL	↓ 10%	Gradual decrease
Potassium (plasma)	3.5–4.5 mEq/L	↓ 0.2–0.3 mEq/L	By 20 weeks
Protein (total)	6.5d > 8.5 g/dL	↓ g/dL	By 20 weeks, then stable
Sodium	135–145 mEq/L	↓ 2–4 mEq/L	By 20 weeks, then stable
Urea nitrogen	12–30 mg/dL	↓ 50%	First trimester
Uric acid	3.5–8 mg/dL	↓ 33%	First trimester, increase at term
URINARY CHEMISTRIES			
Creatinine	15–25 mg/kg per day (1-1.4 g/d)	No significant change	
Protein	Up to 150 mg/d	Up to 250–300 mg/d	By 20 weeks
Creatinine clearance	90–130 ml/min per 1.73 m^2	40%–50%	By 16 weeks
SERUM ENZYMATIC ACTIVITIES			
Amylase	23–84 IU/L	↑ 50%–100%	Controversial
Transaminase	5–35 mU/dL	No significant change	Glutamic pyruvic (SGPT)
Glutamic oxaloacetic (SGOT)	5–40 mU/dL	No significant change	
Hematocrit (female)	36%–46%	↓ 4%–7%	Lowest values at 30–34 weeks

(continued)

TABLE 7.4 Common Laboratory Values in Pregnancy (*continued*)

TEST	NORMAL RANGE (NONPREGNANT)	CHANGE IN PREGNANCY	TIMING
Hemoglobin (female)	12–16 g/dL	↓ 1.5–2 g/dL	Lowest values at 30–34 weeks
Leukocyte count	4.8–10.8 x 10³/mm	↑ 3.5 x 10³/mm³	Gradual
Platelet count	150–400 x 10³/mm³	Slight decrease	
Erythrocyte count	4.0–5.0 x 10⁶/mm³	↑ 25%–30%	Begins at 6–8 weeks
SERUM HORMONE VALUES			
Coritsol (plasma)	8–21 mcg/dL	↑ 20 mcg/dL	Peaks at 28–32 weeks, then constant to term
Prolactin (female)	25 ng/dL	↑ 50–400 ng/dL	Gradual, peaks at term
Thyroxine, total (T₄)	5–11 g/dL	↑ 5 mg/dL	Early sustained
Triiodothyronine, total (T₃)	125–245 ng/dL	↑ 50%	Early sustained

C. Nutrition should be discussed with referral to a nutritional service, as needed.

D. Consultation should be arranged as needed for physical or emotional problems discovered during the visit, and the patient should be referred to social services or for medical consultation as needed.

E. The patient should be referred for consultation if she is not within normal limits in any aspect of her medical, gynecologic, or obstetrical status.

F. The patient should be screened briefly with questions in Box 7.5 and instructed to return
   1. 1 to 28 weeks gestation: Every 4 weeks
   2. 28 to 37 weeks gestation: Every 2 weeks
   3. 37 weeks gestation to delivery: Weekly
   4. Centering, or group, prenatal care may be recommended if available

G. The patient should be asked whether there is any further information that she needs to share or questions she wishes to ask before her departure from the visit.

H. The patient should be instructed to call with any questions or problems (see Table 7.5 for warning signs).

BOX 7.5 *Questions to Ask at Each Subsequent Prenatal Visit*

Since your last visit have you had problems with:

Physical symptoms, such as:
Headaches
Eyes (blurred vision, blind spots, flashing lights or lines)
Swelling of face
Swelling of hands
Swelling of legs or feet
Pain in your chest
Pain in your back
Pain in your abdomen
Urination (burning or pain)

Leaking urine
Not being able to wait to use the toilet
Bleeding or spotting from vagina
Leaking fluid from your vagina (watery)
Vaginal discharge or change in discharge
Vaginal burning, itching, or bad smell
Increase in sores or growths in genital area
Illnesses or fever
Exposure to sick children or adults

Signs of labor, such as:
Contractions
Cramping
Any changes in the way the baby moves

Pelvic pressure
Low backache
Any visits to another doctor, midwife, nurse, clinic, or emergency room

Any medicines or substances you have used, including:

Medicines (prescription, vitamins, or over the counter)
"Street" or illegal drugs you have used (if any)
Number of cigarettes you have smoked per day (if any)

Plants or herbs/herbal teas used to help you feel better or treat an illness
Kind and amount of alcohol you have used (if any)
Do you need any prenatal vitamins, iron, or other medicines?

Since your last visit, have you had any accidents, falls, been hit, hurt, or threatened?

There are many common discomforts of pregnancy. If there is one particular thing that is bothering you or that you want information about, or help or suggestions on how to work with or relieve the discomfort, please mark below. If none of these worry or bother you, skip this section.

- Nausea (feeling sick to your stomach)
- Diarrhea
- Hemorrhoids
- Vomiting (throwing up)
- Constipation

- Shortness of breath
- Not feeling hungry
- Breast tenderness
- Heartburn
- Varicose veins

(continued)

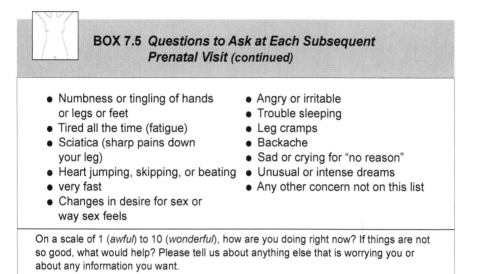

BOX 7.5 *Questions to Ask at Each Subsequent Prenatal Visit (continued)*

- Numbness or tingling of hands or legs or feet
- Tired all the time (fatigue)
- Sciatica (sharp pains down your leg)
- Heart jumping, skipping, or beating
- very fast
- Changes in desire for sex or way sex feels

- Angry or irritable
- Trouble sleeping
- Leg cramps
- Backache
- Sad or crying for "no reason"
- Unusual or intense dreams
- Any other concern not on this list

On a scale of 1 (*awful*) to 10 (*wonderful*), how are you doing right now? If things are not so good, what would help? Please tell us about anything else that is worrying you or about any information you want.

I. Any medication should be weighed for its benefits versus its potential hazards in pregnancy.
J. Inform the patient about prepared childbirth classes.
    1. These classes are readily available throughout the country.
    2. Provide the patient with valuable knowledge about labor and delivery to decrease anxiety.

TABLE 7.5 Warning Signs During Pregnancy

DANGER SIGN OR SYMPTOM	POTENTIAL CAUSE
Marked decrease in fetal movement	Fetal compromise, anoxia
Vaginal bleeding; abdominal pain or cramping	Impending miscarriage, spontaneous abortion, or ectopic pregnancy
Leakage of fluid from the vagina	Premature rupture of membranes (PROM)
Persistent headache	Preeclampsia or pregnancy-induced hypertension
Dizziness	
Spots before the eyes	
Swelling of the hands or face	
Elevated blood pressure	
Fever or chills	Infection
Recurrent vomiting	Hyperemesis gravidarum

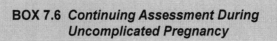

BOX 7.6 *Continuing Assessment During Uncomplicated Pregnancy*

Schedule of Return Visits
Once monthly, 1 to 28 weeks gestation
Every 2 weeks, 27 to 36 weeks gestation
Once weekly, 37 to 40 weeks gestation

Weeks gestation	Assessment	Rationale
Every visit	Weight	Evaluate fetal growth, screen for maternal edema, pregnancy-induced hypertension (PIH), under- and overnourishment
	Blood pressure (BP)	Screen for PIH
	Fundal height (McDonald's Rule)	Evaluate fetal growth
	Leopold's maneuvers after 32 weeks gestation	Determine fetal position
	Fetal heart rate (FHR) after 10 weeks gestation	Evaluate fetal well-being with Doppler after 10 weeks gestation, with fetoscope if desired after 20 weeks gestation
	Edema	Screen for PIH, fluid retention
	Symptoms	Identify problems, discomforts
	Adjustment	Identify problems, provide support
	Nutrition	Determine adequacy of diet
	Urinalysis	Glucose screen for gestational diabetes, protein screen for PIH
6 to 12 weeks	Chorionic villus sampling*	Detect fetal chromosomal abnormalities
10 to 12 weeks	Ultrasound if indicated	Determine fetal age, development
	Hemoglobin (Hgb) electrophoresis*	Detect sickle cell, thalassemias, other hemoglobinopathies
15 to 20 weeks	α-Fetoprotein	Screen for fetal neural tube defects

(continued)

BOX 7.6	*Continuing Assessment During*	
	Uncomplicated Pregnancy (continued)	

	Amniocentesis*	Detect fetal genetic abnormalities
	Ultrasound if indicated	Determine fetal age, development, screen for anomalies
24 to 28 weeks	Glucose 50 mg	Detect gestational diabetes
28 to 34 weeks	Hematocrit/Hgb	Detect anemia
37 to 42 weeks	Group B strep (GBS) screening	Identify cervical changes preceding labor onset
	Pelvic examination, with sexually transmitted disease (STD) screening, if indicated	Screen for current changes in STD status

*For clients at risk.

---

3. Exercise and toning in preparation for labor makes labor easier for most women.
4. Classes are a good way to help partners or support people be involved with pregnancy.
   K. Additional concerns
   1. Sexual intercourse
      a. May be unrestricted in normal pregnancy as long as the cervix is not significantly dilated.
      b. Avoid if vaginal bleeding, ruptured membranes, or premature labor are present.
   2. Travel
      a. Travel in itself is not necessarily harmful.
      b. Avoid long periods of sitting, which may cause venous stasis.
      c. Patient should consider possibility that competent obstetrical care may not be immediately available in some areas.
      d. Pressurized aircraft pose no additional risk. Airlines may have restrictions on overseas flights related to gestational age.
   L. Box 7.5 lists questions to review at subsequent prenatal visits.
   M. Box 7.6 lists continuing assessments for a complicated pregnancy.

Bibliography

Food and Drug Administration. (1979). Content and format for labeling for human prescription drugs. *Federal Register, 44*, 37434–37467.

Yaffe, S. J. (1990). Introduction. In R. K. Briggs, R. K. Freeman, & S. J. Yaffe (Eds.). *Drugs in pregnancy and lactation* (p. xiii). Baltimore, MD: Williams and Wilkins.

Assessment and Clinical Evaluation of Obesity in Women

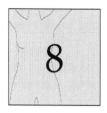

8

Frances M. Sahebzamani
and Yolanda R. Hill

I. **Obesity in women**
   A. Obesity is recognized as a complex, multifactorial, chronic disease whereby excess body fat is accumulated through complex interactions between the environment, genetic predisposition, human metabolism, neuroendocrine, and behavioral factors. Obesity disproportionally and differentially affects women's health across a spectrum of physical, psychological, and social conditions.
      1. Although obesity is generally thought to be attributable to an imbalance between chronic overnutrition and lower caloric expenditure, current research has shown that obesity is influenced and regulated by the hormonal and metabolic function of adipocytes (Kushner, 2012).
      2. Body fat is comprised of both subcutaneous adipose tissue (gluteo–femoral weight distribution) and visceral adipose tissue (fat cells deposited into skeletal muscle and the viscera) (Figure 8.1).
      3. Over the past decade, research has led to a better understanding of the role of visceral adipose tissue as an active regulator of whole-body homeostasis through the production of more than 50 adipokines, hormones, and other molecules that directly affect a wide variety of psychological and physiological processes. Adipokines perform essential regulatory roles in appetite and food intake, mood, energy expenditure, reproduction, cell viability, immunity, and inflammation and cardiovascular function.

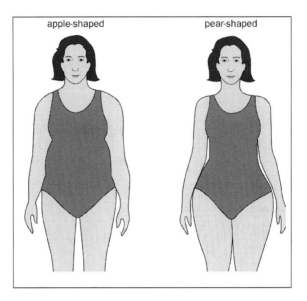

FIGURE 8.1 Apple-shaped and pear-shaped body habitus.

4. Adipokines release proinflammatory peptides (e.g., tumor necrosis factor [TNF]), high-sensitivity C reactive protein (hs-CRP), interleukin 6 (IL-6), plasminogen activator inhibitor 1 (PAI-1), and vascular endothelial growth factor (VEGF) and secrete hormones (adiponectin, leptin, resistin) that contribute to a chronic low-grade inflammatory response. This chronic low-grade inflammatory state promotes metabolic aberrations highly associated with the development of atherosclerosis, autoimmune inflammatory diseases, and further weight accumulation.
5. In the clinical setting, ranges for normal weight, overweight, and obesity are determined using weight and height to calculate a surrogate measure of percentage of body fat called the body mass index (BMI) (Table 8.1).

II. **Measures of obesity**
   A. BMI is calculated when height and weight are entered into a formula known as the Quetelet index (weight [kg]/height [m²]).
   B. BMI is used in the clinical setting to assess risk for the development of obesity-related diseases and as a metric for determining treatment interventions (see Section IX in this chapter on obesity-focused physical exam).
   C. As BMI increases, risk for visceral adiposity, metabolic dysregulation, the development of functional disorders, chronic disease

TABLE 8.1. Table of Body Mass Index Measurements

	120	130	140	150	160	170	180	190	200	210	220	230	240	250
4'6"	29	31	34	36	39	41	43	46	48	51	53	56	58	60
4'8"	27	29	31	34	36	38	40	43	45	47	49	52	54	56
4'10"	25	27	29	31	34	36	38	40	42	44	46	48	50	52
5'0"	23	25	27	29	31	33	35	37	39	41	43	45	47	49
5'2"	22	24	26	27	29	31	33	35	37	38	40	42	44	46
5'4"	21	22	24	26	28	29	31	33	34	36	38	40	41	43
5'6"	19	21	23	24	26	27	29	31	32	34	36	37	39	40
5'8"	18	20	21	23	24	26	27	29	30	32	34	35	37	38
5'10"	17	19	20	22	23	24	26	27	29	30	32	33	35	36
6'0"	16	18	19	20	22	23	24	26	27	28	30	31	33	34
6'2"	15	17	18	19	21	22	23	24	26	27	28	30	31	32
6'4"	15	16	17	18	20	21	22	23	24	26	27	28	29	30
6'6"	14	15	16	17	19	20	21	22	23	24	25	27	28	29
6'8"	13	14	15	17	18	19	20	21	22	23	24	25	26	28

Note: White = underweight, BMI < 18.5
Dark gray = normal, BMI 18.5–24.9
Medium gray = overweight, BMI 25–29.9
Light gray = obese, BMI 39–39.8

and premature death increases. As BMI approaches or exceeds 35, women have a 92-fold increased risk for the development of type 2 diabetes, compared with a 42-fold increased risk for men.

D. Research has shown that a weight loss as low as 3% to 5% of total body weight can improve health outcomes and reduce risk for the development of obesity-related comorbidities (Table 8.2).

E. BMI provides an approximation of mortality and morbidity risk for obesity and is used because it correlates with the amount of body fat but *it is not* a measurement of body fatness. An adult who has a BMI

TABLE 8.2. Medical Complications of Obesity

Diabetes mellitus (type 2)	Hypertension
High cholesterol levels	Coronary heart disease
Congestive heart failure	Angina pectoris
Stroke	Asthma
Osteoarthritis	Musculoskeletal disorders
Gallbladder disease	Sleep apnea
Respiratory problems	Gout
Bladder control problems	
Cancer	

between 25 and 29.9 is considered overweight. An adult who has a BMI of 30 or higher is considered obese.

F.   BMI measures are not gender specific.

II.   **Prevalence of obesity**

A.   Based on the most recent data from the National Health and Nutrition Examination Survey, in the year 2011 to 2012, 35.8% of Americans were overweight (BMI greater than or equal to 25 kg/m^2) and 35.7% of adult Americans met the BMI diagnostic criteria for obesity (BMI greater than or equal to 30 kg/m^2). The age-adjusted prevalence of obesity in men was 35.5% and 35.8% in women.

B.   Although the proportion of adults with a BMI greater than or equal to 30 kg/m^2 has remained stable between 2009 and 2012, the proportion of obese adults with severe obesity is increasing (Figure 8.2). Severe obesity is defined as a BMI greater than or equal to 40 kg/m^2 (class 3 obesity) or a BMI greater than or equal to 35 kg/m^2 with obesity-related comorbidities (class 2 obesity). Among adults classified as obese, women represent the greatest proportion of adults with severe obesity. Of women of reproductive age (20–39 years), 7.5% meet the diagnostic criteria for class 3 obesity. The prevalence of women with a BMI greater than or equal to 35 is 17.2%.

C.   Severe obesity increases the risk of premature death in women and the risk for serious pregnancy complications, including an increased risk for birth defects, fetal adiposity, and the development of childhood obesity in the offspring (Table 8.3).

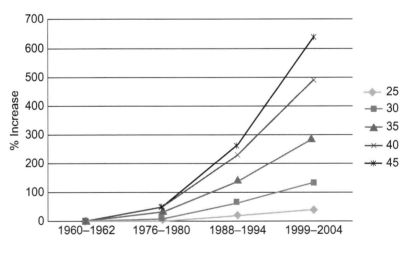

FIGURE 8.2 Prevalence of severe obesity.
Source: Kral (2012).

TABLE 8.3 Reproductive Complications of Severe Obesity

Maternal

Gestational diabetes mellitus (GDM)

Preeclampsia

Eclampsia

Pseudotumor cerebri

Acute cholecystitis

Caesarian section

Postpartum wound infection

Operative vaginal delivery

Metabolic disturbances
  Elevated free fatty acids
  Hyperglycemia

Fetal/Neonatal

Spontaneous abortion

Stillbirth

Fetal monitoring and imaging problems

Premature birth secondary to obstetrical and medical complications

Intrauterine growth restriction (IUGR) second to problems such as preeclampsia

Congenital malformations

Low Apgar score

Large for gestational age (LGA)

Increased fetal adiposity

Hypoglycemia

Neonatal/Infant/Child

Difficulty breastfeeding

Risk of low IQ

Aggressive eating style

Risk of pediatric obesity

Type 2 diabetes

Metabolic syndrome
  Impaired glucose tolerance
  Dyslipidemia
  Hypertension
  Fatty liver

(continued)

TABLE 8.3 Reproductive Complications of Severe Obesity *(continued)*

Neonatal/Infant/Child
Asthma
Depression
Orthopedic disorders
Truancy

Source: Kral (2012).

D. The rates of obesity are disproportionate in ethnic groups. There is a higher prevalence of obesity among African American and Hispanic women than among White women. Among non-Hispanic Black adults, 56.6% of women are obese compared with 37.1% of men. In 2011–2012, the prevalence of obesity was higher among non-Hispanic black (47.8%), Hispanic (42.5%), and non-Hispanic white (32.6%) adults than among non-Hispanic Asian adults (10.8%) (Table 8.4).

III. **Gender differences in obesity**
   A. Gender differences in obesity and overweight are related to biologic, psychological, and social issues (i.e., differences in anatomy, hormonal influences, mood disorders, stressors, and quality-of-life issues).
   B. Women are vulnerable to weight gain during reproductive milestones (puberty, pregnancy, postpartum, and menopause). Female sex hormones, specifically progesterone, as well as changes in hormones related to estrogen deficiency with menopause, influence food intake, body composition, and energy expenditure (Table 8.5).
   C. Obesity has been linked to disorders of menstruation and to infertility in women. Exogenous hormones for contraception or symptoms

TABLE 8.4 Prevalence of Obesity Among U.S. Women According to Age

AGE (y)	PREVALENCE (%)
20 – 39	54.3
40 – 59	66.1
≥ 60	68.1

Note: Women are more likely to become overweight (BMI ≥ 25) as they become older.

TABLE 8.5 Hormonal Influences Affecting Obesity Expression in Women

PREMENOPAUSAL AND EARLY POSTMENOPAUSAL YEARS	PERIMENOPAUSE, MENOPAUSE, AND POLYCYSTIC OVARY SYMDROME
Estradiol primary source of estrogen, which promotes gluteo–femoral adipocyte distribution	Estrone is the primary source of estrogen (Estradiol is apporximately one tenth of premenopausal levels)
Estrogen receptor β more prominent in subcutaneous fat	Visceral adipocyte distribution pattern
Not associated with decreased adiponectin levels, IR, inflammatory or prothrombic factors	Estradiol deficiency promotes a shift to a reduced lean body mass
	Reduced functional activity levels
	Androgen receptors more prominent
	Highly associated with decreased adiponectin levels, IR, FFA, dyslipidemia, prothrombic and proinflammatory potential, and glucose intolerance

of menopause have been shown to affect weight. Most women in developed countries live substantial portions of their lives in a postmenopausal state.

D. In the American culture, slimness is valued and rewarded. These cultural norms may promote social stigma, body image dysfunction, and eating disorders in women.

E. Obesity affects quality and quantity of life (Table 8.6).

TABLE 8.6 National Institutes of Health Guidelines for the Management of Obesity by Body Mass Index

TREATMENT	BMI CATEGORY				
	25–26.9 kg/m^2	27–29.9 kg/m^2	30–34.9 kg/m^2	35–39.9 kg/m^2	≥ 40 kg/m^2
Diet, exercise, behavior therapy	With comorbidities	With comorbidities	+	+	+
Pharmacotherapy		With comorbidities	+	+	+
Surgery				With comorbidities	+

IV. Genetic causes of obesity

A. Approximately 112 candidate genes have been identified and associated with obesity.

    1. Obesity has been shown to be primarily polygenic with each gene candidate contributing to the phenotype and with multiple genes interacting with environmental influences. Gene mutations, deletions, single nucleotide polymorphisms (SNPs), and epigenetic differences are all known to contribute to the development of obesity. Inherited genetic variations have been shown to significantly influence body mass and how the body responds to physical activity and nutrition.

    2. Current research on the epigenetics of obesity is investigating the influence of behavioral and environmental factors on genetic expression.

B. Mongenetic obesity is rare and usually associated with extreme obesity, the conditions of which necessitate special care and appropriate referrals for further genetic assessment, treatment, and counseling. Mongenetic causes of obesity may be identified by associated physical characteristics

    1. Prader–Willi syndrome: Short stature, hypogonadism, short extremities

    2. Angleman's syndrome: Normal stature, movement disorder, happy affect

    3. Down syndrome: Short stature, typical facial features, cardiac malformation, hypotonia

    4. Bardet–Biedl syndrome: Normal/short stature, rod–cone dystrophy, polydactyly, renal structural defects

    5. Alstrom syndrome: Normal/short stature, deafness, cardiomyopathy, rod–cone dystrophy

    6. Albright's osteodystrophy: Normal/short stature, bradydactyly [short fingers], subcutaneous ossification

    7. Cohen syndrome: Normal/short stature, distinctive facial features, retinochondrial dystrophy, granulocytopenia

    8. Carpenter syndrome: Short stature, acrocephaly, polydactyly, hypogonadism

V. Medical causes of obesity

A. Hypothalamic obesity

    1. Hypothalamic obesity is rare, and results from hypothalamic damage from traumatic insult to the central nervous system (CNS). Affected structures include bilateral injury to the ventromedial hypothalamus, the paraventricular hypothalamus, or the amygdala. The pathophysiology resulting from damage to the hypothalamic structures results in the simulation of a relative state of CNS starvation through the inability to transduce afferent hormonal signals of adiposity.

2. Symptoms consist of increased intracranial pressure (headache, vomiting, blurred vision), hypopituitarism, and neurologic problems (seizures, coma, somnolence, temperature dysregulation).

3. Hypothalamic obesity is caused by an increase in the secretion of insulin and adipogenesis (Lustig, 2008).

B. Endocrine causes of obesity
1. Insulin resistance: The metabolic dysregulation associated with insulin resistance, prediabetes, and type 2 diabetes results in insulin resistant subcutaneous adipocytes and increased visceral adipocyte accumulation, increased risk for cardiometabolic disease, and perpetuation of weight gain.

C. Hypothyroidism
1. Women have a twofold increased risk for hypothyroidism with risk increasing with age. Although the prevalence of hypothyroidism is low in obese individuals, overweight and obesity are associated with high normal thyroid stimulating hormone (TSH) and low normal fT4, fT3 and total T3 levels in euthyroid individuals.

2. High normal TSH levels have been associated with increased visceral adiposity, elevated waist circumference, and triglyceride levels. The mechanism linking high TSH levels within the normal range is not well understood. Hypotheses include the increased TSH and elevated peripheral thyroid hormone levels (fT3 and total T3) may be an adaptation process to increase energy expenditure in order to reduce further weight gain. Basal metabolic rate, total energy expenditure, and sleeping energy expenditure are positively correlated with the serum total T3 or fT3 concentrations.

3. Changes in thyroid hormone concentrations may be regarded as a consequence rather than a cause of obesity. Decline in TSH has been reported after caloric restriction leading to a 10% weight loss or following bariatric surgical procedures.

D. Adrenal syndrome
1. Cushing's syndrome is characterized by central obesity, hypertension, and "moon faces" and associated with chronic exposure to elevated cortisol levels. Elevated cortisol levels can result from disease that results in excess cortisol, adrenocorticotropic hormone (ACTH), or corticotropin-releasing hormone (CRH) or from long-term use of glucocorticoid medications.

2. Common physical characteristics include central obesity, thin extremities, and abnormal fat deposition along the collarbone or neck (buffalo hump).

E. Polycystic ovary syndrome (PCOS) is the most prevalent heterogeneous endocrine disorder in women and is characterized by hyperandrogenism, menstrual irregularities, central adiposity, insulin resistance, and polycystic ovaries.

1. The prevalence of PCOS is estimated at 15% to 20% of women. Of women with PCOS, 30% to 50% are overweight or obese.
2. Clinical manifestations include oligomenorrhea or amenorrhea, hirsutism, infertility, and mood disorders, including depression, anxiety, and binge eating disorder (BED).
3. Insulin resistance affects 50% to 70% of women with PCOS, resulting in multiple cardiometabolic comorbidities, including metabolic syndrome, diabetes, dyslipidemia, and hypertension.
4. Weight loss has been shown to improve menstrual irregularities, fertility, and symptoms of androgen excess.
5. In addition to the management of cardiovascular risk factors, the clinical management of PCOS includes the use of oral contraceptives to normalize menstrual irregularities and reduce hirsutism and the use of spironolactone and finasteride to reduce androgen excess.
6. Proper diagnosis and management of PCOS is essential to the prevention of metabolic, endocrine, reproductive, and cardiovascular complications.

VI. Eating disorders

A. Women manifest a 2:1 higher prevalence of eating disorders than men. Common eating disorders found in overweight and obese women include BED, night eating syndrome (NES), and bulimia.
B. BED is thought to be a compensatory response to chronically high stress levels with subsequent heightened responsiveness to high-calorie, hyperpalatable foods. Approximately 45% to 60% of obese individuals meet the *Diagnostic and Statistical Manual of Mental Disorders (DSM-5)* diagnostic criteria for BED.
   1. NES is characterized by morning anorexia, evening hyperphagia, insomnia, and depressed mood. Prevalence of NES is estimated at 9% to 15% of obese outpatients and 54% to 64% of individuals with severe obesity (class 2 or 3 obesity) (Table 8.7).
   2. Bulimia nervosa is characterized by frequent episodes of binge eating followed by inappropriate behaviors, such as self-induced vomiting, to avoid weight gain. *DSM-5* criteria include the criteria for BED and include compensatory behaviors. Current inappropriate compensatory behaviors in order to prevent weight gain are described as self-induced vomiting; misuse of laxatives, diuretics, or other medications; fasting; or excessive exercise.
C. Treatment of BED, NES, and bulimia may include psychotherapy, antidepressants, and neuroleptics.

TABLE 8.7 Proposed Diagnostic Criteria for Night Eating Syndrome (NES)

A. Daily eating pattern of evening/nighttime hyperphagia of one or both of the following:

  1. At least 25% caloric intake after the evening meal

  2. At least two episodes of nocturnal eating per week

B. Awareness and recall of evening- and nocturnal-eating episodes

C. At least three of the following must be present:

  1. Morning anorexia and/or skipped breakfast four or more mornings per week

  2. Presence of a strong urge to eat between dinner and sleep onset and/or during the night

  3. Sleep onset and/or sleep maintenance insomnia four or more nights per week

  4. Presence of a belief that one must eat to return to sleep

  5. Mood is frequently depressed and/or mood worsens in the evening

D. The disorder is associated with significant distress and/or impairment in functioning.

E. The disordered pattern of eating is maintained for at least 3 months.

F. The disorder is not secondary to substance abuse or dependence, medical disorder, medication, or another psychiatric disorder.

Sources: Milano (2011), Bray (2007), and Gallant (2012).

    D. Psychotherapy can reduce the incidence of BED, but this treatment option has not been useful in reducing body weight.

    E. Pharmacotherapy with antidepressants and appetite suppressants can reduce binge or NES frequency and BMI. Newer generation neuroleptics, such as topiramate and zonisamide, have been associated with weight loss in clinical studies of epilepsy and obesity and have shown promise in the treatment of BED (Table 8.8 and Table 8.9).

    F. Combination therapies to include medication and cognitive behavioral therapy are significantly better than either alone.

VII. Risk factors associated with exogenous obesity

    A. Metabolic syndrome represents a clustering of cardiovascular and metabolic risk factors known to accelerate atherosclerosis and cardiovascular disease (Table 8.10).

      1. Visceral adipocytes and insulin resistance resulting from decreased sensitivity of insulin receptors drive the development of metabolic syndrome.

      2. Women with metabolic syndrome have a threefold to fivefold increased risk for cardiovascular disease and events.

TABLE 8.8 Pharmacotherapeutic Options for the Management of Eating Disorders

MEDICATION	OBESITY	ANOREXIA	BULIMIA	BED	NES
Topiramate	+	Not tested	++	+++	Not tested
Zonisamide	+	Not tested	Not tested	+	Not tested
SSRI	+	+/–	+	+	+
SNRI	++	+/–	+/–	+/–	+/–
Atypical	++	+/–	Not suitable	+	+/–

Source: Milano (2011), Bray (2007), and Gallant (2012).

TABLE 8.9 Effects of Common Antidepressants on Weight

MEDICATION	EFFECT ON WEIGHT
Amitriptyline	Gain
Nortriptyline	Gain
Imipramine	Gain

SSRIs
    Sertraline
    Fluoxetine
    Fluvoxamine
    Paroxetine]
    Citalopram
	Neutral
	Neutral
	Neutral
	Gain
	Neutral

NaSSAs Mitrazapine	Gain

SNRI
    Venlafaxine
    Sibutramine
	Neutral
	Loss

Atypical Buproprion	Loss

Source: Gallant (2012).

3. The increased release of free fatty acids impairs insulin clearance by the liver and alters peripheral metabolism.
4. Adiponectin, a hormone secreted by adipocytes, regulates response and reduces cardiovascular risk. Adiponectin levels are inversely related to adipocyte mass.
5. The National Cholesterol Education Panel (NCEP) Adult Treatment Program (2001, 2004) defines metabolic syndrome as the clustering of three of the following criteria:

    a. Waist circumference more than 88 cm (> 35 in.)

    b. High-density lipoprotein (HDL) less than 50 mg/dL

    c. Triglyceride level greater than 150 mg/dL

    d. Fasting glucose level greater than 110 mg/dL.

    e. Blood pressure (systolic, diastolic, or both) greater than or equal to 130/greater than or equal to 85 mmHg.

  B. Reproductive milestones contributing to risk of obesity in women

    1. Puberty: Has been shown to be a vulnerable period for development of obesity. Studies have shown that the age of onset of menses may contribute to the development of obesity later in life. During menarche, the gonadal steroids exert strong influences on body composition related to adipose tissue growth. Early onset of puberty is associated with high adiposity in adults.

    2. Postpartum: Retention of weight after pregnancy may be a factor in obesity in young women. The weight gain may reflect changes in the lifestyle of the woman rather than the physiologic changes associated with childbirth. After delivery, women may have a higher intake of food, have more accessibility to food during the day, and may experience decreased physical activity levels. Postpartum breastfeeding has been associated with maternal weight loss.

TABLE 8.10 Factors Included for the Metabolic Assessment of Obesity

PARAMETER	MEASUREMENT	CRITICAL VALUE
Obesity	Body mass index	Up to 24.9 = normal 25–29.9 = overweight 30–34.9 = class I obesity 35–39.9 = class II obesity ≥ 40 = class III obesity
Body fat distribution	Waist circumference	Women > 35 in (89 cm)
Fasting lipid profile	High-density lipoprotein (HDL)	Women < 50 mg/dL
	Triglycerides	Women > 150 mg/dL
	Low-density lipoprotein	Women > 100 mg/dL
Insulin resistance	Fasting blood glucose (mmol/L)	> 100 mg/dL HOMA-IR ≥ 5mmol/L
	Fasting insulin	60 pmo/L
Hypertension	Blood pressure	Systolic > 130 mmHg Diastolic > 85 mmHg

Source: Soleymani and Garvey (2013).

3. Postmenopause: Menopause is a period of significant physiological changes that are related to estrogen depletion and cessation of ovarian function and is associated with increased body weight, increased adiposity, and obesity-related diseases.
   a. Estrogen is thought to positively regulate body fat accumulation and weight distribution by reducing lipoprotein lipase levels in tissue and by serving as an anorectic, decreasing appetite, and affecting feeding behavior.
   b. Research evidence of the effects of postmenopausal hormone replacement therapy (HRT) on weight gain, adioposity, and distribution have been mixed, with some studies demonstrating no effect of HRT on weight gain and adiposity whereas other studies demonstrate weight loss and a shift to less android weight distribution with HRT.
   c. Weight gain in postmenopausal women has also been attributed to the rapid decline in resting metabolic rate during menopause and to the slower decline with subsequent aging. Decreased physical activity also contributes to decreases in resting metabolic rate.
C. Menopause
   1. Studies have shown that estradiol deficiency results in a shift to a more atherogenic lipid profile characterized by increases in total cholesterol, low-density lipoproteins (LDL-C), and triglyceride and insulin levels.
   2. Research has shown that menopause is accompanied by an increase in abdominal fat distribution and a decline gluteal–femoral distribution.
   3. Resting metabolic rate declines rapidly during menopause, suggesting an influence of estrogen on resting metabolic rate.
   4. Decreases in metabolic rate may also be associated with a loss of lean tissue mass and the loss of the luteal phase effects on an increase in energy expenditure.
   5. The ratio of androgens to estrogens shifts, thereby increasing visceral adiposity.

VIII. Obesity-focused health history
   A. An obesity-focused history allows the development of tailored recommendations and interventions to maximize treatment outcomes.
   B. Components of the obesity-focused health history in women include
      1. Past and current prescription and over-the-counter medications: Weight gain is a common side effect or adverse effect of medications (Box 8.1).

BOX 8.1 *Medications Associated With Weight Gain*

- Glucocorticoids
- Megace
- Cyproheptadine
- Antidepressants (tricyclic, monoamine oxidase [MAO] inhibitors, selective serotonin reuptake inhibitors [SSRIs], mirtazapine)
- Mood stabilizers (lithium)
- Antipsychotics and phenothizianes (clozapine, olanzapine, risperidone)
- Antiepileptic medications (valproate, gabapentin)
- Hormones (contraceptives, corticosteroids, progestational steroids)
- α-Adrenergic-blocking drugs (beta blockers are really more of an issue; also calcium channel blockers, especially amlodipine, cause ankle edema in women, thus weight gain)
- Antidiabetic agents (sulfonylureas, insulin, thiazolidinediones, and drugs that stimulate insulin release)
- Opiates
- Asthma medications with steroids (Vanceril, Pulmicort, Azmacort, Aero-Bid)
- Osteoporosis treatments (reloxifine)
- Antihistamines including Azelastine (Astelin) and diphenhydramine (Benadryl)

2. History of past and current comorbidities, particularly obesity-related comorbidities
3. History of reproductive milestones and weight gain (menarche, pregnancy, breastfeeding, menopause)
4. Change in lifestyle events. Weight gain is associated with changes in lifestyle events, including marital status, employment status or occupation, illness, or caregiving responsibilities.
5. Sleep patterns and current symptoms of sleep disorders (increased stressor, menopausal symptoms, sleep apnea, restless leg syndrome)
6. Weight gain history and velocity of weight gain (estimation of weight gain over a given period of time)
7. Current physical activity and exercise routines
8. Employment status, type of occupation, and work environment
9. Dietary recall
10. History of tobacco cessation, current use of nicotine or other tobacco products

TABLE 8.11 Effect of Weight Loss on Clinically Significant Versus Cosmetically Significant Outcomes

TYPE OF PROCEDURE	WEIGHT LOSS	CLINICALLY SIGNIFICANT	COSMETICALLY SIGNIFICANT
Diet/ Exercise	10%; from 300 to 270 lbs	Yes	No
	10%; from 200 to 180 lbs	Yes	Probably not
	10%; from 150 to 135 lbs	Yes	Yes
Liposuction	7%; from 220 to 200 lbs	No	Probably not
	7%; from 160 to 149 lbs	No	Yes
Surgery (RYGB/LB)	40%; from 264 to 165 lbs	Yes	Yes

Source: Bray (2007).

11 History of substance abuse (illicit drugs, alcohol)
12. Family history: May provide insights into predisposing genetic factors
13. Social support and financial resources: Assess to obesity-related treatments
14. Assessment of readiness and motivation for weight loss
15. Appropriateness of the patient's expectation and weight-loss goals. Educating patients regarding the differences between weight loss, which will have a cosmetic impact, versus health impact (Table 8.11).

IX. **Obesity-focused physical examination**
   A. Height, weight, and BMI
      1. Height
      2. Weight
      3. Body habitus
         a. Gynoid (pear-shaped body)
            (1) Hips wider than shoulders due to body stores of fat there; lower risk for diabetes and heart problems
         b. Android (apple-shaped body)
            (1) Body fat is stored around middle; higher risk for heart problems
            (2) Common in midlife and menopause due to decreasing levels of estrogen
   B. BMI measurement
      1. BMI should be rounded to the nearest tenth.
         a. Example: 29.85 is expressed as 29.9.
         b. Example: 29.84 is expressed as 29.8.
      2. Example of calculation of BMI for a patient who weighs 130 pounds and is 5 feet 4 inches tall is provided in Figure 8.4.

$$\text{Body mass index} = \frac{\text{Kg of body weight}}{\text{M}^2 \text{ of body height}}$$

FIGURE 8.3 Formula for BMI, also known as the Quetelet index.

1. Convert weight from pounds to kilograms.
   Weight: 130 lb = 59.09 kg (1 lb = 2.2 kg)

2. Convert height from inches to centimeters.
   Height: 5 ft 4 in. = 64 in. × 2.54 = 162.56 cm (1 in. = 2.54 cm)

3. Convert the height to meters by dividing the number of centimeters by 100:
   162.56 cm/100 = 1.6256 (Do not round the value.)

4. Take the square of the resulting number and save it. (Do not round the value.)
   To get the square, multiply the number by itself.
   1.6256 × 1.6256 = 2.6425753

5. To calculate the BMI: Divide the weight by the square of the height calculated in
   No. 4. (Do not round either the weight or the square of the height.)
   59.09 kg ÷ 2.6425753 = 22.36; BMI = 22.4

FIGURE 8.4 Example of how to calculate BMI for a patient who weights 130 pounds
and is 5 feet 4 inches tall.

C. Waist and hip circumference: Provides an indication of trunk or
   visceral obesity, often associated with diabetes and heart disease. To
   determine the circumference
   1. The patient should stand up straight in the upright position
      with feet together.
   2. Instruct patient to relax and stand with arms to the side.
   3. Expose the waist with the undergarments pulled below the waist.
   4. Find the natural waist, which is the narrowest part of the torso.
      This area is midway between the inferior border of the rib cage
      and the superior aspect of the iliac crest.
   5. Place the tape measure at the measuring point and locate the
      point on the tape where the zero aligns with the measuring
      point. Record to the nearest 0.1 cm. Hold tape horizontally.
   6. If necessary, ask the obese patient to elevate any sagging
      abdominal wall.
   7. Take measurement at the end of normal expiration.

X. Physical findings associated with cardiometabolic risk

  A. Funduscopic examination: Hypertensive or diabetic retinopathy, evidence of hyperlipidemia (xanthalasmas, corneal arcus)

  B. Neck: Enlarged circumference

  C. Cardiovascular: Cardiomegaly, carotid or abdominal bruit; a sustained, enlarged (> 3 cm diameter) apical impulse, which may be displaced outside the midclavicular line, is characteristic of isolated left ventriculara hypertrophy (LVH).

  D. Skin: Acanthosis nigricans, acne, hirsutism

XI. Laboratory testing

  A. Fasting blood glucose level: Impaired fasting or impaired glucose tolerance; diagnosis of type 2 diabetes

  B. Lipid panel (total cholesterol, HDL-C, LDL-C, triglycerides , highly sensitive C reactive protein [hs CRP])

  C. Electrocardiography: LVH, evidence of myocardial ischemia

  D. 2D echocardiogram to identify LVH and left ventricular function

  E. Dual-energy x-ray absorptiometry: accurate way to measure total body fat

  F. Computed tomography (CT): Can quantify the amount of visceral fat in the abdomen

XII. Treatment interventions

  A. Assessment of physical symptoms, functional limitations, and metabolic risk

   1. The Edmonton Obesity Staging System provides a systematic approach for determining physical symptoms, functional limitations, and metabolic risk to identify treatment options through a tailored treatment plan based on intensity of risk (Table 8.12).

   2. Provides for a complications-based approach to treatment options

  B. Behavioral strategies

   1. Assess for mood disorders (depression, anxiety, eating disorders, posttraumatic stress disorder [PTSD])

   2. Common recommendations

    a. Coping with stress

    b. Coping with frustration

    c. Compensation strategies

    d. Social environment

    e. Referral to groups

    f. Referral to Internet links or books

    g. Referral for psychotherapy

  C. Nutritional

   1. Evidence-based dietetics practice is the use of systematically reviewed scientific evidence in making food and nutrition practice decisions by integrating best available evidence

TABLE 8.12 Edmonton Obesity Staging System

STAGE	OBESITY-RELATED RISK FACTORS	PHYSICAL SYMPTOMS, PSYCHOPATHOLOGY, FUNCTIONAL LIMITATIONS, AND IMPAIRMENT OF WELL-BEING
0	None (blood pressure, serum lipids, fasting glucose, etc.)	None
1	Subclinical (borderline hypertension, impaired fasting glucose, elevated liver enzymes, etc.)	Mild
2	Established (hypertension, type 2 diabetes mellitus, sleep apnea, osteoarthritis, reflux disease, polycystic ovary syndrome, anxiety disorder, etc.)	Moderate
3	Established end-organ damage (myocardial infarction, heart failure, diabetic complications, incapacitating osteoarthritis, etc.)	Significant
4	Severe disabilities (potentially end-stage disabilities, etc.)	Severe

with professional expertise and patient values to improve outcomes.

2. Common nutritional recommendations
   a. Quality and quantity of food intake
   b. Time of consumption
   c. Impact of daily calories
   d. Specific food recommendations
   e. Implementation strategies
   f. Referral to groups
   g. Referral to Internet links or books
   h. Referral to dieticians
   i. Referral to commercial weight-loss programs
3. Obtain dietary history through 24-hour or weekly recall
   a. Web-based diet diaries (Loseit.com; myfitness.pal)
4. Computation of estimated daily caloric intake (Table 8.13, Table 8.14)
   a. BMI 27–35 decrease in caloric intake of 300 – 500 kcal /d = 10% weight loss in 6 months (0.24–0.45kg/wk)
   b. BMI 35 > decrease in caloric intake of 500 – 1000 kcal /d = 10% weight loss in 6 months (0.45–0.90 kg/wk)

TABLE 8.13 Calculating Daily Caloric Requirements

Step 1

Estimate the recommended individual caloric requirement (kcal per day) by calculating the resting energy expenditure (REE).

For adult women:

REE = 10 × weight (in kg) + 6.25 × height (in cm) − 5 × age (in years) − 161

Example = 10 × 59.09 + 6.25 × 162.56 − 5 × 36 − 161 = 1587.9

$$590.9 \quad + \quad 1016 \quad\quad -19 \ = 1587.9$$

Weight: 130 lbs = 59.09 kgs

Height: 5" 4 = 64 inches **x** *2.54* = 162.56 cm

Step 2

Multiply REE by an activity factor (AF) of 1.5 for women for light activity to estimate daily caloric need or by 1.6 for women for higher activity.

Example = 1587.9 × 1.5 = 2381.85 kcal

REE × AF = estimated total caloric need (kcal per day) to maintain weight
REE = resting energy expenditure

TABLE 8.14. Recommended Average Daily Energy Allowances for Women

POPULATION GROUP	AGE (Y)	KCAL/KG	KCAL/DAY
Women:	11–14	47	2,200
nonpregnant,	15–18	40	2,200
nonlactating	19–24	38	2,200
	25-50	36	2,200
	> 51	30	1,900

Note: This is based on women engaged in light to moderate physical activity, with no underlying medical condition.

    D. Pharmacologic
        1. Many state boards of nursing prohibit the prescription of anti-obesity medication by an advanced practice registered nurse (APRN). Check with your state board of nursing for guidance on anti-obesity medications.
        2. Recommendations for pharmacologic therapies for the management of obesity in patients with metabolic dysregulation compared to metabolically healthy patients (Figure 8.5, Table 8.15)

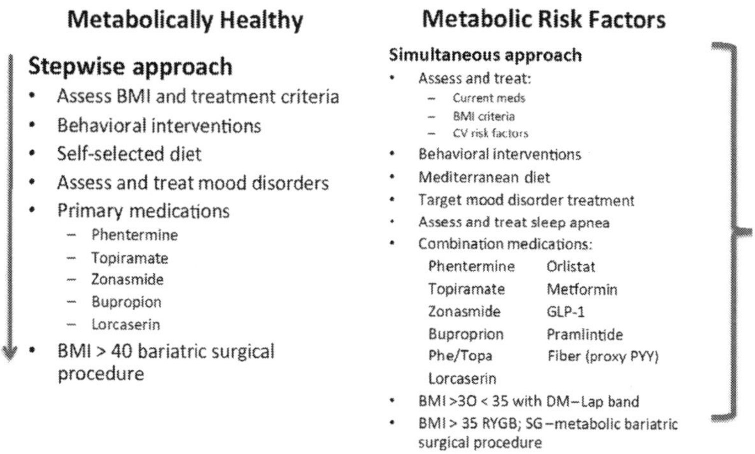

Metabolically Healthy

Stepwise approach
- Assess BMI and treatment criteria
- Behavioral interventions
- Self-selected diet
- Assess and treat mood disorders
- Primary medications
  - Phentermine
  - Topiramate
  - Zonasmide
  - Bupropion
  - Lorcaserin
- BMI > 40 bariatric surgical procedure

Metabolic Risk Factors

Simultaneous approach
- Assess and treat:
  - Current meds
  - BMI criteria
  - CV risk factors
- Behavioral interventions
- Mediterranean diet
- Target mood disorder treatment
- Assess and treat sleep apnea
- Combination medications:

Phentermine	Orlistat
Topiramate	Metformin
Zonasmide	GLP-1
Buproprion	Pramlintide
Phe/Topa	Fiber (proxy PYY)
Lorcaserin	

- BMI >30 < 35 with DM–Lap band
- BMI > 35 RYGB; SG –metabolic bariatric surgical procedure

FIGURE 8.5 Pharmacologic strategies based on assessment of metabolic health: Management strategies for obesity.

TABLE 8.15 Current FDA-Approved Pharmacologic Options

MEDICATION	MECHANISM OF ACTION	OBTAINED
Adipex-P (Phentermine)	Appetite suppressant—similar to amphetamine—acting on the central nervous system	Controlled prescription
Dexedrine (Dextroamphetamine Saccharate)	CNS stimulant—an amphetamine analog	Controlled prescription
Alli (Orlistat)	Reduction in fat absorption via inhibition of pancreatic lipase activity in intestine	Over the counter
Xenical (Orlistat)		Prescription
Qysmia (Phentermine/Topiramate)	Carbonic anhydrase inhibitor, noradrenalin releaser, and anticonvulsant that suppresses appetite, impacts satiety, stimulates thermogenesis	Controlled prescription
Belviq (Lorcaserin)	Selective 5-HT2C receptor agonist	Controlled prescription

E. Surgical procedures

1. Of the approximate 250,000 bariatric surgical procedures performed each year in the United States, 70% are preformed on women.
2. Types of surgical procedures

   a. Restrictive and malabsorptive bariatric procedures (metabolic surgery):

      Laparoscopic gastric bypass (Roux-en-Y)

      Biliopancreatic diversion (BPD)

      Duodenal switch (DS) with BPD

      Sleeve gastrectomy

   b. Restrictive-only bariatric procedures

      Laparoscopic adjustable gastric band (LAGB)

      Gastric stapling procedures

3. The term *metabolic surgery* has emerged to describe procedures intended to treat type 2 diabetes as well as to reduce cardiometabolic risk factors.
4. National Institutes of Health criteria for bariatric surgical procedures include

   a. BMI greater than or equal to 40 kg/m² without coexisting medical problems and for whom bariatric surgery would not be associated with excessive risk

   b. Patients with a BMI greater than or equal to 35 kg/m² and one or more severe obesity-related co-morbidities (Box 8.2)
5. Gender-specific issues related to women and bariatric surgical procedures

---

BOX 8.2 *Common Co-morbidities Considered Medically Necessary by Third-Party Payers for Bariatric Surgical Procedures*

- Type 2 diabetes
- Hypertension
- Hyperlipidemia
- Obstructive sleep apnea (OSA)
- Obesity–hypoventilation syndrome (OHS)
- Pickwickian syndrome (a combination of OSA and OHS)
- Nonalcoholic fatty liver disease (NAFLD)
- Nonalcoholic steatohepatitis (NASH)
- Pseudotumor cerebri
- Gastroesophageal reflux disease (GERD)
- Asthma
- Venous stasis disease
- Severe urinary incontinence
- Debilitating arthritis
- Considerably impaired quality of life

Source: Mechanick (2013).

    a. Estrogen therapy should be discontinued before bariatric surgery (1 cycle of oral contraceptives in premenopausal women; 3 weeks of HRT (see Box 8.3) in postmenopausal women) to reduce the risks for postoperative thromboembolic phenomena.

    b. Weight loss through bariatric surgical proceeds may increase fertility. Women should have counseling for reliable contraceptives and consideration for nonoral contraceptives post restrictive/malabsorption procedures.

    c. Women of childbearing years are at a greater risk for malabsorption anemia post restrictive/malabsorption procedures related to menstruation.

    d. Calcium and vitamin D absorption are decreased following restrictive/malabsorption.

XIII. Development of a weight management plan: An effective weight management plan based on best practice, research, and guidelines is designed to help an overweight or obese person reach and stay at a healthy body weight.

    A. The NHLBI (National Heart, Lung, and Blood Institute) panel recommends treatment for obesity for patients with a BMI of 25 to 29 kg/m^2 and with two or more risk factors and for patients with a BMI of 30 or more with no risk factors.

    B. The overall goals of weight management are to reduce body weight and maintain a lower body weight long-term, prevent further weight gain, and control potential risk factors.

    C. Nurse practitioners should counsel their patients about dietary interventions, increasing the amount of physical activity, behavior therapy, pharmacotherapy, and a combination of all techniques.

    D. The ability to prescribe obesity drugs varies by state. Check with your state board of nursing regarding the rules and regulations

---

BOX 8.3 *Psychosocial Factors Predictive of Poor Long-Term Outcomes of Bariatric Surgery*

- Unrealistically high expectations for weight loss
- Untreated psychological disorders
- Untreated adverse eating patterns: grazing, night eating syndrome, emotional or nonhungry eating, BED...or multiple adverse eating behaviors
- ETOH (alcohol) abuse, addictive and impulsive behaviors
- Poor access to social support

Source: Mechanick (2013).

BOX 8.4 *Selected Internet Resources for Patients*

www.eatright.org
American Dietetic Association offers information on nutrition, healthy lifestyle, and how to find a registered dietician.
www.nal.usda.gov/about/oei/index.htm
National Heart, Lung, and Blood Institute Obesity Education Initiative offers information on selecting a weight-loss program, menu planning, food-label reading, and BMI calculation and interpretation.
www.niddk.nih.gov/health/nutrit/win.htm
Weight Control Information Network has weight-loss articles from the National Institutes of Health.
www.fitday.com
www.myfitnesspal.com
www.loseit.com
www.sparkpeople.com
www.weightwatchers.com
www.nofusa.org (National Obesity Foundation)

Note: fitday.com gives nutritional analysis of calories, fat, protein, carbohydrates, and fiber in table and graph form as well as offering journals, and goal-setting and activity-tracking tools.

---

for prescribing U.S. Food and Drug Administration (FDA) anti-obesity medications (see Table 8.15).

E. The most effective therapy for weight loss and maintenance is a combination of a low-calorie diet, an increase in physical activity, and lifestyle modifications.

F. Using this therapy for at least 6 months and setting a goal for a 5% to 10% reduction in weight should be the initial goal for the patient. A patient's continued participation is the most important outcome in weight management.

G. Results of recent clinical trials suggested that weight management plans should be created according to a woman's current phase of life. The critical reproductive milestones that should be targeted include puberty, pregnancy, postpartum, and during menopause.

H. Internet sources are listed in Box 8.4 for further information.

Bibliography

Bray, G. A., & Greenway, F. L. (2007). Pharmacological treatment of the overweight patient. *Pharmacological Reviews, 59,* 151–184.

Carwel, M. L., & Spatz, D. L. (2011). Eating disorders & breastfeeding. *MCN; American Journal of Maternal Child Nursing, 36*(2), 112–117; quiz 118-9. doi: 10.1097/ NMC.0b013e318205775c

Centers for Disease Control and Prevention. (n.d.). *National Health and Nutrition Examination Survey*. U.S. Department of Health and Human Services.

Chan, J. M., Rimm, E. B., Colditz, G. A., Stampfer, M. J., & Willett, W. C. (1994, September). Obesity, fat distribution, and weight gain as risk factors for clinical diabetes in men. *Diabetes Care, 17*, 961–969. doi:10.2337/diacare.17.9.961

Cho, Y. M., Merchant, C., & Kieffer, T. J. (2012). Targeting the glucagon receptor family for diabetes and obesity therapy. *Pharmacology & Therapeutics, 135*, 247–278.

Colditz, G. A., Willett, W. C., Rotnitzky, A., & Manson, J.E. (1995, April 1). Weight gain as a risk factor for clinical diabetes mellitus in women. *Annals of Internal Medicine, 122*(7), 481–486.

Daniel, S., Soleymani, T., & Garvey, W. T. (2013). A complications-based clinical staging of obesity to guide treatment modality and intensity. *Current Opinion in Endocrinology & Diabetes and Obesity, 20*(5), 377–388.

Davis, C. (2013). A narrative review of binge eating and addictive behaviors: Shared associations with seasonality and personality factors. *Front Psychiatry, 4*,183.

Flegal, K. M., Carroll, M. D., Kit, B. K., & Ogden C.L. (2012, February 1). Prevalence of obesity and trends in the distribution of body mass index among US adults, 1990–2011. *Journal of the American Medical Association, 1, 307*(5), 491–497.

Gallant, A. R., Lundgren, J., & Drapeau. (2012). The night-eating syndrome and obesity. *Obesity Reviews, 13*, 528–536.

Giandilia, A., Russo, G. T., Romeo, E. L., Alibrandi, A., Villari, P., Mirto, A. A., … Cucinotta, D. (2014, January). Influence of high-normal serum TSH levels on major cardiovascular risk factors and visceral adiposity Index in euthyroid type 2 diabete subjects. *Endocrine, 47*(1), 152–160.

Hill, J. O., & Wyatt, H. (2002). Outpatient management of obesity: A primary care perspective. *Obesity Research, 10*(2), 124S–130S.

Jakicic, J. M. (2002). The role of physical activity in prevention and treatment of body weight gain in adults. *Journal of Nutrition* (Suppl.), 3826S–3829S.

Johnson, D. B., Gerstein, D. E., Evan, A. E., & Woodward-Lopez, G. (2002). Preventing obesity: A life cycle perspective. *Journal of the American Dietetic Association, 106*(1), 97–102.

Klauer, J., & Aronne, L. (2002). Managing overweight and obesity in women. *Clinical Obstetrics and Gynecology, 45*, 1080–1088.

Kral, J. G. (2004). Preventing and treating obesity in girls and young women to curb the epidemic. *Obesity Research, 12*(10), 1539–1546.

Kral, J. G., Kava, R. A., Catalano, P. M., & Moore, B. J. (2012). Severe obesity: The neglected epidemic. *Obesity Facts, 5*, 254–269.

Kushner, R. F. (2012).Clinical assessment and management of adult obesity. *Circulation, 126*, 2870–2877. doi: 10.1161/CIRCULATIONAHA.111.075424

Lustig, R. H. (2008). Hypothalamic obesity: Causes, consequences, treatment. *Pediatric Endocrinology Reviews, 6*(2), 220–227.

Lyznicki, J. M., Young, D. C., Riggs, J. A., & Davis, R. M. (2001). Obesity: Assessment and management in primary care. *American Family Physician, 63*, 2185–2196.

Mechanick, J. I., Youdim, A., Jones, D. B. W., Garvey, W. T., Hurley, D. L., McMahon, M. M., … Brethauer, S. (2013). Clinical practice guidelines for the perioperative nutritional, metabolic, and nonsurgical support of the bariatric surgery patient—2013 update; Cosponsored by American Association of Clinical Endocrinologists, the Obesity Society, and American Society for Metabolic & Bariatric Surgery, *Endocrine Practice, 19*(2), 337–372.

Messina, G., Viggiano, A., De Luca, V., Messian, A., Chieffi, S., & Monda, M. (2013). Hormonal changes in menopause and orexin-a action. *Obstetrics and Gynecology International, 2013*, 209812. doi: 10.1155/2013/209812. [Epub June 11, 2013].

Milano, W., De Rosa, M., Milano, L., & Capasso, A. (2011). Night eating syndrome: An overview. *Journal of Pharmacy and Pharmacology, 64*, 2–10.

National Center for Health Statistics. (2009). *Healthy People 2010 conference edition.* Hyattsville, MD: Author. Retrieved from http://www.health.gov/healthypeople

National Research Council. (1989). *Recommended dietary allowances. Subcommittee on the tenth edition of the RDAs, Food Nutrition Board, Commission on Life Sciences* (10th ed.). Washington, DC: National Academies Press.

Norman, R. J., Noakes, M., Wu, R., Davies, M. J., Moran, L., & Wang, J. X. (2004). Improving reproductive performance in overweight/obese women with effective weight management. *Human Reproduction Update, 10*(3) 267–280.

Ogden, C. L., Carroll, M. D., Kit, B. K., & Flegal, K. M. (2013, October). Prevalence of obesity among adults: United States, 2011–2012. *NCHS Data Brief* (131), 1–8.

Østbye, T., Peterson, B. L., Krause, K. M., Swamy, G. K., & Lovelady, C. A. (2012, February). Predictors of postpartum weight change among overweight and obese women: Results from the Active Mothers Postpartum study. *Journal of Women's Health, 21*(2), 215–222. doi: 10.1089/jwh.2011.2947 [Epub November 17, 2011].

Ruiz-Tovar, J., Boix, E., Galindo, I., Zubiaga, L., Diez, M., Arroyo, A., & Calpena, R. (2013, December 18). Evolution of subclinical hypothyroidism and its relation with glucose and triglycerides levels in morbidly obese patients after undergoing sleeve gastrectomy as bariatric procedure. *Obesity Surgery, 24*(5), 791–795.

Ryan, D., & Stewart, T. (2004). Medical management of obesity in women: Office-based approaches to weight management. *Clinical Obstetrics and Gynecology, 47*(4), 914–927.

WebMD. (n.d.). *Weight loss clinic, parenting & childhood obesity.* Retrieved December 2, 2005, from http://www.weightlossmd.com/parenting_and_child_obesity.asp

Wing, R. R., & Hill, J. O. (2001). Successful weight loss maintenance. *Annual Review of Nutrition, 21*, 323–341.

Lesbian Health (Don't Ask . . . Won't Tell: Lesbian Women and Women Who Have Sex With Women)

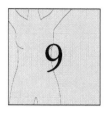

9

Yvette Marie Petti

I. **Introduction and overview**
   A. Lesbians experience health disparities in terms of prevention screening and desired health outcomes as compared to heterosexual women.
   B. Often, lesbian women avoid care due to perceived and lived experiences of homophobia from health care providers and health care institutions and systems.
   C. Lesbian women are less likely to seek out care due to
      1. Stigma associated with being identified as lesbian
      2. Previously experienced negative encounters with health care providers
   D. Lesbian women are at further risk for delayed care and reduced health care screening related to variables such as
      1. Lack of health insurance
      2. Lack of provider awareness
      3. Provider ignorance
      4. Lack of understanding of their own health risks
      5. Health system design issues
   E. One of the largest gaps identified in the literature that contributes to reduced screening and provider bias is the lack of curriculum addressing the health care needs of lesbian women.

II. **Screening recommendations for sexual-minority women (lesbian, bisexual, and women who have sex with women)**
   A. Breast cancer screening
      1. Lesbian women have lower rates of mammograms and higher rates of breast cancer than heterosexual women.

2. This has been cited as a lack of access to care because of a lack of insurance coupled with health behaviors such as smoking, null parity, obesity, and alcohol consumption.
3. Lesbian women have been found to participate less often than heterosexual women in self-breast awareness, so be inclusive in your offerings of mammography and in reviewing self-breast awareness with your lesbian patients as a standard of care.
4. Exploring any misgivings that your lesbian patient may have about self-touch and her risk for the development of breast cancer is your opportunity to offer her appropriate education and screening.
5. Be familiar with community resources offering support for screening as many lesbian women are underinsured or have no insurance.

B. Cervical cancer screening and human papillomavirus (HPV): The facts
1. Lesbian women's rates for cervical cancer screening are lower than those for heterosexual women due to
   a. Barriers to access to care
   b. Provider naïvety
   c. Fear of examination
   d. Other system barriers
2. A significant percentage of lesbian women have reported a history of having intercourse with a male partner at some time and many continue to have intermittent intercourse with bisexual men.
3. Lesbian women are at greater risk for higher rates of abnormal Pap smears due to delayed screening and intervention
4. Lesbian women and women who have sex with women are not immune to HPV and other factors leading to cervical cancer.
5. The current Pap smear screening guidelines should be applied when providing care to lesbian women and women who have sex with women.
6. Be sensitive to the likely possibility that your lesbian patient has had sexual trauma and/or negative provider experience by conveying a compassionate and safe environment for her to participate in this recommended screening examination.

C. Screening for sexually transmitted infections (STIs)
1. Lesbian women and women who have sex with women have exposures to sexually transmitted infections such as trichomoniasis, gonorrhea, chlamydia, genital herpes, human papilloma virus, hepatitis C, syphilis, and HIV, so screen for these.
2. Exposure to STIs (like all women) is dependent on sexual practices, partner's risks, and number of partners. Box 9.1 lists high-risk sexual practices of lesbian women and women who have sex with women.

BOX 9.1 *Listing of High-Risk Sexual Practices of Lesbian Women and Women Who Have Sex With Women*

- Oral to vaginal contact
- Tribadism: Genital to genital contact
- Digital stimulation
- Oral to anal contact
- Sharing of sex toys

3. Lower risk sexual practices include kissing and rubbing genitalia on her partner's body. Lesbians do not always know their own risks for STIs and hence do not always take precautions; this provides an opportunity for education.
4. Lesbian women and women who have sex with women can transmit trichomoniasis and other infections to one another.
5. Including a thorough sexual history of gender of partner, number of partners, and type of sexual practices, and including an oral/pharyngeal external (or internal as needed) rectal examination during the screening for HPV is critical due to the association of HPV with oral and rectal cancers.
6. Include discussion of whether she and her partner(s) use condoms and/or dental dams and practice washing their hands and sex toys after penetrative sexual contact.
    a. Offer and discuss screenings for STIs candidly with your lesbian patients.
7. Understand your own comfort level when having candid discussions with your patients regarding sexual practices and behaviors.
8. Use inclusive language and communicate in a neutral, matter-of-fact manner.

III. **Using inclusive language**
   A. Use words that "open the door," are neutral, and are expressed in an unbiased manner.
   B. When asking about socioeconomic profile, the use of the word "partnered" conveys openness to the patient.
   C. When asking about partners, deliver the question in a manner that gives control back to the patient, and in a neutral tone ask "male," "female," or " both male and/or female."
   D. Avoid using the term "sexually active" as this may have an ambiguous meaning. Rather, ask the patient, "Are you having sex with males, females, or both?"

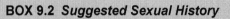

BOX 9.2 *Suggested Sexual History*

I am going to ask the following questions not to judge you but to identify your care needs.

- Have you ever had sex forced on you by your partner, partners, or anyone?
- Do you have a sexual partner or partners at this time? Are they male, female, or both?
- Do you feel safe in your relationship with your partner or partners at this time?
- Do you have any concerns about your sexual relationship with your partner or partners at this time?
- Do you participate in oral to vaginal contact with your partner or partners?
- Do you participate in oral to anal contact with your partner or partners?
- Do you participate in penile to vaginal intercourse with your partner or partners?
- Do you have any difficulty reaching orgasm with your partner or partners?
- Do you use sex toys (vibrators, strap-on penis, pelvic balls)? If so, do you share these with your partner or partners?
- Have you ever had a sexually transmitted infection, such as trichomoniasis, gonorrhea, chlamydia, genital herpes, genital warts, HPV, HIV, hepatitis C, syphilis, pelvic inflammatory disease (PID)?

E. Use the following to preface the beginning of your inquiry regarding her sexual history: "I am going to ask you some questions about your sexual health. These questions are not intended to embarrass you or to judge you, but rather to provide information that will help me identify what health screening and care you may need."

F. Ask, "Are you having sex with males, females, and/or both males and females?"

G. Do not presume that your patient is having sex with only one person, so use "partner" and "partners" sequentially when you are asking about the patient's sexual history.

H. Be sure to include a question during the sexual history interview regarding safety. An example of how to assess the safety of your patient with her partner(s) is to ask, "Do you feel safe in your relationship with your partner (s)?"

I. Many self-identified lesbians have experienced physical, emotional, and sexual assault during their lives, and the health screening examination provides an opportunity to assess for domestic and other encounters of violence by your patient.

J. Examples of questions to include in your sexual history with lesbian women and women who have sex with women are presented in Box 9.2.

> **BOX 9.3** *Definitions for Selected Sexual Acts*

- Giving face or going down: Oral to genital/vaginal contact
- Fisting: Using a fist and/or several fingers introduced into the vagina and/or rectum for digital stimulation
- Rimming: Rectal/anal stimulation with partner's tongue

IV. **Approach to patient and provider communication**
  A. Variables identified in the literature as barriers to the promotion and health screening of self-identified lesbians: Lack of trust of provider and/or health care system, lack of health insurance, provider insensitivity, and biases of traditional health care delivery systems
  B. Three main influences related to sexual minority women's disclosure to their providers: Sexual identity experience, perceived risk of disclosure, and the quality of relationship to provider
  C. Make your language inclusive to convey a neutral and safe environment for your lesbian patient to discuss her health and sexual history.
  D. Use a nonjudgmental and neutral tone when asking about sexual practices and/or addressing sexual concerns. Box 9.3 lists some terminology used among lesbian women to describe their sexual practices.

V. **Risk assessment and reduction**
  A. The Gay and Lesbian Medical Association's (GLMA's) health and behavioral topics that all lesbian women should discuss with their provider
    1. Breast cancer
      a. Have higher rates disproportionately to heterosexual women
    2. Depression/anxiety
      a. Have higher rates of mental distress and depression
        (1) Due to chronic stress related to barriers to disclosure of sexual orientation/practices
        (2) Due to lack of social support
        (3) Due to social and institutional discrimination
      b. Fewer care-seeking behaviors
      c. Include depression screenings.
        (1) The Patient Health Questionnaire-2 (PHQ-2)
        (2) The Patient Health Questionnaire-9 (PHQ-9)
    3. Heart health
      a. Ask about physical activity participation.
      b. Screen fasting lipids and glucose.

      c. Include alcohol, substance, and tobacco use.

      d. Include family history of heart disease.

   4. Gynecologic cancer

      a. Lesbian and bisexual women are at higher risk for ovarian and endometrial cancer.

         (1) Thought to be due to higher rates of obesity, smoking, and lack of adequate screening

         (2) Ask about last date and results of Pap smear screening.

      b. Educate about importance of yearly well-women examination, which includes pelvic examination.

   5. Fitness

      a. Rates of physical activity have been identified as being lower than heterosexual women in some populations of lesbian women.

      b. Include physical activity participation and tolerance in assessment.

   6. Tobacco and alcohol use

      a. Rates of tobacco and alcohol use are higher among lesbian and bisexual women.

      b. Offer tobacco-cessation intervention.

   7. Substance use

      a. Rates of substance use/abuse are higher among young self-identified lesbians and bisexual women.

   8. Intimate partner violence

      a. Lesbian women, bisexual women, and women who have sex with women experience intimate partner violence.

      b. Include questions about safety in your assessment.

      c. Resources are sited in Box 9.4 for women identified at risk.

   9. Sexual health

      a. Ask about sexual practices, partner(s) gender.

      b. Ask about history of sexual trauma.

      c. Ask about history of STIs.

      d. Ask about sexual concerns (vaginal dryness, dyspareunia, inorgasmia, changes in libido).

      e. Ask about use of sex toys.

         (1) Ask about shared sex toys with partner(s).

         (2) Ask how they clean and store sex toys.

B. Other age/subpopulation screenings

   1. Osteoporosis

      a. Include dietary assessment of calcium intake and vitamin D.

      b. Ask about family history of osteoporosis.

      c. Ask about prolonged use of Depo-Provera/Mirena, corticosteroids.

      d. Ask about early menopause/surgical menopause.

      e. Order a dual-energy x-ray absorptiometry (DXA) scan as appropriate by presentation and history.

BOX 9.4 *Resources*

- Gay and Lesbian Medical Association: www.glma.org
  http://www.glma.org/_data/n_0001/resources/live/Top%2010%20forlesbians.pdfp
- Top Ten Things Lesbian Women Should Discuss with their Providers (GLMA)
- Domestic Violence Resource: info@thenetworklared.org
  1-800-799-SAFE (7233)
  24 hours in English and Spanish
  TDD: 800-787-3224

---

2. Colorectal cancer screening
   a. Ask about family history.
   b. Ask about anal receptive intercourse with men (risk of HPV associated with development of colorectal cancer).
   c. Offer the national recommended screenings to all women—including fecal occult blood testing and/or colonoscopy screening as appropriate.
   d. Offer a list of community resources for these screenings.

Bibliography

Agenor, M., Krieger, N., Austin, S. B., Haneuse, S., & Gottlieb, B. R. (2013). Sexual orientation disparities in Papnicolau Test among US women: The role of sexual and reproductive health services. *American Journal of Public Health, 16,* e1–e6. doi:10.2105/AJPH2013.30154

Blosnich, J., Foynes, M. M., & Shipherd, J. C. (2013). Health disparities among sexual minority women veterans. *Journal of Women's Health, 22*(7), 631–636.

Breiding, M. J., Chen, J., & Walters, M. L. (2013*). National Intimate Partner and Sexual Violence Survey (NISVS): 2010 findings on victimization by sexual orientation.* Supported by the National Center for Injury Prevention and Control–U.S. Division of Violence Prevention. Retrieved from http://stacks.cdc.gov/view/cdc/12362

Brown, J. P., & Tracy, J. K. (2008). Lesbians and cancer: An overlooked health disparity. *Cancer Causes Control, 19,* 1009–1020.

Douglas-Brown, L. (2013). CDC: Lesbian, gay domestic violence rates same or higher than heterosexuals. *Gay Voice, 11*(3). Retrieved from http:// www.thegavoice.com/news

Eliason, M. J. (2009). *Best practices of lesbian/bisexual women with substance use disorders* (funded report from the State of California Department of Alcohol and Drug Programs Contract No. 07-00135. Lesbian, Gay, Transgendered, Bisexual Treatment and Recovery Improvement, Statewide Technical Improvement Resources. Retrieved from http://gilgerald.com/storage/reserach-papers/09%20 report %20women.pdf

Fredriksen-Golden, K. I., Kim, H. J., Barkan, S. E., Muraco, A., & Hoy-Ellis, C. P. (2013). Health disparities among lesbian, gay, and bisexual older adults: Results from a popular based study. *American Journal of Public Health, 103*(10), 1802–1809. doi:10.2105/AJPH2012.30110. Epub June 2013.

Gruskin, E. P., Hart, S., Gordon, N., & Ackerson, L. (2001). Patterns of cigarette smoking and alcohol use among lesbians and bisexual women enrolled in a large health maintenance organization. *American Journal of Public Health, 91*(6), 976–979.

Hutchinson, M. K., Thompson, A. C., & Cederbaum, J. A. (2006). Multisystem factors contributing to disparities in preventive health care among lesbian women. *Journal of Obstetric, Gynecologic, and Neonatal Nursing, 35*(3), 393–402.

Johns, M. M., Pingels, E. S., Youatt, E. J., Soler, J. H., McClelland, S. I., & Bauermeister, J. A. (2013). LGBT community, social network characteristics, and smoking behaviors in young sexual minority women. *American Journal of Community Psychology, 52*(1-2), 121–154. doi 10.1007/s10464-013-9584-4

McNair, R. P., Hegarty, K., & Taft, A. (2012). From silence to sensitivity: A new Identity Disclosure Model to facilitate disclosure for same-sex attracted women in general practice consultations. *Social Science Medicine, 75*(1), 708–716. doi: 10.1016/j.socscimed.2012.02.037

Morrazzo, J. M., Coffey, P., & Bingham, A. (2005). Sexual practices, risk perception, and knowledge of sexually transmitted disease among lesbian and bisexual women. *Perspectives on Sexual and Reproductive Health, 37*(1), 6–12.

Mosack, K. E., Brouwer, A. M., & Petroll, A. E. (2013). Sexual identity, identity disclosure, and health care experiences: Is there evidence of differential homophobia in primary care practice? *Women's Health Issues, 23*(6), e341–e346. doi 10.1016/j.whi2013.07.004

Polek, C., & Hardie, T. (2010). Lesbian women and knowledge about human papillomavirus. *Oncology Nursing Forum, 37*(3), E191–E197.

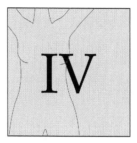

Evaluation of the Menopausal Woman

Assessment of Menopausal Status

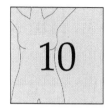

10

Diane Todd Pace and R. Mimi Secor

I. **Menopause explained**
  A. Spontaneous or natural menopause is marked by the end of the reproductive stage of a women's life. It is a period of transition, and for most women is a normal, physiological, and developmental life event often perceived differently across various cultures.
    1. Personal attitudes, lifestyle, and even social and demographic factors may influence one's perception of menopause. Many studies have found that attitudes toward menopause overall are mostly positive or neutral than negative.
    2. This change in reproduction has often been medicalized, and indeed some women have symptoms that affect their quality of life (QOL). It is mainly these women who seek out interventions from their primary care provider. However, in several studies, women experiencing menopause reported no decrease in QOL, and only about 10% of peri- and postmenopausal women reported feelings of despair, irritability, or fatigue during this transition time.
  B. The U.S. Census Bureau estimates that 6,000 women reach menopause every day.
    1. There were estimated to be 52 million postmenopausal women in the United States in 2010, and numbers are rapidly increasing as baby boomers continue to reach midlife and beyond.
    2. Today a woman of age 54 can expect to reach age 84.3 and spend one third of her life in the period known as postmenopause.
  C. A woman's health evaluation around the time of menopause should be similar to her health evaluation throughout her life span. There is no single menopause syndrome, and it is important to stress

individualization with each woman as an important focus when assessing and developing a plan of care. At the time of the initial visit
1. Determine menopausal status.
2. Discuss her view of menopause and her desire for intervention of symptoms affecting her QOL.
3. Counsel on healthy behaviors such as smoking cessation, weight management, and exercise.
4. Discuss health promotion/risk reduction.
5. Consider pharmacological interventions, both hormone therapy/estrogen therapy and nonhormone therapy options for managing symptoms.
6. Discuss nonpharmacological options for managing symptoms.
D. Definition: Menopause is the permanent cessation of menses after 12 consecutive months of amenorrhea, or when follicle stimulating hormone (FSH) levels (greater than 30 mIU or mIU/mL) are consistently elevated in the absence of other obvious pathologic causes.
1. This event usually results from loss of ovarian follicular function due to aging or can be induced by medical intervention, such as surgery (hysterectomy with bilateral oophorectomy), chemotherapy, or radiation.
2. On average, natural menopause occurs around age 51 but may range between 40 to 58 years of age.
3. Menopause-related definitions are summarized in Table 10.1.
E. The menopause transition represents the time when menstrual cycle, endocrine, and central nervous system changes occur.

TABLE 10.1 Menopause-Related Definitions

Perimenopause /Menopause transition	Occurs around menopause, beginning in the early transition, ending 12 months after the final menstrual period (FMP)
Premature menopause	General term used to describe menopause occurring before 40 years of age. It may occur spontaneously or be induced as a result of a medical intervention, such as oophorectomy, chemotherapy, or radiation therapy.
Early menopause	Natural menopause occurring well before the average age, equal to or less than 45 years of age. Includes premature menopause
Menopause	Permanent cessation of menses after 12 consecutive months of amenorrhea, or consistently elevated FSH (greater than or equal to 30 mIU) in absence of other obvious pathologic causes
Postmenopause	From FMP (natural or induced) extending through late menopause ending with death

1. In 2001 a group of scientists from multiple countries and disciplines met to propose nomenclature to stage the reproductive aging cycle in a female's life to the time of menopause (Stages of Reproductive Aging Workshop [STRAW+10]. Model may be viewed in executive summary accessed at http://www. menopause.org/docs/default-document-library/straw10.pdf? sfvrsn=2). In 2010, STRAW+10 reconvened to review the advances in the changes in the hypothalamic–pituitary–ovarian function and update the criteria. In view of the continuing lack of international standardization of biomarker assays for clinical diagnosis, the scientists considered the menstrual cycle criteria to remain the most important criteria for staging.

2. Further delineation of the early postmenopausal years, stages +1a, +1b, +1c, were extended because research indicates FSH levels continue to increase and estradiol levels continue to decrease till approximately 2 years after the final menstrual period (FMP) when levels begin to stabilize. Symptoms, most commonly vasomotor flushes, are reported during these stages.

3. Stage +1c represents a period of stabilization for most women. The usual time frame of the early postmenopause period for most women averages 5 to 8 years.

4. Late postmenopause in which further endocrine changes occur is named stage +2. During this stage the processes of aging such as vaginal dryness and urogenital atrophy are more prevalent.

5. The menopause transition may be further divided into stages according to the nomenclature summarized in Table 10.2.

TABLE 10.2 STRAW+10 Stages of Menopause

−2 Stage = Early perimenopause	Onset of menstrual variability Duration: Variable Menstrual cycle: Variable
−1 Stage = Late perimenopausal transition 0 = Final menstrual period	Significant menstrual variability Duration: 1–3 years Menstrual cycle: Interval of amenorrhea of greater than 60 days Symptoms: Vasomotor symptoms likely
+1a Stage = Early postmenopause	Duration: FMP–1 year Symptoms: Vasomotor symptoms most likely
+1b Stage = Early postmenopause +1c Stage = Early postmenopause	Duration: 1 year Duration: 3–6 years
+2 Stage = Late postmenopause	Remaining life span until death

II. **Physiology of menopause**
   A. The menopause transition, also referred to as perimenopause, is associated with fluctuating hormone secretion causing irregular menstrual cycles and finally permanent cessation of menses.
   B. At birth, women have 1 to 2 million follicles. Accelerated follicular atresia (egg death) occurs in perimenopause and by menopause only a few hundred to a few thousand follicles remain.
   C. A year before the final menstrual period a marked increase in FSH (more than 30 mIU/mL) occurs and plateaus within 2 years of the FMP. This is due to the rapid loss of follicles, resulting in reduced inhibin B, which increases FSH levels.
   D. For a brief period, higher levels of FSH produce more follicles, causing overproduction of estradiol. This may cause a range of perimenopausal symptoms, including irritability, bloating, mastalgia, menorrhagia, growth of fibroids, and endometrial hyperplasia.
   E. Irregular cycles and reduced fertility are associated with the menopause transition. However, it is critical to note and discuss with the woman that pregnancy is possible until menopause occurs (12 months since FMP).
   F. The ovary is the major source of estrogen (during the reproductive years), with reductions occurring in the late menopausal transition, and major reductions in estrogen secretion throughout the first year of postmenopause (first 12 months after FMP). After this, a gradual decline occurs over the following several years.

III. **Menopause introduction and clinical issues**
   A. Women often will present to the clinic requesting baseline and/or intermittent hormone testing to determine whether they are menopausal.
      1. This visit provides an opportune time to discuss the nature of menopause as being a time of gathering a careful history and examining her menstrual and symptom history.
      2. Menopause is actually a diagnosis made by viewing retrospectively for 12 months without consecutive occurrence of menses.
      3. Baseline testing is seldom necessary and unwarranted and is often financially challenging unless the results would truly affect the interventions.
      4. In most cases the interventions can be initiated based on the presentation of symptoms and the desire of the woman following an in-depth history and physical.
   B. Only two major early symptoms are directly attributed to menopause: Change in menstrual cycles and vasomotor symptoms.
      1. Menstrual changes
         a. Variability in increasing flow and frequency leading to amenorrhea is considered the hallmark change of

menopause. Approximately 90% of women will experience this change in menstrual cycle for a period of 4 to 8 years before the FMP.
b. Changes vary from light bleeding, heavy blood loss, increased duration of bleeding, skipped cycles, to no changes until a final cycle.
c. Until menopause is reached, pregnancy can still occur and should be considered during assessment in perimenopausal women not using contraception.
d. Endometrial hyperplasia and carcinoma are more prevalent with age. Any bleeding in a postmenopausal woman always warrants further evaluation.
2. Vasomotor-related symptoms (VMS) is a global term referring to hot flashes, hot flushes, and night sweating.
a. The second most frequently reported symptoms of menopause transition, VMS are experienced by up to 75% of all perimenopausal women in the United States.
b. On average, women experience flashes for 6 months to 2 years, and some up to 5 years. Some studies have shown women report VMS for 10 or more years.
c. Fluctuations in estrogen and progesterone occurring in perimenopause and early menopause are commonly associated with vasomotor symptoms.
d. VMS are thought to result from these fluctuations in estrogen and progesterone, but the precise mechanism and trigger of these symptoms is still not fully understood.
e. Hot flashes are transient, recurrent symptoms of flushing and a sudden sensation of heat usually involving the upper body and face and often followed by chills. Heart rate increases of about 7 to 15 beats per minute occur at approximately the same time. Night sweats occurring during sleep hours are often associated with excessive perspiration, feeling overheated, and disrupted sleep.
f. Frequency of hot flashes varies widely among women, ranging from occurring multiple times an hour, hourly, daily, weekly, or monthly. Within a 24-hour period, the greatest number of hot flashes occurs during the early evening hours. Individual episodes of hot flashes usually range from 1 to 5 minutes.
g. Most hot flashes are mild to moderately severe; however, 10% to 15% of women have severe and/or very frequent hot flashes.
h. Prevalence varies among ethnic and racial groups as follows: African American (46%), Hispanic (35%), White (31%), Chinese (21%), Japanese (18%).

BOX 10.1 *Differential Diagnosis of Vasomotor Symptoms*

- Hyperthyroidism
- Autoimmune disorders
- Cancer
- Hypertension (new onset)
- Cardiovascular disease (new risk)
- Medications such as tamoxifen, raloxifen
- Tuberculosis, infection, lymphoma

---

   i. Surgically induced menopause is associated with potentially severe and frequent VMS. This is due to the sudden drop in estrogen from removal of the ovaries.

   j. Nearly 25% of U.S. women experience significant symptoms and seek intervention from their health care provider.

   k. Available pharmacological/nonpharmacological options offer symptomatic relief. The goal of therapy is to individualize options to the woman's needs after assessment for treatment-related risks and to evaluate her personal attitudes about menopause and treatment options. For women choosing hormone/estrogen therapy as an option, it should be noted that VMS may reoccur or worsen once hormone therapy is stopped.

C. Although VMS are common during menopause, it is important to rule out other medical conditions that may mimic VMS and not be associated with menopause (Box 10.1). Clinical evaluation of VMS should be conducted as a part of the clinical evaluation of the menopausal patient described below.

D. Additional physical and psychological symptoms associated include moodiness, anxiety, headaches, memory changes, sleep disturbances, anxiety and depression, urinary symptoms, dry eyes, vaginal and vulvar irritation, dyspareunia, sexual concerns (i.e., desire, arousal, and orgasm), hair and/or skin changes, weight gain, and joint pain.

E. Potential changes and possible late-onset symptoms include
   1. Vulvovaginal atrophy (see Chapter 12, "Atrophic Vaginitis, Vulvovaginal Atrophy")
   2. Osteoporosis (see Chapter 11, "Osteoporosis and Evaluation of Fracture Risk")

F. Additional differential diagnoses should be considered during the initial assessment because other health issues may resemble menopausal symptoms
   1. Thyroid disorders
   2. Diabetes
   3. Cardiovascular disease

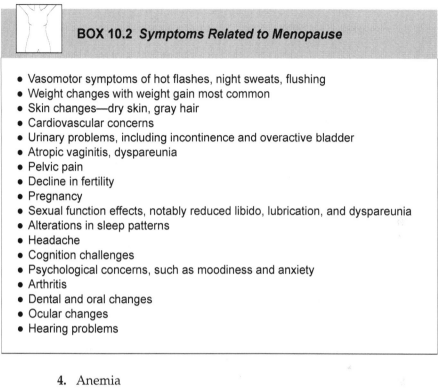

BOX 10.2 *Symptoms Related to Menopause*

- Vasomotor symptoms of hot flashes, night sweats, flushing
- Weight changes with weight gain most common
- Skin changes—dry skin, gray hair
- Cardiovascular concerns
- Urinary problems, including incontinence and overactive bladder
- Atropic vaginitis, dyspareunia
- Pelvic pain
- Decline in fertility
- Pregnancy
- Sexual function effects, notably reduced libido, lubrication, and dyspareunia
- Alterations in sleep patterns
- Headache
- Cognition challenges
- Psychological concerns, such as moodiness and anxiety
- Arthritis
- Dental and oral changes
- Ocular changes
- Hearing problems

4. Anemia
5. Depression
6. Cancer

G. Symptoms and potential concerns that may be addressed during the workup are summarized in Box 10.2.

H. Disease risks, including cancer risks and modifiable risk factors, should be identified by the clinician and addressed with the patient.

IV. **The goal of the clinical health evaluation is to identify menopause and age-related health issues; provide preventive care, anticipatory guidance, education, counseling, and support; and to diagnose and manage health problems.**

A. A comprehensive nine-page menopause health questionnaire to assist clinicians in assessing the menopausal patient is available at the North American Menopause Society (NAMS) website: http://www.menopause.org/edumaterials/questionnare.pdf

B. Regular health examinations are recommended and should include
   1. Comprehensive health, past medical, psychosocial, and family history
   2. Complete physical examination including, vital signs, height, weight, body mass index (BMI), thyroid, breast, pelvic and rectovaginal examinations
   3. Laboratory testing as indicated

      4. Other age- and risk-appropriate tests (bone density, mammogram, skin and colon cancer screening, visual and auditory screening)

C. Comprehensive history

    1. Symptom history

      a. Menopause-related symptoms should be elicited and evaluated regarding frequency, severity, and duration. Also, note any associated symptoms.

      b. Ask detailed questions about symptoms such as vasomotor symptoms of hot flashes, night sweats, flushing, and sleep disturbances.

      c. Other symptoms, both menopause and age related, may include moodiness, anxiety, depression, urinary symptoms, sexual issues such as low libido, dyspareunia, hair/skin changes, weight gain, joint pain, and memory problems.

      d. Ask about patient's management options used till present (i.e., self-care interventions [exercise, yoga, acupuncture], medications, over-the-counter medications, level of coping).

    2. Gynecologic history

      a. Menstrual history, age of menarche, menses pattern over the years, perimenopausal menstrual pattern, last menstrual period (LMP), first menstrual period, abnormal vaginal bleeding, vaginal discharge or pruritus, urinary symptoms

      b. Gynecological issues, including a history of ovarian cysts, polycystic ovarian syndrome (PCOS), fibroids, infertility, endometriosis, premenstrual syndrome (PMS), premenstrual dysphoric disorder (PMDD), sexually transmitted infections (STIs), Pap history, DES (diethylstilbestrol) exposure in pregnancy, and gynecologic surgery

      c. The dates of last breast and Pap exams, and other screening tests, including mammogram, bone density, and most recent lab results

      d. Sexual history

        (1) Sexuality is an important topic to address at midlife, and it is often not a topic initiated by the woman. To obtain a complete sexual history requires the clinician to interact with the woman in a comfortable, nonjudgmental conversation, placing the patient at ease so she can discuss her concerns openly. The sexual history should not assume a heterosexual bias and should be conducted in a supportive, confidential manner. The question could be posed, "Are you currently involved in a sexual relationship and are you having sex with men, women, or both?"

        (2) Include the date of last sexual activity/coitus, number of lifetime sexual partners, history of sexually transmitted infections, complaints of low libido, dyspareunia, history of unprotected sex, orgasm issues.

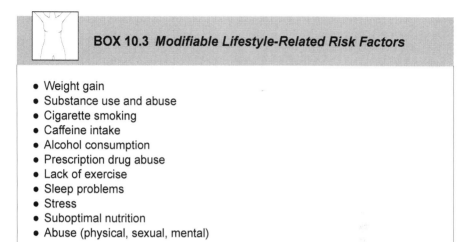

BOX 10.3 *Modifiable Lifestyle-Related Risk Factors*

- Weight gain
- Substance use and abuse
- Cigarette smoking
- Caffeine intake
- Alcohol consumption
- Prescription drug abuse
- Lack of exercise
- Sleep problems
- Stress
- Suboptimal nutrition
- Abuse (physical, sexual, mental)

(3) Inquire whether patient or partner are having any sexual difficulties or concerns about sex they would like to discuss. Preface these questions with information that many women often experience vaginal dryness and changes in sexual desire around the time of menopause.

    e. Contraceptive history: If LMP is less than 12 months ago

      (1) Even though a decline in fertility, varying fluctuations in hormones, and changes in menstrual cycles may diminish the chances for a pregnancy, until menopause has been confirmed by no menstrual periods for 12 consecutive months, an unplanned pregnancy is still possible. Unprotected coitus and current use of contraceptives, duration of use, doses, effectiveness, side effects, and reason for stopping should be discussed. Options to prevent an unintended pregnancy should be investigated.

3. Obstetric history

    a. Number of pregnancies, full-term births, premature babies, abortions, living children, age of first birth, complications during pregnancy or childbirth, current age of children

4. Medical history

    a. Emphasis on cardiovascular disease (CVD), diabetes mellitus (DM), cancer, osteoporosis, and other relevant significant medical conditions, including hospitalizations

    b. Identify modifiable risk factors (Box 10.3) and educate regarding measures to prevent or decrease symptoms of menopause.

    c. Assess for potential risk of developing medical conditions that may be exacerbated during menopause (Box 10.4). Screen where appropriate.

> ### BOX 10.4 *Complications of Menopause*
>
> - Gallbladder disease
> - Cardiovascular conditions such as heart attack or stroke
> - Asthma
> - Cancers of the reproductive tract
> - Sexually transmitted infections
> - Pregnancy/infertility
> - Incapacitating VMS symptoms
> - Diabetes mellitus—metabolic syndrome
> - Adverse effects of traditional and alternative therapies

5. Surgical history
   a. Surgeries and any complications
   b. Hysterectomy; note with ovarian conservation or with oophorectomy
6. Medication history
   a. Current prescription medications (doses, routes, and timing). Discuss patient's adherence. Investigate patient's past use of relative hormones.
   b. Over-the-counter medications, supplements (e.g., black cohosh, ginkgo, soy, yams)
   c. Complementary therapies (acupuncture, yoga, tai chi)
   d. Allergies
7. Psychological history
   a. History of psychotherapy, mental health issues especially depression, anxiety, sleep issues, mood-related conditions, PMS, PMDD, postpartum depression, personality type, coping skills
   b. Developmental challenges include adolescent and/or college-aged children, empty nest, midlife crises, aging parents, retirement, grandchildren, changing spousal relations and roles
   c. Attitude and beliefs about menopause
8. Social history
   a. Occupation, marital status, living situation, financial status, and abuse, including current or past history of verbal, physical, or sexual abuse
   b. Nutritional history
      (1) Calcium, vitamin D, fruit, vegetable, protein, carbohydrate intake, including fiber, junk food, high fat, types of fat, omega-3 fatty acid intake, alcohol, soda, artificial sweeteners, herbal preparations, and vitamins

     c. Lifestyle
        (1) Exercise, sleep, work, recreation, stressors, spirituality, and social network of family and friends

  9. Family history
     a. Age of menopause in female relatives, such as mother, older sisters, and aunts
     b. Osteoporosis, heart disease, cancers (especially history of breast, ovarian, and colon), Alzheimer's disease, coagulopathies, and other significant conditions

10. Review of system update with focus on menopausal health concerns

11. Diagnostic and laboratory testing
     a. As previously discussed, menopause is a clinical diagnosis based on cessation of menses for 12 months (FMP). At present, there is no single test of ovarian function that will predict or confirm menopause. Usually, a woman's medical and menstrual history and symptoms are sufficient to confirm menopause. Serum hormone level testing is not recommended for determining menopausal status.
     b. Laboratory confirmation may be considered if natural menses has been interrupted by hormonal contraceptives.
        (1) FSH is recommended if using hormonal contraceptives that interfere with normal menses. Test day 7 of pill-free interval. If results are unclear, repeat 1 month after discontinuing contraceptive.
        (2) Recommend condom use until lab results are known.
        (3) FSH greater than 30 mIU/mL suggests menopause.
           • Not necessary to diagnose menopause
        (4) Effective contraception should be used for an additional 12 months at which point FSH should be repeated. If still elevated, then contraception may be discontinued and the patient is considered menopausal.
        (5) Estradiol less than 20 pg/mL suggests menopause.
           • Not necessary to diagnose menopause
        (6) Testosterone
           • Indicated if rapidly virilizing symptoms, or suspected tumor, or pathology
           • Not indicated for routine menopausal screening or for low libido
     c. Routine diagnostic tests
        (1) Fasting lipid profile
        (2) Cervical cancer screening/Pap smear (see Chapter 30, "Cervical Cancer Screening")
        (3) Thyroid testing
        (4) Blood glucose

- **(5)** Urine screening
- **(6)** Hepatitis C virus (HCV)
  - **d.** Age and risk-related screenings
    - **(1)** Bone density: Screen for osteoporosis in women age 65 years or older; per the U.S. Preventive Services Task Force (USPSTF), women whose fracture risk is greater than or equal to that of a 65-year-old woman without risk factors (see Chapter 11, "Osteoporosis and Evaluation of Fracture Risk"; see FRAX at http://www.shef.ac.uk/FRAX).
    - **(2)** Mammogram (see Chapter 6, "The Female Breast")
    - **(3)** Skin assessment (see Chapter 5, "Assessment of the Skin")
    - **(4)** Colon cancer screening
    - **(5)** Appropriate cultures or smears with suspicion of infection
    - **(6)** Glaucoma
    - **(7)** Hearing testing
    - **(8)** Immunization update
  - **e.** Other testing as appropriate for the evaluation of health concerns. Endometrial biopsy if irregular menses and heavy bleeding should occur, particularly if it has been more than a year since last menses (see Chapter 33, "Sonohysteroscopy [Fluid Contrast Ultrasound]")
- **D.** Physical examination of the menopausal patient
  1. Height
  2. Weight and BMI (see Chapter 8, "Assessment and Clinical Evaluation of Obesity in Women")
  3. Blood pressure
  4. HEENT (head, eye, ear, nose, and throat)
  5. Lungs
  6. Cardiac/neck for carotids/extremity pulse evaluation
  7. Breast exam
  8. Abdomen
     - **a.** Note tenderness, rebound, and other abnormalities.
  9. Pelvic examination
     - **a.** External genitalia
       - **(1)** Thinning and/or graying of hair, loss of landmarks, tissue pallor, erythema, lesions, fissures, tenderness, urethral caruncle, introital shrinkage or laxity, cystocele, and rectocele
     - **b.** Vagina
       - **(1)** Introital laxity and loss of tone with Kegel and Valsalva maneuver (note cystocele, rectocele, and grade of condition)
       - **(2)** Erythema, pallor, flattening of rugae, abnormal discharge (scant to variable), infection, lesions, shortening of vagina, loss of elasticity, and tenderness.

      c. Cervix
        (1) Erythema, lesions, friability, bleeding, tenderness, flattening, shortening, and stenosis of cervical os (small)
      d. Uterus
        (1) Size, shape, especially asymmetry (associated with fibroids that usually shrink in menopause), diffuse enlargement associated with pregnancy or pathology such as hyperplasia, tenderness, sometimes fibroids, and so forth
      e. Pelvic floor
        (1) Note cystocele, rectocele, introital tone with Kegel and Valsalva maneuver (see Chapter 17, "Pelvic Organ Prolapse").
      f. Ovaries
        (1) In menopause, ovaries should not be palpable.
        (2) If ovaries are palpable a workup is indicated.
  10. Colorectal evaluation
      a. Rectocele, lesions, hemorrhoids, bleeding, tarry stools, guaiac testing
  11. Extremities
      a. Including feet
  12. Skin
      a. Note new or changing lesions
      b. Evaluate yearly, especially with a history of excessive sun exposure.

V. Intervention options
  A. Non-pharmacological options
    1. Although there have been no randomized control studies to validate effectiveness, the following options have been found to be effective in relieving VMS for some women:
      a. Dress in cool layers.
      b. Avoid smoking, which has some effect on estrogen metabolism and increases risk of flushes.
      c. Avoid personal hot-flash triggers (hot drinks, caffeine, spicy foods, ETOH [alcohol], emotional reactions).
      d. Use devices such as cooling pillows (Chillow Pillow®), Bed Fan®, or wicking clothing/pajamas, wicking sheets/pillowcases.
    2. In small, limited studies, exercise, yoga, and acupuncture have shown some improvements in hot flashes and sleep disturbances.
    3. Herbals, such as black cohosh and phytoestrogens, have been found effective for some women in relieving symptoms. Further information may be found at National Center for Complementary and Alternative Medicine (http://nccam.nih.gov/health/menopause).

4. Approximately one third of women will experience vaginal symptoms such as vaginal irritation, dryness, and dyspareunia during menopause often related to the loss of estrogen. Patients can be referred to the NAMS website (http://www .menopause.org) for information on sexuality or to http://www .MiddlesexMD.com for clinician-guided blogs and information and purchase of safe products.

5. Pharmacological options: The decision of which intervention to use is dependent on various factors
   a. Risk/benefit evaluation
   b. Patient preference
   c. Costs of intervention
   d. Side/adverse effects

6. Menopausal hormone therapy is the most effective pharmacological treatment for vasomotor symptoms associated with menopause.

7. Terminology: The term *hormone replacement therapy* is no longer used as appropriate terminology because it is consider a misnomer. The FDA (Food and Drug Administration) declared the word "replacement" can no longer be used by the marketing industry of products in the United States because postmenopausal levels of hormone therapy do not replace premenopausal hormonal levels. The correct terminology for therapies are listed below
   a. HT: Hormone therapy (encompassing both estrogen therapy and combined estrogen–progestogen therapy)
   b. ET: Estrogen therapy only
   c. EPT: Combined estrogen–progestogen therapy
   d. Progestogen: Encompassing both natural progesterone and synthetic progestins

8. A complete list of "Hormone Products for Postmenopausal Use in the United States and Canada" is available for review on the NAMS website (www.menopause.org/docs/professional/ htcharts.pdf?sfvrsn=6), which contains names of products and dosages.

9. Benefits of HT/ET are more likely to outweigh risks for symptomatic women before the age of 60 years or within 10 years after menopause.

10. The option of HT/ET is an individual decision in terms of QOL and health priorities as well as personal risk factors such as age, time since menopause, and the risk of venous thromboembolism, stroke, ischemic heart disease, and breast cancer.

11. Non hormonal pharmacological options, such as antidepressants, antihyperhypertensives, and anticonvulsants, are available for management of vasomotor symptoms although most are not FDA approved for this purpose.

Bibliography

Alexander, I. M., & Andrist, L. C. (2013). Menopause. In K. D. Schuiling & F. E. Likis (Eds.). *Women's gynecologic health* (2nd ed., pp. 285–328). Burlington, MA: Jones & Bartlett Learning.

Ayers, B., Forshaw, M., & Hunter, M. S. (2010). The impact of attitudes towards the menopause on women's symptom experience: A systematic review. *Maturitas, 65,* 28–36.

Centers for Disease Control and Prevention. (n.d.). *Adult immunization schedules—United States, 2013.* Retrieved December 1, 2013, from http://www.cdc.gov/vaccines/schedules/hcp/adult.html

FRAX®. (n.d.). WHO Fracture Risk Assessment Tool: Welcome to FRAX. Retrieved December 1, 2013, from http://www.shef.ac.uk/FRAX

Harlow, S. D., Gass, M. L. S., Hall, J. E., Lobo, R. A., Maki, P., Rebar, R. W., ... de Villiers, T. J. (2012). Executive summary of the stages of reproductive aging workshop + 10: Addressing the unfinished agenda of staging reproductive aging. *Menopause: The Journal of The North American Menopause Society, 19*(4), 387–395.

North American Menopause Society (NAMS). (2010). *Menopause practice: A clinician's guide* (4th ed.). Cleveland. OH: Author.

Stuenkel, C. A., Gass, M. L. S., Manson, J. R., Lobo, R. A., Pal, L., Rebar, R. W., & Hall, J. E. (2012). A decade after the Women's Health Initiative: The experts do agree. *Menopause: The Journal of The North American Menopause Society, 19*(8), 846–847.

Osteoporosis and Evaluation of Fracture Risk

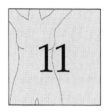

11

R. Mimi Secor, Nancy R. Berman,
Richard Pope, and Cathy R. Kessenich

I. **Scope of the problem**
   A. Osteoporosis is a disease of low bone mass and compromised bone strength that leads to increased risk of fracture.
   B. Low bone mass can be quantified through bone density testing and is reported along a continuum from mild to severe.
   C. Fracture risk is significantly increased when low bone mass reaches the severity of osteoporosis, but the majority of fractures occur in women with mild to moderate low bone density (osteopenia) as there are more women in that range.
   D. Bone density testing will identify women with osteoporosis who should be treated for fracture prevention. This is in accordance with the National Osteoporosis Foundation (NOF) and the World Health Organization (WHO).
   E. Additionally, women will be identified with low bone mass who should also consider preventative therapy for fracture prevention.
   F. Because most women with osteoporosis will not have symptoms, bone densitometry is an attempt to establish some means of recognizing those women who have the potential to develop fractures and those who will not.
   G. Bone mass measurements provide a quantitative value so that a low bone density diagnosis can encourage the patient to modify her lifestyle, diet, and consider the option of approved medications for treatment.
   H. Central dual-energy x-ray absorptiometry (DXA) scanning is the accepted methodology. It is highly reproducible and accepted by multiple organizations, including WHO, NOF, and the American Association of Clinical Endocrinology (AACE).

    I.   Bone mass densitometry (BMD) predicts the risk for fracture even more accurately than hypertension predicts risk for stroke.

    J.   Many clinicians will be treating women with increased fracture risk. It is imperative that they understand the indications for BMD and the implications of treatment.

II. **Osteoporosis explained**

    A. Definition

        1. Osteoporosis is defined as a skeletal disorder characterized by compromised bone strength predisposing a person to increased risk for fracture.

        2. It is a condition of porous bones that is underdiagnosed because it is a silent disease process.

        3. Most serious fractures are those of the hip because they contribute substantially to morbidity rate, mortality rate, and health care costs.

        4. There is an increased risk for osteoporosis with advancing age; it begins at the wrist and progresses to the vertebrae and last to the hip.

        5. Osteoporosis is a generalized disease that affects all skeletal sites.

        6. Osteoporosis as defined by DXA scanning with a T-score of under –2.5; a significant risk for fracture.

        7. Low bone density in and of itself is not a risk for fracture but rather an important marker for potential risk over time.

    B. Related statistics

        1. Osteoporosis causes approximately 2.3 million fractures annually at a cost of more than $23 billion in the United States and Europe.

        2. One in two women over 50 years of age will suffer a fracture secondary to osteoporosis, or nearly 25 million postmenopausal American women are affected.

        3. Seventy-five percent of women between the ages of 45 and 75 years have never talked to their doctor about osteoporosis.

        4. A woman's relative risk for hip fracture is equal to her combined risk for breast, uterine, and ovarian cancers.

        5. Vertebral fractures are the most common (700,000 annually), whereas the occurrence of hip fractures is 300,000 annually.

        6. All races and ethnic groups can be affected, including African Americans, Mexicans, and Asians, in addition to Caucasians.

    C. Guidelines from the NOF and the North American Menopause Society (NAMS) recommend when to initiate bone density testing and how often to repeat this testing. It is prudent to screen women at risk for osteoporosis (Box 11.1).

    D. Some facts related to hip fractures

        1. Equal in number to wrist fractures

        2. More expensive than wrist fractures because of immobility and prolonged hospitalization

> ### BOX 11.1 *Risk Factors for Osteoporosis*
>
> - Dietary and weight-related factors
> - Slight build with loss of body fat
> - High caffeine intake
> - Excessive alcohol consumption
> - Lifetime low intake of dietary calcium (lactose intolerance)
> - Lack of weight gain since age 25
> - Eating disorder
> - Estrogen deficiency
> - Early menopause
> - Nulliparity
> - Family history of osteoporosis, including paternal and maternal hip fracture
> - Present smoking
> - Lack of exercise
> - Inability to rise from a chair without using the armrest for support
> - Immobility
> - Other conditions and medications may also increase risk such as hyperthyroidism or hyperparathyroidism
> - Long-term steroid therapy (prednisone 5 mg or more for greater than 3 months) especially in those women with rheumatoid arthritis or chronic lung disease
> - Heparin treatment
> - Intestinal malabsorption such as gastric bypass surgery, celiac disease, and other conditions
> - Cushing's disease
> - Type 1 diabetes

3. The mortality rate associated with hip fractures is 12% to 20% during the year after injury.
4. Fewer than 50% of patients with a hip fracture ever return to their prefracture level of function.
5. One in seven women experiences osteoporosis-induced hip fractures.

E. Some facts related to vertebral fractures
   1. They are twice as common as hip fractures.
   2. They are less readily diagnosed because up to two thirds are asymptomatic and painless.
   3. Successive fractures lead to a loss in height.
      a. A loss of 1.5 inches is suggestive of osteoporotic spinal fractures.
      b. Figure 11.1 visually shows how fractures can lead to loss of height throughout the life span.

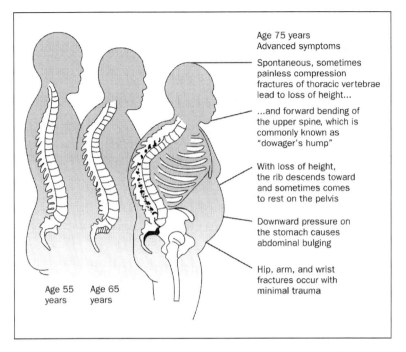

Age 75 years
Advanced symptoms

Spontaneous, sometimes painless compression fractures of thoracic vertebrae lead to loss of height...

...and forward bending of the upper spine, which is commonly known as "dowager's hump"

With loss of height, the rib descends toward and sometimes comes to rest on the pelvis

Downward pressure on the stomach causes abdominal bulging

Hip, arm, and wrist fractures occur with minimal trauma

Age 55 years Age 65 years

FIGURE 11.1 Silent vertebral fractures can lead to loss of height and related symptoms.

III. Measurement of bone density

A. Bone density is measured in grams per square centimeter.

    1. Bone density differs throughout the body due to variations in cortical and trabecular bone distribution

    2. Used to define osteoporosis in terms of standard deviations from the average peak bone mass

    3. *Standard deviation* is a statistical term used to express the average amount by which an individual's bone density varies from the norm.

    4. Values are matched against average bone density for young adult women when bone mass generally is at its peak.

B. Parameters for diagnosis: Both the WHO and NOF categorize a patient's bone density using standard deviation (SD).

    1. The WHO scale

        a. Low risk of osteoporotic fracture: Patients with an SD of 0 to –1.0 below peak bone density is normal.

        b. Greater risk of fracture: Patients with an SD between –1 and –2.5 are diagnosed with osteopenia (low bone mass).

        c. Have osteoporosis: Patients with an SD greater than 2.5 are diagnosed with osteoporosis, even though they have not had a bone fracture.

    d. Using these criteria, the WHO classifies 30% of postmenopausal women in the United States as having osteoporosis.

    e. The WHO and NOF recommend that all individuals who are categorized with osteoporosis should be treated.

  2. NOF scale

    a. An SD of 0 to –1.0 below peak bone density is normal, the same as that used by WHO.

    b. Osteoporosis: –2.5 SD or less than that of a young adult reference population

    c. NOF criteria would classify 45% of postmenopausal women as osteoporotic.

  3. Low BMD at spine, hip, or forearm is sufficient for a diagnosis of osteoporosis.

  4. One SD at the spine or hip increases the risk of fracture approximately twofold.

C. T-score: The report of the BMD when compared to a young adult average in standard deviations. See Table 11.1 for a summary of the SD categories of bone density.

  1. Normal: –1.0 and above

  2. Low bone mass (osteopenia): T-score between –1.0 and –2.5

  3. Osteoporosis: T-score at or below –2.5

  4. Severe or established osteoporosis: T-score at or below –2.5 with one or more fractures

D. Vertebral imaging

  1. Vertebral fracture assay (VFA) can be performed at the same time as BMD on certain machines.

    a. This is a scan of the spine that evaluates vertebral height and has no increase in risk of radiation. Also known as *lateral vertebral assay* (LVA)

    b. If VFA is not available, then a dorsal spine and/or lumbar spine x-ray is helpful to identify compression fractures.

TABLE 11.1 Summary of Bone Density T-Score Categories

DIAGNOSIS	BMD T-SCORE: NUMBER OF SD BELOW MEAN IN HEALTHY YOUNG WOMEN*
Normal	No lower than −1
Osteopenia (low bone mass)	Between −1 and −2.5
Osteoporosis	−2.5 or less
Severe osteoporosis	−2.5 or less with fragility fractures

     c. These tests should be ordered when there is height loss of more than 1.5 inches and can be performed easily at the time of DXA scanning.

E. Diagnosis and therapeutic intervention can be based on this assessment. In addition to BMD testing, vertebral imaging is recommended in individuals with a risk of vertebral fracture.
  1. Individuals at risk for vertebral fracture include
    a. All women age 70 and older
    b. Women age 65 to 69 if BMD T-score is –1.5 or below
    c. Postmenopausal women age 50 to 64 with specific risk factors
      (1) Low trauma fracture
      (2) Historical height loss of 1.5 inches or more (4 cm)
      (3) Recent or ongoing long-term glucocorticoid treatment

IV. The procedure

A. Assess and monitor various disease states and conditions.
  1. Evaluate those women at risk for fracture who are unsure whether to initiate therapy.
  2. Detect osteopenia and assess its severity.
  3. Evaluate patients with metabolic bone disease that affects the skeleton including comorbid conditions associated with risk for fractures. These secondary causes of bone disease include hyperparathyroidism, vitamin D deficiency, and other conditions.
  4. Monitor the effectiveness of prevention or treatment measures for osteoporosis.
  5. Monitor a patient undergoing long-term glucocorticoid therapy.
  6. Evaluate a patient with a hip, radial, or vertebral compression fracture.
  7. Establish baseline BMD for future measurements in those with prior osteoporotic fracture.

B. Contraindications to BMD evaluation
  1. Pregnancy is the only absolute contraindication.
  2. Spinal deformity. Use radius and hip. The diagnosis can be established by testing the wrist. For patients with hyperparathyroidism the wrist is best used for diagnosis and monitoring.
  3. The presence of orthopedic hardware. Use another location away from hardware. Note: BMD results can be affected by the presence of metal objects such as a belt, button, or corset. It also can be affected by the patient's recent ingestion of calcium-containing tablets.

C. Accuracy: Generally good (90%–95%)

D. The DXA scan
1. When BMD is indicated, central DXA is the preferred technique, not peripheral.
2. DXA measures the density of bone at major sites.
   a. Hip
   b. Spine
   c. Forearm
3. Accuracy: Within 3% to 5%
4. Precision: Within 0.5% to 2.0%
5. Best correlation to predict the risk of fractures at the hip
6. Process takes 10 to 15 minutes, with the woman lying on a table while an imager passes over her body.
7. A computer calculates the density of the patient's bones and compares with normal bone at peak mass, as well as the average bone density for the patient's age.
8. Results are expressed in grams per square centimeter in SD of peak value of matched controls.
9. Bones with normal mineralization produce a higher reading in grams per centimeter than does osteoporotic bone.
10. Limitations of the DXA
    a. There is a precision error that is part of the test. Be sure that regular testing of phantoms are performed and the software is up to date. The testing center will be able to provide this information.
    b. Same machine, same location, same technologist are preferred. Measuring patients on different machines and/or different manufacturers can be misleading as error rates are difficult to calculate.
E. Diagnosis at single or multiple bone sites: Controversial
1. Some studies have determined that there is not a great difference in bone density at different sites.
2. Other studies reported that BMD at several sites increased the predictive accuracy.
F. Biochemical tests: Blood and urine tests measure the rate of bone remodeling.
1. These tests indicate a high rate of bone turnover, which may indicate rapid bone loss.
2. Commonly used in research but not in clinical practice except in uncommon instances.

V. Diagnostic assessment
1. NOF diagnostic guidelines for BMD testing
   a. In women age 65 and older and men age 70 and older, recommend bone mineral density testing.

     b. In postmenopausal women and men age 50 to 69, recommend BMD testing based on risk-factor profile.

     c. Recommend BMD testing and vertebral imaging to those who have had a fracture, to determine degree of disease severity.

     d. Note: BMD testing should be performed at DXA facilities using accepted quality assurance.

VI. Lifetime monitoring recommendations

  A. The NOF recommends follow-up intervals for bone density testing.

     1. Perform BMD testing 1 to 2 years after initiating therapy to reduce fracture risk and every 2 years thereafter. More frequent testing may be warranted in certain clinical situations.

     2. Every 2 to 5 years in untreated postmenopausal women

  B. Dietary recommendations (Table 11.2).

  C. Women who are diagnosed with osteoporosis should be treated to prevent fracture.

     1. BMD T-scores greater than –2.5 or worse should be treated.

     2. Guidelines for treatment choices are available from NOF and NAMS.

  D. Preventative therapy may be indicated for women at high risk of fracture who do not have T-scores of –2.5 or worse. Examples include those on long-term steroid therapy, those with rheumatoid arthritis, or other inflammatory arthridities.

    The Fracture Risk Assessment Tool (FRAX) was developed to identify those individuals who would benefit from treatment.

     1. The FRAX tool was developed by the WHO to evaluate the fracture risk for patients.

     2. It is based on individual patient models to integrate the risks associated with clinical risk factors and BMD at the femoral neck.

     3. FRAX is a calculation tool that incorporates patient demographics and the bone density at the femoral neck in a computer calculation.

TABLE 11.2 Daily Recommendations for Dietary Supplements

SUPPLEMENT	AGE (YEARS)	DAILY REQUIREMENTS
Calcium	< 50	1,000 mg
Calcium	> 50	1,200 mg
Vitamin D	< 50	400–800 IU
Vitamin D	> 50	800–1,000 IU

4. FRAX addresses factors such as age, height, weight, family history of hip fractures of either parent, history of previous fracture as an adult, current smoking, glucocorticoid use, and chronic disease, such as rheumatoid arthritis, that contribute to fracture risk. The calculator also provides a list of other medical causes of secondary osteoporosis that are associated with high risk for fracture.
5. FRAX recognizes that the risk of fracture may be greater than the T-score suggests and allows for consideration of initiation of therapy for high-risk individuals.
6. The algorithms give the 10-year probability of fracture.
   a. Recommends that the patient be treated if the risk of major osteoporotic fracture is 20% or greater, even if the BMD is not –2.5 or greater (osteoporosis).
   b. Recommends that the patient be treated if the risk of a hip fracture is 3% or greater, even if the BMD is not –2.5 or greater.
7. The tool is found at http://www.shef.ac.uk/FRAX.

Bibliography

International Society for Clinical Densiometry. (2012). *Osteoporosis screening guidelines.* Retrieved from http://www.iscd.org/publications/osteoflash/osteoporosis-screening-guidelines

National Osteoporosis Foundation. (2013). *Clinician's guide to prevention and treatment of osteoporosis.* Washington, DC: Author. Retrieved from http://nof.org/hcp/clinicians-guide

Nelson, H. D., Haney, E. M., Chou, R., Dana, T., Fu, R., & Bougatsos, C. (2010). Screening for osteoporosis: Systematic review to update the 2002 U.S. Preventive Services Task Force Recommendation. Evidence Synthesis No. 77. *AHRQ Publication No. 10-05145-EF-1.* Rockville, MD: Agency for Healthcare Research and Quality.

North American Menopause Society. (2010a). Management of osteoporosis in postmenopausal women: 2010 position statement of the North American Menopause Society. *Menopause, 17*(1), 25–54. doi: 10.1097/gme.0b013e3181c617e6

North American Menopause Society. (2010b). *Disease risk in menopause practice: A clinician's guide* (4th ed.). Mayfield Heights, OH: Author.

Siris, E., & Delmas, P. D. (2008). Assessment of 10-year absolute fracture risk: A new paradigm with worldwide application. *Osteoporosis International, (19)*4, 383–384. doi: 10.1007/s00198-008-0564-8

Szulc, P., & Delmas, P. D. (2008). Biochemical markers of bone turnover: Potential use in the investigation and management of postmenopausal osteoporosis. *Osteoporosis International, 19*(12), 1683–1704. doi: 10.1007/s00198-008-0660-9

Wagner, E. H., Williams, C. A., Greenberg, R., Kleinbaum, D., Wolf, S. H., & Ibrahim, M. A. (2009). Simply ask them about their balance—Future fracture risk in a national cohort study of twins. *American Journal of Epidemiology, 169,* 143. doi: 10.1093/aje/kwn379

World Health Organization Collaborating Center for Metabolic Bone Diseases. (n.d.).*"FRAX" tool, online.* Retrieved from www.shef.ac.uk/frax

Atrophic Vaginitis, Vulvovaginal Atrophy

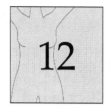

R. Mimi Secor

I. **Atrophic vaginitis explained**
    A. Statistics
        1. Statistics indicate that 45 million women are menopausal and that this number is growing as baby boomers reach menopause and beyond.
        2. Three years after the onset of menopause, almost 50% of women will experience vaginal dryness.
        3. Atrophic vaginitis is also known as vulvovaginal atrophy (VVA) and genital atrophy (GA), which is the new preferred term according to the North American Menopause Society (NAMS). Also referred to as *urogenital atrophy* and *atrophism*.
    B. Some facts
        1. Symptoms of VVA/GA are commonly associated with menopause when estrogen levels drop, causing thinning of the vulvovaginal epithelium.
        2. Urogenital atrophy is the most inevitable consequence of menopause.
        3. Atrophic changes are reversible with estrogen therapy.
        4. Conditions associated with low estrogen are summarized in Box 12.1.

II. **Pathophysiology**
    A. Atrophic urogenital changes can occur during perimenopause, often well in advance of cessation of menses. Vaginal mucosal tissues contain many estrogen receptors that are commonly affected by lower levels of estrogen.

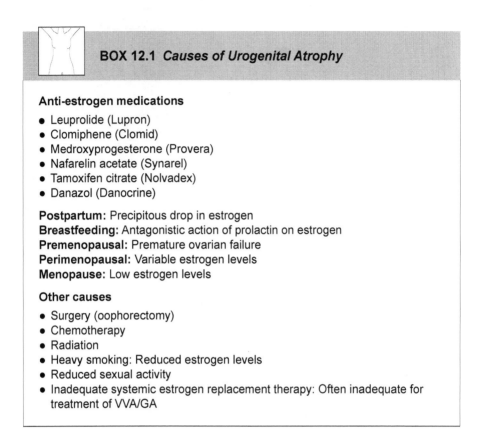

BOX 12.1 *Causes of Urogenital Atrophy*

Anti-estrogen medications
- Leuprolide (Lupron)
- Clomiphene (Clomid)
- Medroxyprogesterone (Provera)
- Nafarelin acetate (Synarel)
- Tamoxifen citrate (Nolvadex)
- Danazol (Danocrine)

Postpartum: Precipitous drop in estrogen
Breastfeeding: Antagonistic action of prolactin on estrogen
Premenopausal: Premature ovarian failure
Perimenopausal: Variable estrogen levels
Menopause: Low estrogen levels

Other causes
- Surgery (oophorectomy)
- Chemotherapy
- Radiation
- Heavy smoking: Reduced estrogen levels
- Reduced sexual activity
- Inadequate systemic estrogen replacement therapy: Often inadequate for treatment of VVA/GA

B. As the vaginal walls become thinner, there is decreased support of the pelvic organs, adjacent muscles, and ligaments.

C. The drop in estrogen causes a decrease in glycogen reducing lactobacilli resulting in an elevation in vaginal pH (from acid to alkaline). This is frequently associated with overgrowth of various pathogenic bacteria such as *Gardnerella vaginalis,* mycoplasma, streptococci, and other bacterial organisms (see Figure 12.1).

D. Reduced estrogen may also result in a reduced blood flow, loss of collagen, elasticity, and muscle tone. Thinning of the urogenital epithelium and/or atrophism leads to various symptoms associated with VVA/GA, including dyspareunia and pruritus.

E. Similar tissue changes may involve the urinary tract contributing to dysuria, incontinence, urinary frequency, and increased risk of urinary tract infections.

F. Symptoms and signs of genitourinary atrophy may develop slowly, over many months or years, or may be of more rapid onset.

G. Symptoms vary and are influenced by factors such as an individual's estrogen levels and response to these levels.

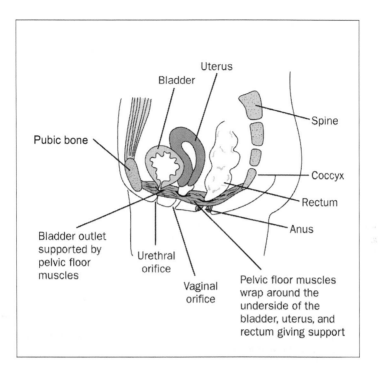

FIGURE 12.1 Side view of bladder and related structures.

III. Indications for evaluation
A. The complaint of urogenital symptoms is an indication for a thorough workup.

IV. Assessment
A. A history of symptoms may include the following
  1. Vulvovaginal symptoms
     a. Vulvar dryness, lack of lubrication, pruritus, irritation, and vaginal discharge
  2. Vaginal bleeding
     a. Due to tissue thinning and friability, vaginal spotting is often a presenting symptom. The source of bleeding must be determined and, if necessary, a biopsy and/or ultrasound should be performed.
     b. Bleeding may be noticed after sex or after wiping with toilet tissue.
  3. Dyspareunia
     a. Also known as painful intercourse, dyspareunia may result from stretching or tearing of the thin, narrowed introital mucosa, or from stretching of the dry, less elastic, thinner, and shorter vagina.

        b. These changes are less likely to occur if sexual relations are maintained during perimenopause and beyond (the "use it or lose it" phenomenon).

    4. Low libido and other sexual complaints, such as lack of lubrication, dyspareunia, and distress, may be associated with atrophic and/or sexual complaints.

    5. Urinary symptoms

        a. The lower urinary tract and pelvic musculature are under the influence of estrogen and share a common embryologic origin with the vagina.

        b. Squamous epithelium of the trigone and urethra becomes thin and blood flow decreases when estrogen levels are low.

        c. Urinary symptoms related to low estrogen levels include dysuria, hematuria, frequency, nocturia, urinary incontinence (usually stress type), sensation of a dropped bladder, and history of frequent urinary tract infections.

    6. Hematuria is commonly associated with atrophism and must be thoroughly evaluated as it can, uncommonly, be a symptom of bladder cancer.

  B. Gynecologic history may include

    1. Menstrual history including last menstrual period (LMP), first menstrual period (FMP), abnormal bleeding, history of hot flashes, night sweats, or flushing

    2. Age of biologic mother or sisters at menopause

    3. Date of last Pap test, results, history of abnormal Pap, and management

    4. Sexual history including dyspareunia, dryness, sexual partner (gender), date of last sex, use of lubricants, distress related to symptoms

    5. Total hysterectomy is often associated with moderate to severe VVA/GA and symptoms may be severe due to the sudden reduction in estrogen levels.

 V. **Medical, surgical, and family history; lifestyle; and medications, including use of over-the-counter preparations. (Box 12.2 summarizes the characteristic symptoms of urogenital atrophy.)**

  A. External genitalia exam

    1. Note thinning of hair and tissues, pallor, erythema, lesions, fissures, loss of architectural landmarks, introital shrinkage, vulvar atrophy, pallor, erythema (diffuse versus focal), and tenderness.

    2. Vulvar dryness and/or positive "sticky glove" sign, which occurs when the examiner's glove adheres temporarily and is thought to be diagnostic for VVA/GA.

BOX 12.2 *Summary of Characteristics of Urogenital Atrophy*

Labia (majora and minora)

- Less prominent, flattened
- Fusion of labia minora
- Lax and wrinkled (lack of subcutaneous fat)
- Thinning cell layer
- Prominent sebaceous glands
- Positive "sticky glove" sign
- Easily traumatized (fissures, erythema, excoriations)
- Irritation due to continuous use of pads for urinary incontinence

Clitoris

- Less prominent
- Retracts beneath the prepuce
- Slight atrophy

Subcutaneous fat

- Diminished

Pubic hair

- Thinning
- Less coarse

Vaginal wall epithelium

- Thin (a few layers thick)
- Friable
- Shiny
- Small ulcerations
- Patches of granulation tissue
- Petechial spots (resemble trichomoniasis)
- Fissures
- Ecchymotic areas from exposed capillaries (mottling appearance)
- Loss of rugae
- Decreased vascularity (pale)
- Less lubrication (dryness)
- Loss of distensibility, elasticity
- Decreased discharge

Vagina

- Introital stenosis (less than two fingers in diameter)
- Shortened
- Shrinkage of fornices
- Less elasticity
- Possible cystocele, rectocele, or pelvic prolapse

(continued)

> **BOX 12.2** *Summary of Characteristics of Urogenital Atrophy (continued)*

Discharge
- Variable quantity and quality
- Watery to thick, white, yellow/green
- May be serosanguineous from friable surfaces

Maturation index
- Predominance of parabasal and basal cells, few superficial cells

Vaginal wet mount/microscopy
- Elevated pH
- Negative amine/KOH (potassium hydroxide) whiff test
- Reduced lactobacilli, increased white blood cells (WBCs), negative for clue cells, trichomoniasis, yeast

Cervix
- Shrinks, flattens into vaginal wall
- Os becomes tiny
- Squamo–columnar junction recedes up the cervical canal
- Atrophied crypts and ducts in canal

Uterus
- Smaller
- Endometrium thins—less glandular, atrophic
- Uterine stripe less than 4 mm
- Fibroids may shrink

Perineum
- Minor fissures or superficial lacerations within the posterior fourchette, perineum

Urethra
- Caruncle—red, berry-type protrusion, often friable
- Atrophy
- Polyps
- Prolapse/eversion of urethral mucosa

Pelvic floor
- Muscle tone diminishes
- Cystocele
- Rectocele

Ligaments and connective tissue
- Lose of strength and tone

Bladder mucosa and urethra
- Decreased tone

   3. Urethral caruncle
      a. Small friable polyp of urethral mucosa that protrudes from the inferior border of the urethral meatus (Figure 12.2)
      b. Associated with symptoms of dysuria, frequency, and may be the cause of vaginal bleeding in the menopausal woman
B. Vaginal exam
   1. Cystocele, rectocele, and grade (see Chapter 17 "Pelvic Organ Prolapse")
   2. Introital laxity, tension, loss of tone with Kegels, and/or Valsalva maneuver
   3. Tenderness with palpation or during speculum insertion and/or exam
   4. Note vaginal pallor, erythema, loss of rugae (flattening), lesions, shortening of vagina, loss of elasticity, tenderness
   5. Discharge: Variable quantity ranging from scant to copious, and variable quality ranging from thin to thick, and varying color from white to yellow/green and possibly malodorous.

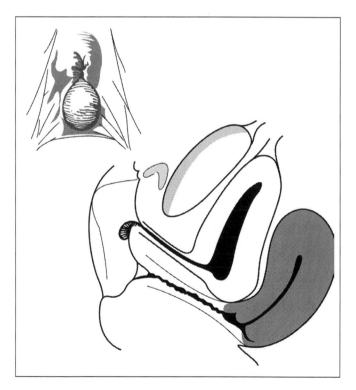

FIGURE 12.2 Small polyp of urethral mucosa in sagittal section and shown protruding from the inferior border of the urethral meatus.

6. Abnormal discharge may mimic trichomoniasis or other sexually transmitted infection (STI), associated discharge
7. Cervix
   a. Erythema, lesions, friability, bleeding, tenderness, flattening and shortening, stenosis of cervical os (small)
C. Bimanual exam
   1. Uterus
      a. Size, shape, especially asymmetry (associated with fibroids that usually shrink in menopause), diffuse enlargement associated with pregnancy or pathology such as hyperplasia, tenderness, sometimes fibroids
   2. Pelvic floor (see Chapter 17 "Pelvic Organ Prolapse")
      a. Note cystocele, rectocele, introital tone with Kegels, and Valsalva maneuver.
   3. Ovaries
      a. In menopause, ovaries should *not* be palpable.
      b. If ovaries are palpable, a timely and thorough workup is indicated.

VI. **Diagnostic testing and differential diagnosis**
   A. Differential considerations (Table 12.1)
      1. Vaginal pH
         a. Atrophic vaginitis is associated with a significantly elevated vaginal pH, usually above 5.
            (1) A normal vaginal pH (4.0 to 4.5) indicates normal circulating estrogen levels and rules out VVA/GA.
            (2) A high pH is due to the lack of lactobacilli, which make lactic acid.
         b. Many factors can alter the vaginal pH results (Box 12.3).
      2. Amine testing with potassium hydroxide (KOH)
         a. If negative, bacterial vaginosis (BV) is unlikely, and VVA/GA must be considered especially if the vaginal pH is also elevated.
      3. Vaginal microscopy (see Chapter 10, "Assessment of Menopausal Status").
         a. Note reduced or absent lactobacilli (LB).
         b. Note immature epithelial cells indicating low estrogen.

TABLE 12.1 Differential Considerations in the Diagnosis of VVA/GA

DIFFERENTIAL	pH	KOH	MICROSCOPY
VVA/GA	≥ 5.0	Negative	Few lactobacilli (LB), WBCs variable, immature epithelial cells (ECs)
Trichomoniasis	> 5.0	Negative	Trichomonads, WBCs, immature ECs, few LB
BV	> 4.7	Positive	Clue cells, few WBCs, few LB

BOX 12.3 *Factors Affecting Vaginal pH*

- Menses (pH 7.2)
- Semen (pH ≥ 7)
- Cervical mucus (pH ≥ 7)
- Lubricant from speculum and/or gloves
- Intravaginal medication
- Tap water

---

    c. Rule out trichomoniasis. If microscopy is equivocal for the identification of *trichomoniasis*, a trich culture or office test (i.e., Affirm or Osom tests) should be done. *Trichomoniasis* may be asymptomatic for decades and reactivate in perimenopause or postmenopause. The clinical presentation may mimic that of VVA/GA.

    d. Rule out genital herpes with herpes select serology immunoglobulin G (IGG) type 2 testing. HSV 2 (herpes simplex virus) may be latent and/or asymptomatic for decades, activating in perimenopause or menopause. Genital HSV 2 is very common, and prevalence increases with age, affecting one out of three women older than age 30. Adding to the diagnostic challenge is that most clinical presentations are atypical, further evading easy diagnosis.

    e. If WBCs are noted, this is most likely related to atrophic effects resulting in secondary vaginal infection, which will resolve when local estrogen is administered and maintained. Initial treatment is daily for 2 to 6 weeks, and then may be tapered to two to three times a week depending on patient response. If symptoms recur, frequency of treatment may need to be increased to daily, and then gradually decreased again after 2 to 6 weeks of daily treatment.

    f. STIs must be ruled out (see Chapter 21, "Sexually Transmitted Infections"), especially if WBCs are noted. STIs are increasing in older adults, so assessing risk is important and should include clinical assessment (history and exam), determining age of sexual partners, use of condoms, and sexual behaviors.

  4. Refer to Chapter 32, "Maturation Index," for more information on performing this diagnostic test.

VII. Treatment considerations

  A. Local estrogen is preferred to systemic estrogen as it is more effective for the treatment of atrophic vaginitis and is thought to be safer due to lower systemic absorption compared to oral administration.

B. Systemic estrogen is not recommended for treatment of atrophic symptoms and if it is given for VMS (vasomotor symptoms) additional local estrogen may be necessary to adequately treat atrophic symptoms.

C. Only the intravaginal estrogen ring "FemRing" is effective for the treatment of both hot flashes and atrophic vaginitis/VVA/GA.

D. Local estrogen therapy begins with daily intravaginal treatment for 2 to 6 weeks then may be tapered to three times weekly then twice a week as needed thereafter.

E. Applying a small pea-sized amount of local estrogen cream to the introital area may relieve dyspareunia. Daily application is recommended initially, then two or three times weekly as needed thereafter.

F. Less effective than estrogen, non-prescription over-the-counter lubricants may help relieve dyspareunia and vaginal dryness.

G. If bacterial vaginosis (BV) is present with atrophic vaginitis/VVA/GA, either local estrogen alone may be used, or BV may be treated initially then followed by treatment with local estrogen. If estrogen has been stopped and BV recurs, local estrogen should be restarted and used daily for 2 to 6 weeks, then twice weekly as maintenance long term to prevent BV. Estrogen supports the regrowth and maintenance of lactobacilli, which is thought to help prevent recurrent BV infections and recurrent VVA/GA.

H. If vulvar skin lesions do not resolve within 6 weeks, a skin biopsy should be considered (see Chapter 32, "Maturation Index").

I. A new nonestrogen, oral selective estrogen receptor modulator (SERM), ospemifene (Osphena) is approved for the treatment of VVA/GA and is similar in efficacy to local estrogen. The dose is 60 mg and is taken orally once a day with food. Absorption is enhanced by fatty foods. The side effect profile is favorable; however, warnings and contraindications contained in the package insert should be reviewed with the patient when considering this new medication.

VIII. Follow-up

A. Follow-up visits may range from 2 weeks to 3 months based on the severity of the patient's problem, response to therapy, and clinician recommendation.

Bibliography

Bachman, G., Bouchard, C., Hoppe, D., Ranganash, R., Altomare, C., Viewag, A., ... Helzner, E. (2009). Efficacy and safety of low-dose regimens of conjugated estrogen cream administered vaginally. *Menopause, 16*(4), 719–727.

Chism, L.A. (2012). Overcoming resistance and barriers to the use of local estrogen therapy for the treatment of vaginal atrophy. *International Journal of Women's Health, 4*, 551–557.

Dorr, M. B., Nelson, A. L., Mayer, P. R., Ranganath, R. P., Norris, P. M., Helzner, E. C., & Preston, R. A. (2010). Plasma estrogen concentrations after oral and vaginal estrogen administration in women with atrophic vaginitis. *Fertility and Sterility, 94*(6), 2365–2367.

Kingsberg, S. A., & Krychman, M. L. (2013). Resistance and barriers to local estrogen therapy in women with atrophic vaginitis. *Journal of Sexual Medicine, 10,* 1567–1574.

Portman, D. J., Bachmann, G. A., Simon, J. A., & Ospemifene Study Group. (2013). Ospemifene, a novel selective estrogen receptor modulator for treating dyspareunia associated with postmenopausal vulvar and vaginal atrophy. *Menopause, 20*(6), 623–630.

Robb-Nicholson, C. (2007). Is vaginal estrogen safe? *Harvard women's health watch* (p. 7). Retrieved November 27, 2013, from http://www.harvard.edu

Rozenberg, S., Vandromme, J., & Antoine, C. (2013). Postmenopausal hormone therapy: Risks and benefits. *National Reviews in Endocrinology, 9,* 216–227. doi:10.1038/ nrendo.2013.17.

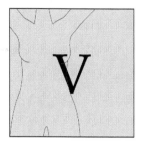

Gynecologic Abnormalities

Assessment of Pelvic Pain

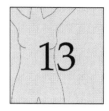

13

Amy M. O'Meara

I. Pelvic pain

   A. Definition

      1. Refers to pain in the region of a woman's internal reproductive organs

      2. Pelvic pain may be a symptom of infection or may arise from pain in the pelvic bone or in nonreproductive internal organs, such as the bladder or colon.

      3. Pelvic pain can very well be an indication that there may be a problem with one of the reproductive organs in the pelvic area (uterus, ovaries, fallopian tubes, cervix, or vagina).

      4. It is important to do a thorough health history and focused physical exam (see Chapter 3, "The Health History," and Chapter 4, "The Physical Examination").

II. Pelvic pain assessment

   A. Symptom review (Box 13.1)

      1. Location of pain

      2. Description of pain: Sharp, dull, throbbing, intermittent, continuous

      3. Does pain radiate?

      4. What activities, if any, make the pain worse?

      5. What measures, if any, relieve the pain?

      6. Any unintentional or recent weight gain or loss?

      7. Rate pain on a scale of 1 to 10, 10 being the worst.

      8. Has similar pain occurred before?

      9. Presence of urinary or gastrointestinal symptoms

         a. Diarrhea or blood in stool or urine

     10. Vaginal bleeding or discharge

     11. Pain with intercourse

     12. Timing in relation to menses, change in character

> **BOX 13.1 Pelvic Pain Assessment: COLDERR**
>
> - Character: What does the pain feel like? (sharp, dull, crampy)
> - Onset: Does the pain come on suddenly or gradually? Is it cyclic or constant?
> - Location: Is the pain localized or diffuse?
> - Duration: How long has the pain been present and how has it changed over time?
> - Exacerbation: What activities or movements make it worse?
> - Relief: What medication, activities, and positions make it better?
> - Radiation: Does the pain radiate anywhere? (back, groin, flank, shoulder)

13. Sexual history
    a. Exposure to sexually transmitted infections
    b. Change in sexual partner
    c. Unprotected intercourse
    d. Change in contraception
    e. Use of sex toys
14. Pelvic surgery in past 12 to 24 months

B. Abdominal assessment
    1. Scars: Indicate previous surgery or injury. Penetration of the peritoneum my result in adhesions (see Section IV. C; Pelvic adhesions).
    2. Bowel sounds: May be altered by paralytic ileus, peritonitis, intestinal obstruction, diarrhea
    3. Percussing
       a. Tympany may suggest intestinal obstruction.
       b. Dullness may suggest enlarged liver or spleen, distended bladder, pregnancy, or tumor.
    4. Palpation
       a. Light palpation: Persistent involuntary muscle spasm with relaxation suggests peritoneal inflammation (acute abdomen).
       b. Deep palpation: Sources of masses include tumors, pregnant uterus, bowel obstruction, abdominal aortic aneurism.
    5. Pain mapping: A process by which the patient and provider identify and document the exact location and intensity of pain. Patients may also do this outside of the office visit if pain is not active at that time.

C. Pelvic examination (see Chapter 4, "The Physical Examination)
    1. Pelvic muscles (see Chapter 17, "Pelvic Organ Prolapse")
    2. Visualize vagina and cervix
    3. Assess uterine size, mobility, cul-de-sac nodularity
    4. Ovaries

D. Cervical motion tenderness (Chandelier sign)
    1. Traditionally associated with pelvic inflammatory disease (PID) May also be seen in

       a. Twenty-eight percent of patients with appendicitis (note, usually limited to right side with appendicitis, and is bilateral with PID)

       b. Ectopic pregnancy

       c. Endometriosis

       d. Ovarian cysts

       e. Degenerating uterine fibroids

       f. Ovarian torsion

  E. Rectal exam

     1. Assess for masses, lesions, tenderness, discharge.

  F. Figure 13.1 shows the pain sites within the abdominal and pelvic cavities.

III. **Acute pelvic pain (APP). Most common type of pelvic pain, often experienced by patients after surgery or other soft tissue traumas. It tends to be immediate, severe, and short lived.**

  A. Pregnancy related

     1. Spontaneous abortion

       a. Inevitable abortion: Cervix is dilated, bleeding, and cramping is typically worse

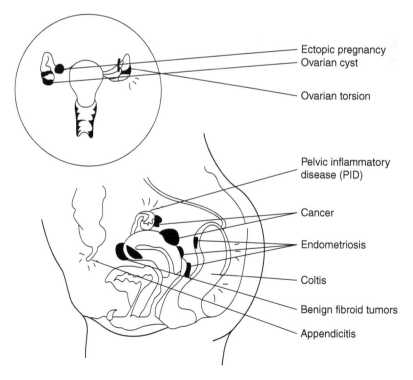

FIGURE 13.1 Pelvic pain sites.

      b. Incomplete abortion: Heavy bleeding and cramping. Passage of products of conception (POC).

      c. Complete abortion: Cramping and bleeding decreased, cervix closes

      d. Missed abortion: Amenorrhea only symptom; no cramping, bleeding, cervical changes

      e. Septic: Abortion with upper genital tract infection

      f. Labs/Imaging: Ultrasound, serial beta hCG, Rh, complete blood count (CBC) as indicated

  2. Ectopic pregnancy

      a. Should *always* be in differential for acute pelvic pain

        (1) Risk factors

- History of PID
- Prior tubal surgery
- Current intrauterine contraception (IUC) use
- Prior ectopic pregnancy
- If patient has had one ectopic, chance of a second is 10% to 20%

      b. Imaging/Labs

        (1) Ultrasound: Gestational sac should be visible by ultrasound at 5.5 weeks and/or beta hCG of 1500 to 2400 mIU/mL.

        (2) Serial beta hCG: Levels should increase by at least 50% every 2 days.

B. Gynecologic, infectious

  1. PID

      a. Treat all women with pelvic or lower abdominal pain who, on exam, have cervical motion tender tenderness *or* uterine tenderness *or* adnexal tenderness.

        (1) Leukocytes in vaginal secretions (most women with PID will have this). Its absence argues strongly against PID.

        (2) Cervical exudates

        (3) Cervical friability

        (4) Temp greater than 101°F (38.3°C)

        (5) Labs:

- Elevated sedimentation rate
- Elevated C-reactive protein
- Gonorrhea and chlamydia

  2. PID indications for hospitalization

      a. Surgical emergency (e.g., appendicitis) cannot be ruled out

      b. Patient is pregnant

      c. Patient does not respond to oral antibiotics

      d. Patient unable to follow or tolerate oral medications

      e. Severe illness with high fever, nausea, vomiting

      f. See Tubo-ovarian abscess, which follows

g. NOTE: Advisability of routine removal of intrauterine device (IUD) with PID has not been established and is not currently recommended practice by the Centers for Disease Control and Prevention (CDC).

3. Tubo-ovarian abscess
   a. Occurs in 15% to 34% of cases of PID
   b. May spread to other structures, such as the bladder
   c. Diagnosis by bimanual, ultrasound, or laparoscopy
   d. Surgical management indicated
4. Endometritis: Pregnancy-related inflammation of endometrium
   a. Occurs post–normal spontaneous vaginal delivery (NSVD) 1% to 3%, post caesarian 13% to 90%
   b. Unlike PID, not associated with infertility or chronic pelvic pain (CPP)
   c. Presentation
      (1) Fever, usually within 36 hours of delivery (100.4+°F) F within 10 days of delivery, 101.6+°F within first 24 postpartum hours
      (2) Uterine tenderness
      (3) Lower abdominal pain
      (4) Foul-smelling lochia
      (5) Abnormal vaginal bleeding and/or discharge
      (6) Malaise
5. Dysmenorrhea
   a. Recurrent, crampy, subrapubic pain during first few days of menses
   b. Typically occurs for the first time within 2 years of menarche
   c. More commonly a cause for chronic pelvic pain than acute pelvic pain
   d. Caused by overproduction of or heightened response to endometrial prostaglandins
   e. Dysmenorrhea after years of pain-free menses suggestive of endometriosis
      (1) Dysmenorrhea treatment
         • Nonsteroidal anti-inflammatory drugs (NSAIDs): 800 mg ibuprofen every 6 hours for up to 2 days. Take with food.
         • Combined oral contraceptives
         • Exercise
      (2) Major causes of secondary dysmenorrhea
         • Endometriosis
         • Adenomyosis
         • PID
         • Adhesions
         • Uterine fibroids
         • Cervical stenosis (stenosis without obstruction is a very rare cause)

- Inflammatory bowel disease
- Irritable bowel syndrome (IBS)
- Psychogenic disorders
- Uterine polyps

6. Uterine fibroids
    a. Most commonly present with pain after age 35
    b. Present in about 20% to 25% of women of reproductive age
        (1) Typically presents as chronic pressure. May be acute pain with fibroid degeneration or torsion of pedunculated fibroid.
        (2) On exam, uterus may feel firm, nontender, irregularly enlarged, textured.
        (3) Ultrasound is diagnostic.

7. Ovarian cysts
    a. Physiologic cysts
        (1) Should not cause pain unless there is rupture, torsion, or hemorrhage. Most physiologic cysts will resolve spontaneously in 1 to 2 months.
    b. Ovarian cysts, rupture
        (1) Release of fluid from a follicular cyst
        (2) Fluid may irritate the peritoneum.
        (3) Pain onset may be sudden and severe, but resolves spontaneously.
    c. Ovarian cysts, hemorrhage
        (1) Rupture of a corpus luteum cyst
        (2) Highly vascular, may lead to severe hemorrhage and pain similar to that of ectopic pregnancy
        (3) May be managed by watchful waiting, or surgery may be indicated

8. Adnexal torsion
    a. Presents as sudden unilateral, colicky, lower abdominal pain. Nausea and vomiting in two thirds of cases.
    b. Enlarged, tender adnexa in 90% of patients
    c. Adnexa twists along utero–ovarian ligament, may involve fallopian tube as well.
    d. Typically proceeded by enlargement of ovary by cyst or neoplasm.

9. Gastrointestinal, acute
    a. Appendicitis
    b. Gastroenteritis
    c. Diverticulosis/diverticulitis
    d. See IBS, Section IV. E (about 49% of chronic pelvic pain as well)
    e. Inflammatory bowel disease
    f. Bowel obstruction
    g. Mesenteric lymphadenitis
    h. Constipation
    i. See Section IV. C; Pelvic adhesions

10. Urinary tract, acute
    a. See Chapter 35, "Urinalysis"
    b. Interstitial cystitis
    c. Pyelonephritis
    d. Nephrolithiasis
       (1) Symptoms
           • Pain of differing degrees that comes and goes in waves
           • Pain with urination
           • Frequent urge to urinate
           • Pink, red, or brown urine
           • Nausea and vomiting
           • Foul smelling, cloudy urine
C. Box 13.2 summarizes the differentials in the diagnosis of acute pelvic pain.

IV. **CPP: To be considered chronic, pelvic pain must last for 6 or more months. Fifteen percent to 20% of women age 18 to 50 have chronic pelvic pain for 1 or more years. Box 13.3 lists those historical factors that increase the risk for CPP.**
A. Endometriosis
   1. The number one leading cause of gynecologic pelvic pain
   2. Occurs in 7% to 10% of women in the United States; 4 out of 1,000 hospitalized annually
   3. The presence of endometrial mucosa implanted in sites other than uterine cavity
   4. The tissue responds to normal hormonal cycling, causing bleeding, an inflammatory response, and so forth
   5. Implants found on ovaries, fallopian tubes, inside and outside bowel, inside and outside urinary bladder, kidney, spleen, nasal mucosa, spinal canal, breast
   6. The amount of ectopic tissue does not appear to have any correlation with severity of symptoms.
   7. Risk factors
      a. Delayed childbearing
      b. Long menses
      c. Short menstrual cycle
      d. Early menarche
      e. Family history (tenfold increased incidence)
      f. Structural defects
      g. Iron deficiency
      h. Because it is estrogen dependent, primarily seen previous to menopause
      i. Seen in 20% to 50% of infertile women

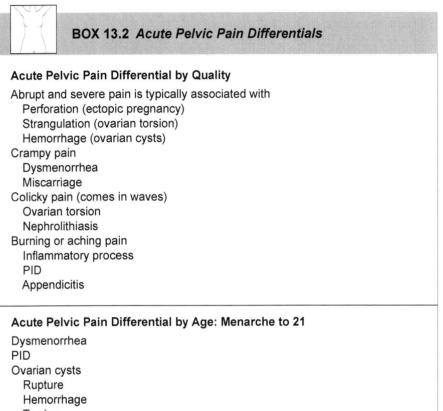

BOX 13.2 *Acute Pelvic Pain Differentials*

Acute Pelvic Pain Differential by Quality

Abrupt and severe pain is typically associated with
  Perforation (ectopic pregnancy)
  Strangulation (ovarian torsion)
  Hemorrhage (ovarian cysts)
Crampy pain
  Dysmenorrhea
  Miscarriage
Colicky pain (comes in waves)
  Ovarian torsion
  Nephrolithiasis
Burning or aching pain
  Inflammatory process
  PID
  Appendicitis

Acute Pelvic Pain Differential by Age: Menarche to 21

Dysmenorrhea
PID
Ovarian cysts
  Rupture
  Hemorrhage
  Torsion
Pregnancy
  Miscarriage
  Ectopic pregnancy
Appendicitis
IBS

Acute Pelvic Pain Differential by Age: 21 to 35

Ovarian cysts
  Hemorrhage
  Torsion
  Rupture
Endometriosis
Pregnancy
  Miscarriage
  Ectopic pregnancy
PID
IBS

(continued)

BOX 13.2 *Acute Pelvic Pain Differentials* (continued)

Acute Pelvic Pain Differential by Age: 35 to Menopause

Uterine fibroids
Endometriosis
Ovarian tumor benign or malignant
Pregnancy
   Miscarriage
   Ectopic pregnancy
Nephrolithiasis
IBS
Diverticulitis
Hernias
PID

Acute Pelvic Pain Differential by Onset: Seconds to Minutes

Ovarian cysts
   Rupture
   Hemorrhage
   Torsion
Tubo–ovarian abscess
Abdominal aortic aneurysm
Ectopic pregnancy
Aortic dissection
Nephrolithiasis
Appendicitis

Acute Pelvic Pain Differential by Onset: Hours to Days

Diverticulitis
Herpes zoster
Gastroenteritis
Mittelschmertz
Primary dysmenorrhea
Miscarriage

Acute Pelvic Pain Differential by Onset: Days to Weeks

Neoplasms
Cystitis
Pyelonephritis
Ectopic pregnancy
PID
Diverticulitis
Miscarriage
Abdominal aortic aneurysm

(continued)

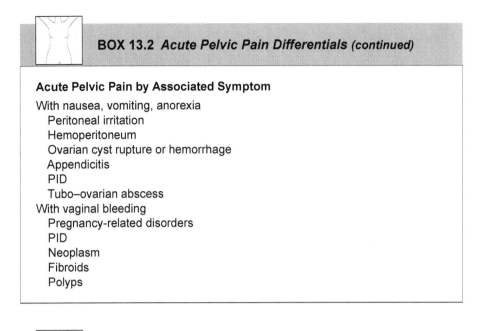

BOX 13.2 *Acute Pelvic Pain Differentials (continued)*

Acute Pelvic Pain by Associated Symptom
With nausea, vomiting, anorexia
    Peritoneal irritation
    Hemoperitoneum
    Ovarian cyst rupture or hemorrhage
    Appendicitis
    PID
    Tubo–ovarian abscess
With vaginal bleeding
    Pregnancy-related disorders
    PID
    Neoplasm
    Fibroids
    Polyps

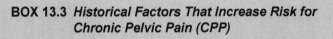

BOX 13.3 *Historical Factors That Increase Risk for Chronic Pelvic Pain (CPP)*

- **Physical or sexual abuse** (40%–50% of women with CPP have a history)
- **PID** (18%–35% of women with PID will develop CPP)
- **Endometriosis** (seen laparoscopically in 33% of women with CPP)
- **Interstitial cystitis (IC)** (38%–85% of women with CPP may have IC)
- **IBS** (symptoms seen in 50%–80% of CPP)

    j. Occurrence may be as high as 80% of women with chronic pelvic pain
    k. Endometriosis found in 20% to 50% of asymptomatic women
  8. Symptoms
    a. New onset dysmenorrhea
    b. Dyspareunia
    c. Pain with urination and bowel movements
  9. Endometriosis, exam
    a. Fixed, retroverted uterus
    b. Nodularity and/or tenderness in the cul-de-sac and uterosacral ligaments
    c. Ovarian enlargement
      (1) Surgery diagnostic

B. Adenomyosis: Endometrial tissue within the myometrium
   1. Most often asymptomatic
   2. Average onset 40 years of age
   3. Increased parity may be a risk factor.
   4. May cause: Long heavy periods, dyspareunia, dyschezia, dysmenorrhea
      a. Uterus diffusely enlarged, soft, tender during menses; movement of uterus not restricted
C. Pelvic adhesions
   1. Webs of intra-abdominal scar tissue
   2. Most often have history of previous pelvic surgery or injury
   3. Noncyclic pain may be increased with intercourse or activity.
   4. Chronic pain may be related to restriction of bowel mobility, distention, and even bowel obstruction.
      a. Treatment: Surgical lysis of adhesions
D. Pelvic congestion
   1. Varicosities of pelvic veins
   2. Signs and symptoms
      a. Bilateral abdominal and back pain, secondary dysmenor-rhea, dyspareunia, chronic fatigue, IBS
      b. Uterus may be bulky, and ovaries enlarged with multiple cysts
      c. Tenderness of pelvic ligaments
      d. Labs/imaging: Trans-uterine venography, pelvic ultrasound, MRI, laparoscopy
E. IBS
   1. Accounts for 60% of referrals for pelvic pain
   2. 35% of people with IBS have chronic pelvic pain
   3. Diagnosis (Box 13.4)
   4. IBS treatment
      a. High placebo response rates
      b. Reassurance
      c. Education
      d. Stress reduction
      e. Bulk-forming agents
      f. Tricyclic antidepressants
      g. Elimination of food triggers (i.e., caffeine, lactose, sorbitol, alcohol, fat, fructose)
      h. Short-term antispasmodics
      i. Probiotics
G. Interstitial cystitis/painful bladder syndrome (IC/PBS)
   1. Number one GU (genital/urinary) cause of chronic pelvic pain
   2. There are currently no biological markers for use in diagnosis. The diagnosis remains one of exclusion.

BOX 13.4 *Diagnosis for IBS*

Rome Criteria for IBS
- Recurrent abdominal pain or discomfort* at least 3 days/month in the last 3 months. Associated with two or more of the following:
  - Improvement with defecation
  - Onset associated with a change in frequency of stool
  - Onset associated with a change in form (appearance) of stool
  - Criteria must be fulfilled for the prior 3 months with symptom onset at least 6 months prior to diagnosis.

Interstitial cystitis clinical management principles (American Urological Association, 2010)
- Treatments must be from most to least conservative; surgery is the last intervention.
- Initial treatment depends on severity of symptoms, patient preference, and clinical judgment.
- Multiple treatments may be offered concurrently.
- Ineffective treatments should be stopped.
- Pain management should be implemented throughout therapy while minimizing side effects.
- Diagnosis should be reconsidered if no improvement is noted.

*Discomfort means an uncomfortable sensation not described as pain.

---

3. Symptoms commonly start in a woman's 30s and may not be diagnosed until her 40s.
4. Associated with remissions and exacerbations. May spontaneously disappear in 9 months (50%).
5. Symptoms
   a. Pelvic pain, pressure, or discomfort related to the bladder, typically associated with a persistent urge to void or urinary frequency, in the absence of infection or other pathology
      (1) Urinary frequency is usually more than eight times the normal rate
      (2) Nocturia
   b. Present for more than 6 weeks
   c. Pain often increases with bladder filling; may diminish during voiding.
   d. Worse before or during menstruation
   e. Flares with intercourse, either during or 1 to 2 days after
   f. Women with IC also may suffer from seasonal allergies.
   g. Palpable bladder tenderness

6. Etiology
   a. Abnormal bladder epithelial permeability ("leaky bladder theory")
   b. Neurogenic abnormalities
   c. Inflammatory process—mast cells released
   d. Autoimmune disorders
7. Rule out labs and procedures as indicated
   a. Urinalysis, culture—usually negative
   b. Urine cytology, particularly in the presence of hematuria and smoking to rule out bladder cancer
   c. Post void residual—capacity is usually less than 350 cc's
      (1) Imaging
      (2) Simple cystometrogram (CMG) (see Chapter 36, "The Simple Cystometrogram") to rule out overactive bladder
      (3) Vaginal and cervical culture to rule out PID, herpes
      (4) Potassium sensitivity test
      (5) Cystoscopy to assess for Huhner's ulcers (present 10% of the time) and rule out bladder cancer

Bibliography

American Urological Association Education and Research, Inc. (2010). Interstitial cystitis treatment algorithm.

Bickley, L. (2011). *Bates' guide to physical examination and history-taking.* New York, NY: Lippincott Williams & Wilkins.

Centers for Disease Control and Prevention. (2010). *Morbidity and mortality weekly report.* Atlanta, GA: U.S. Department of Health and Human Services.

Chandrashekar, K. B., Fulop, T., & Juncos, L. A. (2012). Medical management and prevention of nephrolithiasis. *The American Journal of Medicine, 344–347.*

Dalrymple, J., & Bullock, I. (2008). Diagnosis and management of irritable bowel syndrome in adults in primary care: Summary of NICE Guidance. *British Medical Journal,* 586–558.

Drossman, D. A. (2006). The functional gastrointestinal disorders and the Rome III process. *Gastroenterology,* 1377–1390.

Falcone, T., & Lebovic, D. I. (2011). Clinical management of endometriosis. *Obstetrics and Gynecology, 118*(3), 691–705.

Hawkins, J. W., Roberto-Nichols, D. M., & Stanley-Haney, J. L. (2011). *Guidelines for nurse practitioners in gynecologic settings* (10th ed.). New York, NY: Springer Publishing Company.

Levine, D., Brown, D., Andreotti, R., Benacerraf, B., Brewster, W., Coleman, B., … Smith-Bindman R. (2010). Management of asymptomatic ovarian and other adnexal cysts imaged at U.S. Society of Radiologists in Ultrasound Consensus Conference Statement. *Radiology, 256*(3), 943–954.

Mao, A. J., & Anastasi, J. K. (2010). Diagnosis and management of endometriosis: The rose of the advanced practice nurse in primary care. *Journal of the American Academy of Nurse Practitioners,* 109–116.

Roberts, S. C., Hodgkiss, C., DiBenedtto, A., & Lee, E. C. (2012). Managing dysmenorrhea in young women. *The Nurse Practitioner, 37*(7), 47–52.

Schuiling, K. D., & Likis, F. E. (2011). *Women's gynecologic health* (2nd ed.). Burlington, MA: Jones & Bartlett.

Scott, J. R., Gibbs, R. S., Karlan, B. Y., & Haney, A. F. (2003). *Danforth's obstetrics and gynecology* (9th ed.). Philadelphia, PA: Lippincott, Williams & Wilkins.

Varney, H., Kriebs, J. M., & Gegor, C. L. (2003). *Varney's midwifery* (3rd ed.). Burlington, MA: Jones & Bartlett.

Zenilman, J. M., & Shahmanesh, M. (2011). *Sexually transmitted infections: Diagnosis, management, and treatment.* Burlington, MA: Jones & Bartlett.

Assessment of Vulvar Pain and Vulvodynia

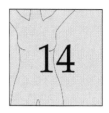

14

Deborah A. Lipkin

I. **Vulvar pain**
   A. In the late 1880s, Skene identified "excessive sensitivity" of the vulva, but it was not until the early 1980s that vulvar pain was covered in the literature. Vulvar pain was officially recognized by the International Society for the Study of Vulvovaginal Disease (ISSVD) in 1976. The term "burning vulva syndrome" was used.
   1. The ISSVD, in 2003, divided vulvar pain into two major groups
      a. Vulvar pain related to a specific disorder
      b. Vulvar pain in the absence of relevant visible finding or clinically identifiable disease. This is termed "vulvodynia," and can be further divided into the categories of provoked, unprovoked, or mixed vulvodynia.
   2. Many vulvar conditions can cause soreness, rawness, irritation, and burning.
   3. It is important to recognize that these conditions can be debilitating, physically, but also emotionally. They can have an enormous impact on functioning in everyday activities, as well as psychosexual functioning.
   4. The most successful treatment involves a multimodal approach of one or all of the following: medical management of identifiable underlying conditions, management of pain, psychological support, sexual therapy, and physical therapy.
   B. Demographics
   1. A 2003 study revealed that 1,280 (16%) of 8,000 women 18 to 64 years of age reported a history of chronic burning, knife-like pain, or pain on contact, with or without itching, that lasted for at least 3 months or more.
   2. Incidence may be much higher. Women are reluctant to disclose their symptoms because of embarrassment, shame, lack of

response from multiple clinicians, or well-meaning clinicians who do not have the knowledge to manage or correctly assess these conditions or who diagnose by phone. One study showed that 39% of women who suffer from vulvar symptoms do not seek treatment.

C. Classification

1. In 2003, the World Congress of the ISSVD revised the classification of vulvar pain disorders. This has remained unchanged.
2. There are two major divisions
   a. Pain with a known cause
      (1) Infectious
      (2) Inflammatory
      (3) Neoplastic
      (4) Neurologic
   b. Pain without a underlying, recognizable disease
3. In either case, pain might occur spontaneously or develop as a result of physiologic provocation. Further classification of vulvodynia recognizes generalized pain and local pain, both of which may be provoked, unprovoked, or mixed.

D. Presentation

1. Pain may range from mild to severe and debilitating; it may be chronic, intermittent, provoked, or unprovoked.
2. It may involve other systems; that is, the urinary tract or the bowel.
3. Pain may be described as sharp, burning, shooting, lancinating, or aching.
4. Mild to severe itching may be present.
5. Symptoms may be associated with position (sitting, standing).
6. Irritants may be problematic, including certain types of fabric (e.g., "Lycra"), personal hygiene products, or laundry detergent.
7. Sexually related symptoms are common and include pain to touch and/or penetration.
8. Discharge and/or odor may be present. Complaints of one or both are common, often despite normal wet prep and potassium hydroxide (KOH).
9. Pelvic floor dysfunction (PFD).
   a. Many women with vulvar pain are likely to have contractile characteristics of the pelvic floor musculature. Occasionally, this is the initial source of pain, but more often it is a secondary source of pain. It is common for women to have no awareness of the tension held within the pelvic floor; they can contract their muscles when asked to "Kegel," but they are unable to release or "drop down" the muscles of the pelvic floor.

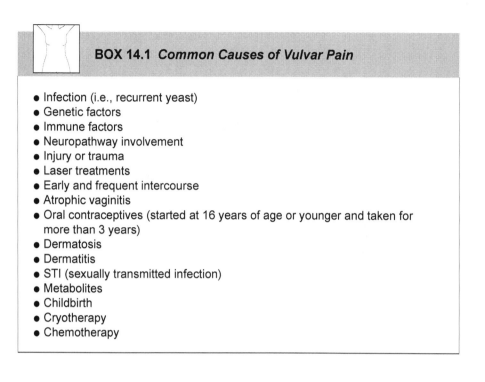

BOX 14.1 *Common Causes of Vulvar Pain*

- Infection (i.e., recurrent yeast)
- Genetic factors
- Immune factors
- Neuropathway involvement
- Injury or trauma
- Laser treatments
- Early and frequent intercourse
- Atrophic vaginitis
- Oral contraceptives (started at 16 years of age or younger and taken for more than 3 years)
- Dermatosis
- Dermatitis
- STI (sexually transmitted infection)
- Metabolites
- Childbirth
- Cryotherapy
- Chemotherapy

    b. Symptoms of PFD include pinching, burning, or aching.
E. Box 14.1 summarizes causes of vulvar pain.
F. What causes the sensation of pain? It may be explained by the following:
    1. Pain is a complex mechanism that may be caused by stimulation of nerve endings, nonmylenated sensory nerve fibers (type C nerve fibers) being responsible for sensations of itching and light pain. Myelinated sensory nerve fibers (type A nerve fibers) are responsible for sensations of deep pain, pressure, and warmth.
    2. Increased numbers of intraepithelial nerve fibers, causing the thresholds for temperature and pain to be lowered, increasing blood flow and erythema
    3. Increased inflammatory substances in the vulvar tissue
    4. Immunologic changes
    5. Genetic susceptibility
    6. Localized vulvodynia: May be due to nociceptors (C-nerve fibers) or neuropathic pain.
        a. Trauma or chronic inflammation of C-nerve fibers may cause the inflammatory cytokines that surround them to fire repeatedly.

BOX 14.2 *Examples of Common Complaints*

"My yearly Pap smear is very painful; please use your smallest speculum."
"I can't use tampons because they hurt too much."
"I cannot have sex anymore" or "my partner is too big."
"It feels like sandpaper."
"I am always aware of my vagina or vulva."
"I have a disgruntled vagina."
"I'm scratching all night long."
"I've had yeast infections/bacterial vaginosis for years."
"It hurts to wear jeans."
Or worse, "My doctor told me to drink more wine—this is all in my head."

---

    b. Mechanoreceptors develop allodynia (pain elicited by nonpainful stimuli) secondary to central sensitization. Neuropathic pain is caused by injury to the sensory nervous system itself.
  7. PFD: Many women with vulvar pain show pelvic floor abnormalities that may be the cause of pain or may worsen existing pain.

II. Assessment of a woman with vulvar pain
  A. History: The patient history may be the most critical piece of the diagnostic tool kit.
    1. A patient with vulvar pain presents with some of the symptoms listed in Box 14.2.
    2. What triggers symptoms? May be provoked or unprovoked, may be constant or associated with intercourse or touch, tight clothing, orgasm.
      a. Was onset gradual or was there one precipitating event?
      b. How long have the symptoms been present and are they constant/intermittent/cyclic?
      c. What are the characteristics of the symptoms? Descriptions might include itching, soreness, sharp, stabbing, prickly, raw, irritated, burning, throbbing.
      d. Is the location general or very specific? In other words, is the pain located over the whole vulva; only at the introitus, anus, or perineum; or elsewhere?
      e. Are there associated skin symptoms, such as bumps, rash, cracks, splitting/fissuring?
      f. Are there associated vaginal symptoms, such as discharge or bleeding?

      g. Which other systems have associated symptoms in particular, urinary tract, bowel, dermatologic, or other gynecologic complaints?

      h. Use of a pain scale will be helpful, especially for reassessment after treatment.

      i. What treatment methods have been tried? What helps? What makes it worse?

  3. Gynecologic history

      a. Gravida/para, types of deliveries, breastfeeding within the last 6 months

      b. Menstrual history

      c. Contraception

      d. Menopausal symptoms

      e. History of abnormal Pap smear

      f. History of sexually transmitted infections

      g. Sexual history, current partner, duration of time with current partner

      h. History of yeast or bacterial vaginosis

      i. Genital injury or trauma

      j. Orgasm: Is the client able to achieve orgasm? Has she ever achieved an orgasm?

      k. History of gynecologic surgery, including urogynecological repairs

  4. Review of systems may reveal a constellation of other, related disorders or autoimmune dysfunction.

      a. Urinary symptoms, especially frequency, urgency, bladder pain

      b. Gastrointestinal symptoms, especially constipation

      c. Dermatologic symptoms

      d. Musculoskeletal symptoms, including back pain

      e. Psychological symptoms, including anxiety related to vulvar symptoms, depression, loss of sleep, and so on

      f. Family history of vulvovaginal symptoms or disorders

  5. Medications: A number of medications may cause vulvar lichenoid processes or fixed medication eruption.

  6. Allergies

  7. Past medical and surgical history

B. Examination

  1. Non-genital exam: General appearance, stature, weight, posture, mouth (looking for ulcers, Wickham's striae, cold sores), skin, nails, thyroid, abdomen, groin, and thighs

  2. Examination of the external pelvic and vulvar structures, beginning anteriorly (closest to abdomen) and progessing posteriorly (toward the anus). *Proceed with gentleness, respect, and caution.* If the patient is unable to tolerate any portion of the exam, consider relaxation techniques, pelvic floor therapy, psychopharmacology consult, cognitive behavioral therapy.

    a. Mons pubis: Note hair distribution and any fissuring or cracking of the skin, especially at the natal cleft.

    b. Labia majora: Note hair distribution, skin changes.
        (1) Skin pigmentation: Observe for whitening, darkening, erythema.
        (2) Lesions: Ulcers, fissures, elevated dark lesions, excoriation, thickened areas (lichenification)

    c. Labia minora
        (1) Architectural changes: Note any agglutination or scarring. Do the labia minora extend fully to the perineum or are they flattened posteriorly? Vulvar dermatoses, such as lichen planus and lichen sclerosus, may cause scarring and/or resorption of the labia minora.
        (2) Pigmentation: Observe for whitening, darkening, erythema.
        (3) Lesions: Ulcers, fissures, elevated dark lesions, excoriation, thickened areas (lichenification)

    d. Clitoris: Does the clitoral hood retract easily over the clitoris? Are the clitoral hood and clitoris scarred? Are they obliterated? Lichen planus and lichen sclerosus both can cause scarring and resorption.

    e. Vestibule
        (1) Pigmentation
        (2) Texture: Is the skin supple, smooth, shiny, tissue-papery?
        (3) Tenderness: Cotton swab exam may produce allodynia, pain elicited by a stimulus that is not normally painful, and/or hyperpathia, when a stimulus causes greater pain than is expected.
        (4) Scarring, or changes in architecture

    f. Perineum: As above, examine for color, texture, and lesions.

    g. Anus: As above, examine for color, texture, and lesions.

3. Examination of the vagina: Use of a virginal speculum is preferred.

    a. Assess discharge color, consistency, and odor.
        (1) Yeast may present as white, thick discharge.
        (2) Bacterial vaginosis discharge may be off-white or gray with a fishy odor. It never causes vaginal mucosal inflammation.
        (3) Inflammatory conditions of the vagina may cause yellow discharge with a sour odor.

    b. Vaginal walls may be a normal pink, pale, or may be inflamed. There may be telescoping or strictures noted during bimanual examination.

    c. Texture of vaginal walls: Supple versus smooth?

    d. Note unusual fissures, lacy patterns, or lesions.

     e. Vaginal tone: Hypertonicity can be noted during speculum and manual examination; however, during manual examination, specific tender spots may be identified.
       (1) It may also be possible to assess involuntary pelvic floor spasms.
       (2) Use caution with evaluation of Kegel; Women with PFD may have difficulty returning to resting tone, resulting in increased pain.
     f. Wet mount, KOH, and pH
       (1) Inflammatory conditions may be assessed with use of microscopy and pH, as they will often present with elevated pH, an increased number of white blood cells, and presence of immature epithelial cells.
       (2) These conditions include vaginal atrophy, desquamative inflammatory vaginitis, lichen planus, and *trichomonas*. Yeast typically presents with a normal pH; however, *yeast is often* not observed by microscopy. Bacterial vaginosis will present with elevated pH and clue cells will be noted by microscope (see Chapter 31, "Vaginal Microscopy").
     g. Yeast culture: Yeast is only observed 30% to 40% of the time by wet mount; therefore, a culture is imperative; it will also speciate, which will guide treatment.
     h. Vulvar biopsy: Biopsy to confirm dermatoses diagnosis and rule out vulvar cancer (see Chapter 39, "Vulvar Cancer and Biopsy").

III. Differential diagnoses: The following list is by no means complete. These are some of the more common disorders. Referral to a vulvovaginal specialist may be necessary.
  A. Vulvodynia: A spontaneous, generalized vulvar pain disorder, which may or may not involve dyspareunia. The pain has no known cause and has lasted for more than 3 months.
    1. Pain may be generalized and provoked, unprovoked, or mixed.
    2. Pain may be localized (for example, the vestibule or clitoris) and provoked, unprovoked, or mixed.
  B. Yeast
  C. Herpes
  D. *Trichomonas*
  E. Inflammatory conditions
    1. Lichen sclerosus: This condition is 10 times more prevalent in women than in men, is often associated with other autoimmune disorders, runs in families, and can occur any time in life.
      a. Lesions can be present on back/shoulders/wrists.
      b. There is a 4% to 5% associated risk for squamous cell carcinoma.

    c. Typical presentation includes itching and the classic whitening (often in the classic "keyhole pattern," surrounding the vulva and anus), dry, tissue-paper appearance; however, it can be more subtle. Excoriations, fissures and lichenification can be observed in women who have been scratching.

    d. Agglutination, a type of scarring, can occur and will present as flattening of labia minora, appearance of synechiae or fusion of minora, clitoris, or other structures.

    e. Diagnosis can be confirmed by biopsy

2. Lichen planus: Vulvar appearance can be reticular or lacy, with Wickham's striae (a reticular, lacy pattern) or erosive (intensely bright red, tender mucosa, typically well demarcated).

    a. Similar to lichen sclerosus, this condition is also present elsewhere on the body.

    b. Diagnosed can be confirmed by biopsy

3. Lichen simplex chronicus: Known as the "itch that rashes" with worsening of symptoms resulting from "itch-scratch-itch" cycling

    a. Skin may appear thickened, but there may also be excoriations and/or fissuring.

    b. Watch for superimposed infection.

    c. Patients may report worsening symptoms with heat, humidity, and irritants.

4. Desquamative inflammatory vaginitis (DIV); also known as lichenoid vaginitis: This is a vaginal inflammatory condition presenting with profuse, yellow, vaginal discharge.

    a. Wet mount will reveal many white blood cells and parabasal cells.

    b. Discharge may or may not be irritating.

    c. DIV may be on a continuum with vaginal lichen planus.

5. Atrophic vaginitis: Lack of estrogen may cause an inflammatory condition.

    a. Presentation may include elevated pH, profuse, yellow discharge; wet mount may reveal many white blood cells and parabasal cells.

    b. This condition is seen in postmenopausal women but also women using medroxyprogesterone (Depo-Provera), breastfeeding mothers, women being treated with gonadotropin-releasing hormone agonists, and, occasionally, oral contraceptive users.

    c. Atrophic vaginitis cannot be distinguished from DIV or inflammatory vaginal conditions either clinically or microscopically.

6. Irritant/contact dermatitis: A response to any exogenous substance
   a. Affected area may appear erythematous with poorly demarcated slightly elevated plaques
   b. Evaluate for chronic versus acute: Many long-used personal hygiene products may be responsible.
7. Psoriasis
   a. Characterized by well-demarcated, thickened red plaques with silvery scaling, common on elbows, knees, scalp, and vulva
   b. Itching is reported, often severe.
F. Neoplastic conditions
   1. Paget's disease: Presents with pruritus as primary symptom; may be eczematous with well-demarcated raised edges
   2. Squamous cell carcinoma: Presents with pruritus as primary symptom; may appear as vulvar plaque, ulcer, or fleshy, nodular or warty mass
   3. Vulvar intraepithelial neoplasia
G. Neurologic conditions
   1. Postherpetic neuralgia: Onset of pain, tingling, or burning more than 4 months after the onset of herpetic lesions
   2. Spinal nerve compression: Symptoms may include sharp pain or burning
   3. Pudendal neuralgia: Burning, constant pain, often relieved only while sitting on a toilet
H. Anatomic/structural conditions
   1. Bartholin's gland: Glands located bilaterally in the vagina at 4 o'clock and 8 o'clock. Pain associated with Bartholin's glands is typically caused by cyst or abscess.
   2. Unruptured or tight hymen: Caused by incomplete degeneration of the central portion of the hymen
   3. Postepisiotomy: Disruption of the nerve pathways may result in pain.
   4. Postsurgical: Disruption of the nerve pathways may result in pain.
I. Table 14.1 summarizes the assessment of the vaginal environment.

IV. **Management: Vulvovaginal complaints are often complex; rarely do they resolve simply. They may require frequent visits with varied trials of treatment before the woman's symptoms are stable and manageable. Psychological support is a cornerstone of all treatment: These women will need understanding and patience. Following is a list of possible options for treatment of vulvar pain and treatment for some of the many possible conditions that cause it. It is, by no means, exhaustive. It should also be noted that many treatments are off-label.**
A. Comfort measures: Gentle care is advised.
   1. Sitz bath/cool soaks
   2. Cool packs, refrigerated (freezing can burn the skin)

TABLE 14.1 Assessment of Vaginal Environment

	CONDITION OF VAGINAL WALLS	ODOR	DISCHARGE COLOR	EPITHELIAL CELLS	WBC/ EPITHELIAL CELL RATIO	pH	CLUE CELLS OR OTHER
Normal	Normal, supple, pink	None	White	Mature appearance	1:1	3.8–4.2	None
Atrophic vaginitis	Smooth, pale, or inflamed	May be strong/ sour	May be scant or yellow	Immature cells are typically present	> 1:1	Elevated	None
DIV/lichenoid vaginitis	Inflamed	May be strong/ sour	Yellow	Immature cells are typically present	> 1:1	Elevated	None
Lichen planus	Inflamed, erosions may be noted	May be strong	Yellow	Immature cells are typically present	> 1:1	Elevated	None
Bacterial vaginosis	Normal	Fishy	Off-white, gray	Mature appearance	1:1	Elevated	Clue cells present
Yeast	May be inflamed	Yeast-like	White/clumpy	Immature cells may be present	Often > 1:1	3.8–4.2	None
Trichomonas	May be inflamed	May be strong	Yellow/green, frothy	Immature cells may be present	Often > 1:1	Elevated	Tricho-monads present, no clue cells

WBC = white blood cell.

   3. Avoidance of irritants (soaps, perfumed soaps/shampoos, perfumed laundry detergent, douching)
   4. "Soak and seal" with petrolatum or vegetable oil to seal in moisture and improved barrier function.
   5. Cotton underwear during the day, no underwear at night
B. Topical treatments for pain
   1. 5% lidocaine; may be applied up to five times daily. It may cause burning or increase in pain. If this occurs, it should be compounded in a neutral base. *Avoid benzocaine, the active ingredient in Vagisil brand, which has been shown to be a contact irritant.*
   2. Dyclonine: Not commercially available, but can be compounded
   3. EMLA: Lidocaine/prilocaine combination cream
   4. Doxepin: Compounding is necessary.
   5. Baclofen/tricyclic antidepressant: Compounded
C. Dietary treatments: A small number of women have found it helpful to lessen or eliminate high-oxalate foods from their diet.
   1. These diets can be restricting, and it may be enough to add calcium citrate to bind oxalates and avoid the worst triggers.
   2. High-oxalate foods include but are not limited to
      a. Berries
      b. Nuts
      c. Legumes, including soy and soy products
      d. Grains, especially wheat
      e. Chocolate
      f. Various vegetables
D. Treatment for yeast: After treatment of active infection, long-term weekly suppression may be necessary. Most patients will tolerate and can safely use fluconazole 150 mg weekly.
E. Treatment for herpes: Long-term suppression with antiviral agents
F. Treatment for *Trichomonas*: Metronidazole
G. Systemic treatment for pain
   1. Tricyclic antidepressants: Start at 10 mg, increase by 10 mg every 3 to 5 days as tolerated; may go as high as 150 mg. These medications can be remarkably helpful in reducing pain but may have significant side effects.
   2. Anticonvulsant medications: Gabapentin—start at 100 mg, increase by 100 mg every 3 to 5 days, as tolerated; may go as high as 3,600 mg; may also be associated with significant side effects. A newer option is pregabalin, or Lyrica (Pfizer Inc.), which may be taken as 100-mg dosages three times a day, with potential for a higher dose.
   3. Selective norepinephrine reuptake inhibitors: Venlafaxine HCl and duloxetine HCl. Both have shown some ability to treat neuropathic pain.

H. Local treatment can include intralesional injections with lidocaine and steroids.
I. Treatment for inflammatory conditions
   1. Superpotent steroid: Clobetasol, halobetasol, or betamethasone diproprionate are the cornerstones of treatment for vulvar inflammation. They can be tolerated for long-term treatment because of the high mitotic rate of the vulvar skin. These medications are sometimes irritating and can be compounded.
   2. Tacrolimus or other immunomodulary medications: These are nearly always irritating, and so are not first-line treatment. They should be used in minuscule amounts as the skin adjusts. Tacrolimus can be very effective in treating otherwise unresponsive lichen planus.
   3. Intralesional triamcinolone can be used for treatment of localized, unremitting lesions. These are very effective for long-term treatment but not well tolerated by patients.
   4. Systemic triamcinolone injections for unrelenting disease
   5. Vaginal estrogen can be used for atrophic conditions.
   6. Vaginal steroid suppository for DIV/lichenoid vaginitis: May begin with commercially prepared 25-mg suppositories (prepared for rectal use) inserted per vagina. If this is ineffective, may try 100-mg compounded hydrocortisone suppositories.
J. Treatment for pelvic floor dysfunction/vaginismus
   1. Pelvic floor physical therapy with biofeedback has been shown to help a significant number of women.
   2. Vaginal valium: Inserted vaginally, diazepam has been shown to reduce pelvic floor muscle spasm in some women.

V. **Patient education and clinician resources**
   A. Stewart, E. G., & Spencer, P. (2002). *The V book: A doctor's guide to complete vulvovaginal health.* New York, NY: Bantam.
   B. Edward, L., & Lynch, P. J. (2011). *Genital dermatology atlas* (2nd ed.). Philadelphia, PA: Wolters Kluwer/Lippincott Williams & Wilkins.
   C. Glazer, H., & Rodke, G. (2002). *The vulvodynia survival guide: How to overcome painful vaginal symptoms and enjoy an active lifestyle.* Oakland, CA: New Harbinger Publications.
   D. International Society for the Study of Vulvovaginal Disease: www.issvd.org
   E. The National Vulvodynia Association: www.nva.org
   F. Wise, D., & Rodney, A. (2011) *A headache in the pelvis* (6th ed.). Occidental, CA: National Center for Pelvic Pain Research.
   G. *UptoDate:* Subscription required; literature reviews with numerous resources for vulvovaginal complaints, authored by experts in the field, and updated every 6 months

H. The Vulval Pain Society: www.vulvalpainsociety.org/vps
I. The University of Michigan Center for Vulvar Pain: http://
obgyn.med.umich.edu/patient-care/womens-health-library/
vulvar-diseases

Bibliography

Bornstein, J., Sideri, M., Tatti, S., Walker, P., Prendiville, W., & Haefner, H. K. (2012). 2011 terminology of the vulvar of the International Federation for Cervical Pathology and Colposcopy. *Journal of Lower Genital Tract Disease, 16*(3) 290–295.

Danby, C. S., & Margesson, L. J. (2010). Approach to the diagnosis and treatment of vulvar pain. *Dermatolgic Therapy, 23*, 485–504.

Edward, L., & Lynch, P.J. (2011). *Genital dermatology atlas* (2nd ed.). Philadelphia, PA: Lippincott Williams & Wilkins.

Groysman, V. (2010). Vulvodynia: New concepts and review of the literature. *Dermatology Clinics, 28*, 681–696.

Haefner, H. K., Collins, M. E., Davis, G. D., Edwards, L., Foster, D. C., Hartmann, E. D., … Wilkinson, E. J. (2005). The vulvodynia guideline. *Journal of Lower Genital Tract Disease, 9*, 40–51.

Harlow, B. L., & Stewart, E. G. (2003). A population-based assessment of chronic unexplained vulvar pain: Have we underestimated the prevalence of vulvodynia? *Journal of the American Medical Women's Association, 58*, 82–88.

Lawton, S., & Littlewood, S. (2013). Vulval skin conditions: Disease activity and quality of life. *Journal of Lower Genital Tract Disease, 17*(2), 117–124.

Lynch, P. J., Moyal-Barracco, M., Scurry, J., & Stockdale, C. (2012). 2011 ISSVD terminology and classification of vulvar dermatological disorders: An approach to clinical diagnosis. *Journal of Lower Genital Tract Disease, 16*(4), 339–344.

Moyal-Barracco, M., & Lynch, P. J. (2004). 2003 ISSVD terminology and classification of vulvodynia: A historical perspective. *Journal of Reproductive Medicine, 49*(10), 772–777.

Rogalski, M. J., Kellog-Spadt, S., Hoffman, A. R., Fariello, J. Y., & Whitmore, K. E. (2010). Retrospective chart review of vaginal diazepam suppository use in high-tone pelvic floor dysfunction. *International Urogynecology Journal, 21*(7), 895–899.

Schlosser, B. J., & Mirowski, G. W. (2010). Approach to the patient with vulvovaginal complaints. *Dermatologic Therapy, 23*, 438–448.

Thorstensen, K. A., & Birenbaum, D. L. (2012). Recognition and management of vulvar dermatologic conditions: Lichen sclerosus, lichen planus, and lichen simplex chronicus. *Journal of Midwifery and Women's Health, 57*(3), 260–275.

Ventolini, G., Swenson, K. M., & Galloway, M. L. (2012). Lichen sclerosus: A 5-year follow-up after topical, subdermal, or combined therapy. *Journal of Lower Genital Tract Disease, 16*(3), 271–274.

Polycystic Ovarian Syndrome

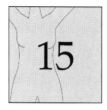

Yvette Marie Petti and R. Mimi Secor

I. **Overview and definition of polycystic ovarian syndrome (PCOS)**
   A. Definition
      1. PCOS is an endocrine disorder and one of the most commonly occurring endocrine disorders in women
      2. Origins of PCOS uncertain but emerging evidence suggests that this is
         a. Genetic disease
            (1) Women with PCOS may have a specific FMR1 sub-genotype.
            (2) Women with a heterozygous-normal/low FMR1 have polycystic-like symptoms of excessive follicle-activity and hyperactive ovarian function.
         b. May be associated with inflammation and an increased level of oxidative stress
      3. PCOS leads to symptoms in 5% to 10% of women of reproductive age 12 to 45 years of age.
      4. Most common cause of female subfertility
   B. Pathophysiology of PCOS
      1. Alteration in hypothalamic–pituitary–ovarian axis due to
         a. Elevated insulin levels, which leads to
            (1) Hyperinsulinemia increases gonadotropin releasing hormone (GnRH) pulse frequency
            (2) Luteinizing hormone (LH) overrides follicule-stimulating hormone (FSH)
            (3) Ovarian-androgen-increased production
         b. Decreased follicular maturation
         c. Decreased SHBG (sex hormone binding globulin) binding
         d. Aromatase is produced by adipose tissue, which changes androstenedione to estrone and testosterone to estradiol.

      e. This creates a negative feedback loop and a paradox of excess androgens and estrogens leading to ineffective feedback mechanism of the effects of FSH.

  2. The principal features are

      a. Anovulation menstruation, leading to irregular menstruation

      b. Overproduction of androgenic hormones, which results in acne and hirsutism

      c. Insulin resistance leading to obesity, type 2 diabetes, and elevated lipids

      d. Insulin resistance is found in normal and overweight women.

      e. Ovaries present as polycystic on ultrasound; however, this does not need to be present to meet criteria of inclusion for PCOS.

      f. Symptoms and severity vary among women.

  3. Ovaries become polycystic when stimulated to produce an excessive amount of male hormones (androgens)—namely, testosterone via one or more of the following

      a. Release of excess LH

      b. Hyperinsulinemia

      c. Decreased levels of sex hormone binding globulin lead to increased free androgens.

  4. The "cysts" that develop are immature follicles; may see a "string of pearls" on ultrasound

  5. Hypothalamic GnRH pulses, which leads to increase in LH/FSH ratio.

C. Impact of PCOS

  1. Endometrial hyperplasia

      a. Increased risk for development of uterine cancer, which is the most common gynecologic cancer in the United States (twofold to threefold increased risk)

      b. Overweight and obesity status contribute to anovulation and irregular or no cycling.

      c. Prolonged or non-cyclic estrogen stimulation can lead to type I endometrial cancers.

      d. This leads to hyperplasia of uterine lining, which places women at risk for development of endometrial/uterine cancer.

  2. Anovulatory cycling

      a. Infertility: Inability to become pregnant after 1 year of intercourse without use of contraception (applies to men and women both)

  3. Psychosocial impact

      a. Emotional distress frequently found in women with PCOS

      b. Higher rates of depression, anxiety

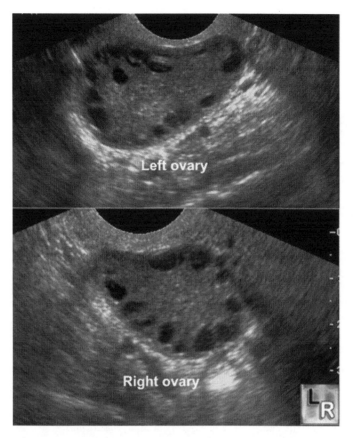

FIGURE 15.1 Classic presentation on ultrasound of the "string of pearls" presentation in PCOS.

From LearningRadiology.com. Used with permission.

    c. Greater fear of negative appearance, lower self-esteem, and higher rates of body dissatisfaction (namely associated with acne, hirsutism, and being overweight)
4. PCOS: Symptoms, signs, and risks
    a. Oligomenorrhea: Highly predictive
    b. Hyperandrogenism: Hirsutism, acne
    c. Obesity: Central obesity
    d. Infertility (25% to 37%) and anovulation
    e. Dysfunctional uterine bleeding (DUB)
    f. Uterine cancer: Increased threefold risk: Endometrial hyperplasia
    g. Insulin resistance, metabolic syndrome, type 2 diabetes
       (1) Threefold to sevenfold increased risk
    h. Heart disease, hypertension, dyslipidemia: 70%
    i. Mental health problems (low allopregnanolone)

II. **Criteria for classification of PCOS**
A. Rotterdam criteria: PCOS present if any two of three criteria present (wider definition)
1. Oligoovulation or anovulation
2. Excess androgen activity
3. Polycystic ovaries (by ultrasound)

III. **Clinical screening**
A. Physical examination
1. Blood pressure, heart rate, temperature, height, and weight (may add measure of adiposity–waist circumference and/or hip-to-waist ratio)
2. Hair distribution: Look for unusual pattern of thinning of hair on crown of scalp, increased facial hair, hair around nipples/over chest, inner legs, and forearms. (Note: Ask patient whether other women in the family have this hair distribution.)
3. Skin: Coarse or dry skin and/or cystic acne over face, chest, and back; examine neck for dark, velvety skin growths (acanthosis nigricans)
4. Eyes: Evaluate for exophthalmos, funduscopic–aterial venous (AV) nicking, and/or blood vessel changes.
5. Neck: Evaluate for thyroid enlargement and/or nodules.
6. Breast exam: Symmetry, skin and/or hair change; nipple discharge; masses
7. Cardiac: Evaluate for tachycardia or bradycardia, rhythm abnormalities, murmurs.
8. Lungs: Breath sounds/wheezing/ronchi
9. Abdomen: Contour, look for purple striae around anterior abdomen, organomegaly, bruits, masses
10. Peripheral: Edema, pulses, loss of vibratory and/or monofilament sensation over extremities
11. Genitalia: Virilization of labia, vaginal atrophy, speculum exam to evaluate vaginal canal and cervix, bimanual exam to evaluate size contour of uterus, also evaluate ovaries
B. Laboratory analysis (see Table 15.1)
1. Ordering of FSH and LH varies depending on the woman's presentation, because an elevated ratio can suggest presence of PCOS but is not diagnostic; should be ordered on day 3 of menstrual cycle.
2. More indicative of presence of PCOS, may be low SHBG levels
3. Serum prolactin (to rule out primary pituitary issue)
4. DHEA-S (dehydroepiandrosterone sulfate level of 700 to 800 mcg dL is likely to indicate adrenal dysfunction); list normal range
5. Free testosterone
6. Estradiol (questionable value)
7. Baseline lipids, HGBA1c, fasting glucose, vitamin D levels, complete blood count (CBC), serum chemistry, thyroid-stimulating hormone (TSH), and free T4

      a. Up to 68% have diabetes

      b. Insulin resistance in overweight and normal weight patients with PCOS

      c. Up to 70% have dyslipidemia (elevated triglycerides and low-density lipoprotein [LDL] cholesterol)

C. Imaging: Transvaginal ultrasound (TVUS)

    1. Evaluate uterine structure: Note on the requisition that you want an endometrial stripe measurement.

    2. Evaluate ovarian status: Note on requisition that you want measurement of ovaries and evaluation.

      a. Polycystic ovaries on ultrasound: 12 follicles 2 mm to 9 mm or increased volume of > 10 ml in one or more ovary

      b. Note that presence of cysts occur in 25% of women without PCOS.

    3. Evaluate endometrial lining

      a. If periods are irregular, which most are, then order anytime.

      b. If periods are at regular intervals, then day 6 through day 10 of menstrual cycle to assure thickening of endometrium is not due to premenstrual physiologic hyperplasia

D. Referral for endometrial biopsy

    1. Based on age, co-morbidities, and TVUS endometrial stripe measurement

    2. Endometrial thickening

      a. Hyperplasia can lead to atypical cellular changes and cancer in the lining of the uterus.

      b. For endometrial stripe greater than 4 mm, endometrial biopsy and/or gynecologic consultation

IV. Clinical intervention

A. Goals of management of PCOS

    1. Lower insulin levels

    2. Restore/preserve fertility

    3. Treat hirsutism and/or acne

    4. Regulate menstruation

    5. Prevent endometrial hyperplasia and hence prevent development of endometrial cancer

    6. Driven decision if the woman is younger or older, as well as her desire for future conception

B. Patient education

    1. If overweight, evaluation of dietary intake and physical activity participation with aim of at least 10% of total body weight reduction to start

      a. Goal is to reduce insulin resistance

      b. Lipid management

      c. Blood pressure management

TABLE 15.1 Summary of Differential Laboratory Workup in PCOS

LABORATORY TESTS	PCOS	PITUITARY DISORDERS DIABETES MELLITUS TYPE 2	NON-CLASSICAL ADRENAL HYPERPLASIA (NCAH)	CUSHING'S SYNDROME	THYROID DISORDERS
2-hour GTT (75 gm load)	≥ 140 and < 200 mg/dL impaired fasting glucose	= 200 mg/dL diabetes mellitus	Check serum 17-hydroxy-orgesterone level; if elevated 2 ng/mL		
HGBA1c	> 6.5 diabetes	≥ 5.6 to 6.4 at risk			
Total testosterone	> 60 PCOS	> 200 tumor			
Free testosterone	Normal range				
FSH/LH ratio	> 3.0 or normal in PCOS		Normal FSH and LH		
Serum prolactin	Normal range (3–27)	If elevated work up			
DHEA-sulfate	Normal range	Elevated	Elevated	Elevated	
Total testosterone	Normal range				
Serum human chorionic gonadotropin (HCG)	Negative				
Serum CBC and CMP (comprehensive metabolic panel)	Normal range				
Serum fasting morning cortisol	Normal range			Elevated	
TSH and free T4	Normal range				Elevated or suppressed

C. Pharmacotherapy (usually done in consultation with gynecologic specialist)
   1. Endometrial protection
      a. Use of progesterone
         (1) Provera challenge
      b. Medroxyprogesterone acetate (MPA): 10 mg by mouth day 1 to day 12, then stop and if bleed occurs, okay; if no bleed then
      c. Combination of oral contraceptives for 1 month, if bleed okay; if no bleed then refer to reproductive endocrinologist
         (1) Cyclical oral progesterone day 1 through day 12 monthly for induction of withdraw bleeding for induction of at least four withdrawal bleeds per year
         (2) Levonorgestrel-releasing intrauterine system (Mirena)
         (3) Etonogestrel implant (Nexplanon)
      d. Use of oral hormonal contraceptives
         (1) Progestin only
         (2) Combined estrogen and progestin (20 mcg preferred due to effects of lipids)
   2. Fertility preservation
      a. If woman in her late 20s/early 30s, refer to fertility specialist if desiring pregnancy, especially if hasn't conceived in 8 to 12 months.
         (1) Metformin: Reduces insulin resistance (not Food and Drug Administration [FDA] approved for use in PCOS but safety and efficacy have been established)
            • Used in combination with chlomiphene or letrozole for clomiphene-resistant (CC-resistant) patients
            • Used with biguanide
            • First-line agent for ovulation
            • Alternative to oral contraceptive (OC) for cycle regulation in PCOS
            • Treatment of PCOS-induced hirsutism
            • Weight loss
            • Reverses insulin resistance
            • Menses induction: 90% in 6 months
            • Category B in pregnancy and lactation; Nonteratogenic
               ▪ 500 to 850 mg up to three times daily
               ▪ May titrate up for effect
               ▪ Avoid if renal disease present
               ▪ Taper up slowly to minimize gastrointestinal (GI) side effects (diarrhea)
      b. Thiazolidinedione: Reduce insulin resistance
         (1) Monitor hepatic function
   3. Treatment of secondary characteristics from hyperandrogenism
      a. Spironolactone: For hirsuitism
         (1) Effective, safe, inexpensive

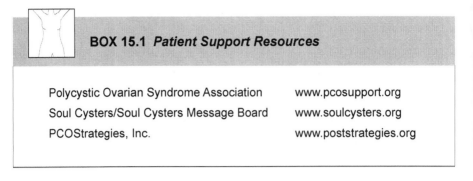

BOX 15.1 *Patient Support Resources*

Polycystic Ovarian Syndrome Association	www.pcosupport.org
Soul Cysters/Soul Cysters Message Board	www.soulcysters.org
PCOStrategies, Inc.	www.poststrategies.org

    (2) Use with caution, contraindicated in pregnancy (must use backup contraception)

    (3) Monitor liver function

    (4) Serum potassium can lead to elevated liver functions and hyperkalemia

  b. Combination hormonal contraceptives may be considered.

D. Pregnancy-related risks

  1. Infertility: 40% in women with PCOS

  2. Spontaneous abortion (SAB): 25% to 73%

  3. Gestational diabetes: Threefold increase

  4. Preeclampsia/hypertension

E. Other considerations

  1. Consider presence of obstructive sleep apnea; assess history; remember PCOS is thought to be related to inflammation and endothelial dysfunction.

F. Surveillance and follow-up

  1. Imperative to set in place clinical follow-up with PCOS patients

  2. Follow-up TVUS if have given cyclical progestin and/or if patient has had D&C (dilation and curettage) to assure endometrial stripe remains suppressed

  3. Important to encourage continued lifestyle modification: Low-carbohydrate and low-fat diet, daily physical activity participation, control of blood pressure

Bibliography

Azziz, R. (2006). Diagnosis of polycystic ovarian syndrome: The Rotterdam criteria are premature. *Journal of Clinical Endocrinology & Metabolism, 91*(3), 781–785. doi: 10.1210/jc2005-2153

Azziz, R., Woods, K. S., Reyna, T. J., Knochenhauer, E. S., & Yildiz, B. O. (2004). The prevalence and features of the polycystic ovary syndrome in an unselected population. *Journal of Clinical Endocrinology & Metabolism, 89*(6), 2745–2749. doi: 10.1210/jc.2003-032046

Balen, A. H., Conway, G. S., Homburg, R., & Legro R. S. (2005). *Polycystic ovary syndrome: A guide to clinical management.* London, UK: Taylor & Francis.

Banaszewka, B., Spaczynski, R. Z., Pelesz, M., & Pawelczyk, L. (2003). Incidence of elevated LH/FSH ratio in polycystic ovary syndrome women with normo- and hyperinsulinemia. *Rocz Akad Med Bialymst, 48*, 131–134. PMID 14737959

Barry, J. A., Kuczmierczyk, A. R., & Hardiman, P. J. (2011). Anxiety and depression in polycystic ovary syndrome: A systematic review and meta-analysis. *Human Reproduction, 26*(9), 2442–2451. doi:10.109/humrep/deq197

Bates, G. W. (2102). Long term management of polycystic ovarian syndrome. *Molecular and Cellular Endocrinology, 373*(1–2), 91–97. doi: 10.10101/j.mce.2012.10.029

DeGroot, P. C., Dekkers, O. M., Rominjn, S. U., & Helmerhorst, F. M. (2011). PCOS, coronary heart disease, stroke, and the influence of obesity: A systematic review and meta-analysis. *Human Reproduction Update, 17*(4), 495–500. doi: 10.1093/humupd/dmr001

De Niet, J. E., de Koning, C. M., Pastoor, H., Dolvenvoorden, H. J., & Laven, J. S. E. (2010). Psychological well-being and sexarche in women with polycystic ovary syndrome. *Human Reproduction, 25*(16), 1497–1503. doi. 10.1093/humrep/deq608

Diamanti-Kandarakis, E., Kandarakis, H., & Legro, R. S. (2006). Role of genes and environment in the etiology of PCOS. *Endocrinology, 30*(1), 19–26. doi: 10.1385/ENDO

Duleba, A. J. (2012). Medical management of metabolic dysfunction in PCOS. *Steroids, 77*(4), 306.

Duleba, A. J., & Dokras, A. (2012). Is PCOS an inflammatory process? *Fertility & Sterility, 97*(1), 7–12.

Gonzalez, F. (2012). Inflammation in polycystic ovary syndrome: Underpinning of insulin resistance and ovarian dysfunction. *Steroids, 77*, 300–305.

Leeman, L., & Acharya, U. (2009). The use of metformin in the management of polycystic ovary syndrome and associated anovulatory infertility: The current evidence. *Journal of Obstetrics and Gynaecology, 29*(6), 467–472. doi: 10.1080/01443610902829414

Legro, R. S., Kunselman, A. R., & Dunaif, A. (2001). Prevalence and predictors of dyslipidemia in women with polycystic ovarian syndrome. *American Journal of Medicine, 111*(8), 607–613.

Moran, L. J., Ko, H., Misso, M., Marsh, K., Noakes, M., Talbot, M., … Teede, H. J. (2013). Dietary composition in the treatment of polycystic ovary syndrome: A systematic review to inform evidence-based guidelines. *Human Reproduction Update, 19*(5), 432. doi: 10.1093/humupd/dmt015

Moran, L. J., Misso, M. L., Wild, R. A., & Norman, R. J. (2010). Impaired fasting glucose tolerance, type 2 diabetes, and metabolic syndrome in polycystic ovary syndrome: A systematic review and meta-analysis. *Human Reproduction Update, 16*(4), 347–363. doi: 10.1093/humupd/dmq001

Murri, M., Luque-Ramirez, M., Insenser, M., Ojeda-Ojeda, M., & Escobar-Morreale, H. F. (2013). Circulating markers of oxidative stress and polycystic ovary syndrome (PCOS): A systematic review and meta-analysis. *Human Reproduction Update, 19*(3), 268–288. doi: 10.1093/humupd/dms059

Nandalike, K., Agarwal, C., Strauss, T., Coupey, S. M., Isasi, C. R., Sin, S., & Arens, R. (2012). Sleep and cardiometabolic function in obese and adolescent girls with polycystic ovarian syndrome. *Sleep Medicine, 13*(10), 1307–1312. doi: 10.1016/j.sleep.2012.02.002

Smith, H. A., Markovic, N., Matthews, A. K., Danielson, M. E., Kalro, B. N., Youk, A. O., & Talbott, E. O. (2011). A comparison of polycystic ovary syndrome and related factors between lesbian and heterosexual women. *Women's Health Issues, 21*(3), 191–198. doi: 10.1016/.whi2010.11.001

Veltman-Verhulst, S. M., Boivin, J. E., Eijkemans, M. J. C., & Fauser, B.J.C.M. (2012). Emotional distress as a common risk in women with polycystic ovary syndrome: A systematic review and meta-analysis of 28 studies. *Human Reproduction Update, 18*(6), 638–651. doi: 10.109/humupd/dms029

Yawn, V. (2012). Polycystic ovarian syndrome. *Advance for NPs & PAs, 3*(12), 11–15.

Abnormal Uterine Bleeding

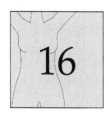

Ivy M. Alexander

I. **Abnormal uterine bleeding (AUB) explained**
   A. Definition
      1. Any uterine bleeding that occurs outside of the normal menstrual parameters for duration of bleeding, amount of flow, cycle length and timing is considered AUB.
         a. Duration under 2 days or over 7 days
         b. Flow of more than 80 mL
         c. Cycle length of under 24 days or over 35 days
         d. Intermenstrual bleeding or postcoital spotting
      2. Multiple different terms have been used historically to describe symptoms or diagnoses of AUB. Terms used to describe AUB are listed in Box 16.1.
      3. Due to this lack of consistency in nomenclature used for AUB, a new classification system was adopted by the Fédération Internationale de Gynécologie et d'Obstétrique (FIGO) in November 2010.
      4. The FIGO classification system was developed by an international workgroup and uses an acronym to identify possible causes for AUB (Box 16.2).
         a. The FIGO classification system guides clinical evaluation and diagnosis for AUB (see Pathophysiology and differential diagnoses, Section III).
         b. PALM etiologies are generally structural problems and the COEIN entities are nonstructural.
         c. The FIGO classification system recognizes that a woman may have one or more entities causing AUB and/or have entities that are symptomatic and do not contribute to the bleeding (e.g., leiomyomas, polyps, adenomyosis).
         d. The workgroup also recommended retiring the terms *menorrhagia, metrorrhagia,* and *dysfunctional uterine bleeding.*

BOX 16.1 *Terms Used to Describe AUB*

- Dysfunctional uterine bleeding (now called "heavy menstrual bleeding")
- Oligomenorrhea
- Menorrhagia
- Intermenstrual bleeding
- Amenorrhea
- Polymenorrhea
- Metrorrhagia
- Menometrorrhagia
- Premenstrual spotting
- Hypermenorrhea
- Hypomenorrhea

BOX 16.2 *PALM–COEIN*

<u>P</u>olyps
<u>A</u>denomyosis
<u>L</u>eiomyoma
<u>M</u>alignancy and hyperplasia

<u>C</u>oagulopathy
<u>O</u>vulatory disorders
<u>E</u>ndometrial disorders
<u>I</u>atrogenic causes
<u>N</u>ot classified

B. Epidemiology
   1. Approximately 1.4 million women report AUB annually.
      a. Prevalence is difficult to estimate accurately due to the variations in nomenclature used for AUB.
   2. The incidence of abnormal bleeding is increased during adolescence and perimenopause.
   3. 10% to 30% of all women report heavy bleeding.
   4. 11% of postmenopausal women have spontaneous bleeding.
   5. AUB is more common among White women, younger women (18 to 30 years), and women who are obese.
   6. Approximately 30% of outpatient office visits in gynecology are related to menstrual problems.

C. Health-related complications associated with AUB
1. AUB is correlated with poorer physical and mental health–related quality of life.
2. Persistent menstrual blood loss of over 80 mL per cycle is associated with anemia.
3. AUB accounts for approximately two thirds of all hysterectomies.
4. Associated with increased health care costs

II. **Clinical evaluation of the woman who presents with AUB**
A. History
1. Establish the onset, duration, severity, and course of the changes in bleeding patterns.
   a. Is this an acute change? Heavy bleeding, need to stabilize the patient?
   b. Is this a chronic problem—persistent pattern (timing, amount, regularity) for most of a 6-month time period?
2. Clarify the women's bleeding pattern
   a. Are her cycles longer, shorter, or irregular?
   b. Is her flow heavier or lighter?
   c. Is she passing clots?
   d. Where does the blood originate?
   e. Are there changes in the pattern of her bleeding (spotting, mid-cycle bleeding, postcoital bleeding, bleeding after exercise)?
   f. Is there a change in the volume of bleeding? Quantify number of pads/tampons used (an increase of two or more pads/tampons per day helps to quantify an increase in blood loss).
3. Has she experienced similar changes in the past?
4. Has she had previous treatment for this or a similar problem?
5. Has she tried any alternative or complementary medicine therapies or other methods for self-care?
6. Does she have symptoms of ovulation?
7. Identify whether she is experiencing any associated symptoms with a review of systems (ROS)
   a. Constitutional—fatigue, malaise, myalgia, chills, fever, weight loss, anorexia
   b. Head, eyes, ears, nose, and throat (HEENT)—dizziness, especially with change in position; gum bleeding
   c. Respiratory—shortness of breath, especially with exertion
   d. Cardiac—tachycardia, palpitations
   e. Gastrointestinal—abdominal pain, cramping, pelvic pain, bloating, elimination changes (constipation, diarrhea, bleeding), flatulence
   f. Genitourinary—urinary urgency, frequency, dysuria, hematuria, odor, color changes, flank pain; genital pruritis, lesions, burning, pain, discharge, odor, dyspareunia
   g. Neurological—dizziness

    h. Skin—rash, bruising

    i. Extremities—arthralgias, joint stiffness, swelling

  8. Complete a full gynecologic history.

    a. Pregnancy history summary including gravida, parous

      (1) How many pregnancies and live births has she had?

      (2) Any problems with bleeding after delivery?

      (3) Has she had any abortions? If yes, were they spontaneous, medical, or surgical?

    b. Menstrual history

      (1) What was her last menstrual period like—normal, late, lighter than normal?

      (2) Age of menarche—What is her usual cycle length, days of flow, flow pattern?

      (3) Does she have any dysmenorrhea? Is it of new onset or worsening?

      (4) If she has a male partner, is she using any form of contraceptive?

      (5) Any history of vaginitis? If yes, how was it treated?

    c. Sexual history

      (1) Partner history—How many currently and over lifetime? Does she have sex with men, women, or both?

      (2) When was her most recent sexual activity?

      (3) What is the frequency and type of sexual activity she engages in? Are there any risky behaviors or activities that correlate with her bleeding?

    d. Sexually transmitted infection (STI) history

      (1) Record any STIs—type, date, treatment

      (2) Date last tested, what tests done, and results

    e. Gynecologic surgery, procedures, problems

    f. Personal hygiene

      (1) Is she douching, using a new type of pads or tampons, or any new products?

  9. Social history

    a. Does she have any history of sexual, physical, or verbal abuse?

    b. What is her lifestyle—diet (any history of eating disorders?), exercise (excessive exercise?), sleep, stressors (excessive stress?), occupation, and recreation, alcohol/drugs, tobacco

  10. Medical history

    a. Identify current or past medical conditions—how managed?

    b. Any personal history of bleeding disorders?

  11. Medications and allergies

    a. Prescription: Borrowed or self-medication

    b. Does she have any allergies to medications, environment, or animals?

    c. Over-the-counter medications

    d. Complementary and alternative medication therapies

12. Family history
    a. Has a sister or mother had similar abnormal bleeding?
    b. Any family history of bleeding disorders?
13. Health screenings
    a. When was her last cervical cytology, pelvic examination, mammogram (if of age), colonoscopy (if of age), lipids and fasting glucose or hemoglobin A1c?
    b. Are her immunizations up to date?
    c. Does she need special testing such as tuberculosis (TB) screening or screening for lung cancer?
B. Physical examination
    1. Vital signs—include orthostatic blood pressures and pulses; include height and weight to calculate body mass index (BMI). Has she lost weight recently?
    2. General appearance and systemic evaluation
        a. Identify level of sexual maturity.
        b. Evaluate body habitus.
        c. Skin and hair—distribution (hirsute?)
    3. HEENT
        a. Mucosal color
        b. Thyroid exam
    4. Breast exam
    5. Cardiac exam
        a. Evaluate for tachycardia, arrhythmias, murmurs.
    6. Abdominal exam
        a. Evaluate for striae, hepatosplenomegaly, tenderness, masses, ascites.
    7. Pelvic exam
        a. Identify source of bleeding—examine external genitalia, vagina, cervix
        b. Assess for cervical motion tenderness.
        c. Collect cervical cytology; STI cultures; vaginal discharge for potassium hydroxide (KOH) test, pH test; wet mount (see Chapter 10, "Assessment of Menopausal Status")
        d. Perform a bimanual exam of her uterus and adnexae— assess for tenderness; uterus size, shape, firmness; adnexa palpability, firmness, fullness or enlargement
        e. Rectal
            (1) Are there any lesions, hemorrhoids?
            (2) Is there any bleeding at the rectum?
            (3) Test stool smear for occult blood.

III. Pathophysiology and differential diagnoses
    A. The FIGO PALM–COEIN acronym (see Box 16.2) provides guidance to the underlying pathophysiology and potential differential diagnoses for AUB in reproductive-aged women.

    B. PALM—structural disorders

       1. Infections—sexually transmitted infections, cervicitis, vaginitis, endometritis

       2. Benign structural abnormalities—polyps, ectropian, cysts, leiomyomata

       3. Premalignant/malignant lesions

       4. Trauma/irritation—intercourse, sexual assault, presence of foreign body

    C. COEIN—nonstructural disorders

       1. Endocrine disorders—hyper-/hypothyroidism, hyperprolactinemia, polycystic ovary syndrome, adrendal hyperplasia/Cushing disease

       2. Hematologic disorders—coagulopathy, leukemia

       3. Renal or liver disorders

       4. Mucosal diseases—Crohn's, Bechet's

       5. Extreme stress

       6. Extreme exercise

       7. Medications—oral contraceptive pills, hormone therapy, selective serotonin reuptake inhibitors, antipsychotics, anticoagulants, corticosteroids

       8. Herbal supplements

       9. Intrauterine devices

      10. Eating disorders

      11. Weight loss

    D. AUB not specified—diagnosis of exclusion, no cause for bleeding identified (organic, structural)

       1. Periodic uterine blood loss of over 80 mL per cycle

       2. Negatively affects her quality of life

    E. Different diagnoses are more common among different age groups. Bleeding in a postmenopausal woman is considered malignant until proven otherwise (Table 16.1).

IV. Diagnostic testing

    A. Diagnostic testing is ordered based on the most likely differential diagnoses and the FIGO PALM–COEIN categorization.

    B. PALM entities are generally structural problems that are identified with direct visualization, imaging (e.g., transvaginal ultrasound, saline infusion sonography), and/or histopathology.

    C. COEIN entities are generally nonstructural problems that are not identified with imaging or direct visualization and other laboratory testing may be warranted.

    D. Consider testing for bleeding disorders if she has two or more of the following symptoms: bruising one to two times per month, frequent gum bleeding, epistaxis one to two times per month, or a family history of bleeding symptoms; or if she has a history of heavy bleeding

TABLE 16.1 Differential Diagnoses for Abnormal Uterine Bleeding Categorized by Age

AGE GROUP	POTENTIAL DIAGNOSES
Neonate	Estrogen withdrawal
Premenarchal	Trauma or foreign body Infection/vulvovaginitis Urologic factors Precocious puberty (rare) Neoplasm (rare)
Early postenarchal	Anovulation/polycystic ovarian syndrome Coagulation disorder Pregnancy Stress/extreme exercise Infection Neoplasm (rare) Trauma
Reproductive years	Anovulation Pregnancy Infection Benign growths Medication Coagulation disorders Endocrine disorders Liver disease Malignancy Trauma Stress/extreme exercise
Perimenopause	Anovulation Medications Malignancy Benign growths
Postmenopause	Malignancy Medications Atrophy Benign growths

since menarche or has had a postpartum hemorrhage, bleeding related to surgery, or bleeding associated with dental work.
   E. Transvaginal ultrasound is used to identify structural abnormalities and the thickness of the endometrial stripe.
      1. An endometrial stripe less than or equal to 4 mm correlates with very low risk for endometrial cancer (1 in 917) and thus endometrial biopsy is not needed.
   F. Endometrial biopsy is needed for all postmenopausal women with bleeding and for women older than age 40.

1. Endometrial cancer risk increases with age
   a. Incidence at age 13 to 18 years is approximately 0.1 out of 100,000 women.
   b. Incidence at age 19 to 34 years is approximately 2.3 out of 100,000 women.
   c. Incidence at age 35 to 39 years is approximately 6.1 out of 100,000 women.
   d. Incidence at age 40 to 49 years is approximately 36.0 out of 100,000 women.
   G. Diagnostic studies to consider for women with abnormal uterine bleeding (Table 16.2)

TABLE 16.2 Diagnostic Studies to Consider for Women With Abnormal Uterine Bleeding

AGE	DIAGNOSTIC TEST
13 to 18 years	• Human chorionic gonadotropin (hCG) to rule out pregnancy • Cultures if sexually active • Coagulation studies: International normalized ratio (INR) or prothrombin time (PT) and partial thromboblastin time (PTT), fibrinogen, von Willebrand factor, ristocetin co-factor • Complete blood count with platelet count to identify coagulation defects, leukemia, anemia
19 to 50 years	• hCG, cervical cytology, cultures • Thyroid-stimulating hormone (TSH)—to identify hypo-/hyperthyroidism, especially if untested in 5 years • Follicle-stimulating hormone (FSH, controversial), maybe with estradiol, progesterone, luteinizing hormone (LH), FSH:LH ratio • CBC (complete blood count) with platelet count and serum iron, blood drawn early in cycle (day 3) • Coagulation studies if screening questions positive • Urine analysis to identify urinary tract infection, renal calculi, bladder cancer • Stool guiac test to identify colon polyps, diverticula, gastrointestinal cancers, ulcer, hemorrhoids, fissures • Ultrasound to identify leiomyomata, structural abnormalities • Endometrial biopsy if 40 years or older and in younger women if any concern for endometrial cancer • Consider fasting serum prolactin test to identify pituitary adenoma if bleeding is infrequent or minimal. • Consider head magnetic resonance imaging to identify pituitary adenoma. • Consider liver function tests and renal function studies to identify systemic illness.

Sources: American College of Obstetrics and Gynecology (2013), Fritz (2011), James (2009), and Munro (2011).

V. Clinical management of AUB

A. Management is tailored to the cause of the bleeding if one can be identified.

B. The goal of therapy (after pregnancy and malignancy have been excluded) is to restore normal menstrual cycles and minimize blood loss and disruption to the woman's life.

C. Management options for heavy menstrual bleeding
  1. Medications
     a. Combined oral contraceptive pills
     b. Progestin-only contraceptive pills
     c. Depot medroxyprogesterone acetate (DMPA)
     d. Levonorgestrel intrauterine device
     e. Nonsteroidal anti-inflammatory drugs (NSAIDs)
     f. Tranexamic acid
  2. Endometrial ablation
  3. Hysterectomy (last resort)

D. Management options for anovulatory bleeding
  1. Medications
     a. Estrogen or progestin to stop bleeding
     b. Combined oral contraceptive pills
     c. Metformin if the woman has insulin resistance

E. Management options for structural causes of bleeding (polyps, leiomyomata)
  1. Medications
     a. Combined oral contraceptive pills
     b. Levonorgestrel intrauterine device
  2. Surgical excision of polyp, leiomyomata
  3. Uterine artery embolization (for leiomyomata)
  4. High-intensity focus ultrasound (for leiomyomata)
  5. Hysterectomy (last resort)

Bibliography

American College of Obstetrics and Gynecology. (2013a). ACOG practice bulletin: Management of abnormal uterine bleeding associated with ovulatory dysfunction. *Obstetrics & Gynecology, 122*(1), 176–185.

American College of Obstetrics and Gynecology. (2013b). ACOG practice bulletin: Management of acute abnormal uterine bleeding in nonpregnant reproductive-aged women. *Obstetrics & Gynecology, 122*(1), 891–896.

Fritz, M. A., & Speroff, L. (2011). *Clinical gynecologic endocrinology and infertility* (8th ed.). Philadelphia, PA: Lippincott, Williams & Wilkins.

James A. H., Kouides P. A., Abdul-Kadir R., et al. (2009). Von Willebrand disease and other bleeding disorders in women: Consensus on diagnosis and management from an international expert panel. *American Journal of Obstetrics and Gynecology, 201*, 12–18.

Matteson, K. A., Raker, C. A., Clark, M. A., & Frick, K. D. (2013). Abnormal uterine bleeding, health status, and usual course of medical care: Analyses using the medical expenditures panel survey. *Journal of Women's Health, 22*(11), 959–965.

Munro, M. G., Critchey, H. O. D., Broder, M. S., & Fraser, I. S. (2011). FIGO classification system (PALM–COEIN) for causes of abnormal uterine bleeding in nongravid women of reproductive age. *International Journal of Gynecology and Obstetrics, 113,* 3–13.

Munro, M. G., Critchley, H. O. D., & Fraser, I. S. (2011). The FIGO classification of causes of abnormal uterine bleeding in the reproductive years. *Fertility and Sterility, 95*(7), 2204–2208.

Tsai, M. C., & Goldstein, S. R. (2012). Office diagnosis and management of abnormal uterine bleeding. *Clinical Obstetrics and Gynecology, 55*(3), 635–650.

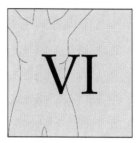

Evaluation of the Pelvic Floor

Pelvic Organ Prolapse

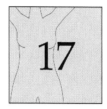

Helen A. Carcio

I. **Pelvic organ prolapse explained**
  A. The pelvis lies at the bottom of the abdominopelvic cavity.
    1. It forms a supportive layer that prevents the pelvic organs from falling through the bony pelvis.
    2. It supports conception and parturition.
    3. It controls storage and evacuation of feces and urine.
  B. Mechanical principles in relation to prolapse of pelvic organs
    1. The uterus and vagina lie suspended in a sling-like network of ligaments and fascial structures attached to the side walls of the pelvis.
    2. Levator ani muscles constrict, forming an occlusive layer on which the pelvic organs may rest.
      a. They consist of strong striated muscle tissue, comprising the iliococcygeus, the pubococcygeus, and the puborectalis (Figure 17.1).
      b. They compress the rectum, vagina, and urethra against the pubic bone, holding them in position.
    3. As long as the pelvic floor musculature functions normally, the pelvic floor is closed and the ligaments and fascia are under no tension.
    4. Problems exist when the pelvic floor muscles relax or are damaged. Risk factors are listed in Box 17.1.
      a. The pelvic floor opens, and the vagina lies between the high intra-abdominal pressure and the low atmospheric pressure, where it must be held in place by ligaments.
      b. Eventually, connective tissue will become damaged and fail to hold the vagina in place.
    5. The increase in intra-abdominal pressure placed on the pelvic floor muscles and ligaments causes the development of a prolapse, rather than problems with the organs themselves.

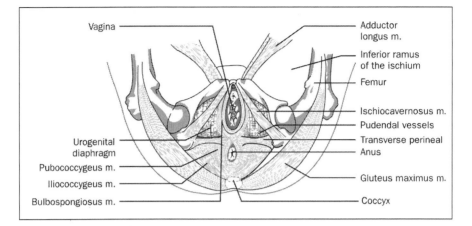

FIGURE 17.1 Muscles of the pelvic floor.

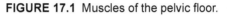

BOX 17.1 *Risk Factors for the Development of Pelvic Floor Relaxation*

- Chronic cough (due to asthma or chronic bronchitis)
- Heavy lifting (prolonged)
- High impact sports
- Obesity
- Pelvic malignancy
- High parity
- White skin color (higher incidence in this population)
- Large uterine or ovarian masses
- Advancing age (estrogen deficiency)
- History of traumatic birth
- Genetic predisposition (less collagen support)
- Previous pelvic or vaginal irradiation
- Multiple anti-incontinence procedures
- Metabolic diseases that affect muscle function
- Failure to reattach the cardinal ligaments at hysterectomy
- Decreased pelvic muscle strength

    C. Urinary continence (see Chapter 18, "Urinary Incontinence")
       1. Depends on support of the urethra
         a. Fascial structures supporting the urethra at the vesical neck
         b. Active muscle contraction
         c. Intact neuromuscular mechanisms
       2. Ability of the urethra to remain closed
       3. Note: Closure pressure of urethra must equal or exceed intravesical pressure.

D. Several factors influence the development of genital prolapse and urinary incontinence.

II. Diagnosis of pelvic organ prolapse
    A. The pelvic examination
        1. Be sensitive to the fact that many of these women may be older and may not have had a pelvic examination in many years.
        2. They may have suffered for months or even years with symptoms and be anxious concerning the cause.
        3. If stress incontinence is present, the woman may be fearful that she will leak during the examination.
        4. It takes a while to develop assessment skills to diagnose correctly the type and extent of a prolapse. It is a good idea to examine all patients for a prolapse, regardless of whether or not they are symptomatic, in order to compare normal and abnormal findings.
        5. Reassure the patient that although pelvic relaxation is slowly progressive, it is unlikely to affect longevity.
        6. The clinician may use a handheld mirror to explain pelvic findings.
    B. Position
        1. Place the patient in a comfortable lithotomy position, with her feet in the stirrups (may be difficult for older women).
        2. She may have to stand and bear down at some point in the examination.
        3. Drape the patient appropriately.
    C. Vital steps in correctly diagnosing a prolapse
        1. The examination must be made with the woman pushing down, as though she is straining at stool; the entire extent of the prolapse must be seen.
            a. Sometimes, women are reluctant to follow through with this part of the examination because they are afraid that they may leak or pass flatus, which would be very embarrassing to them.

TABLE 17.1 Grading Prolapse of the Uterus

DEGREE	DESCRIPTION
Stage 1	Slight to moderate uterine descent with cervix still inside vagina to any distal point 1 cm above the hymen
Stage 2	Uterine descent to 1 cm above or below the hymen
Stage 3	Descent of uterus to a point beyond 1 cm distal to the hymen
Stage 4	Total eversion

b. It is useful to acknowledge what might occur and let the patient know that it is okay.

c. It may be difficult to exert enough pressure in the lithotomy position; the clinician may have to ask the woman to stand and bear down while examining her.

2. The clinician must examine each different structure independently.

D. Once the prolapse is visible, other structures need to be systematically assessed.

1. Focus on the specific defects.

2. Note the severity of the prolapse.

E. Identify the extent that the vaginal wall, cervix, and posterior walls have descended.

1. Examine the anterior and posterior walls by retracting the opposite wall with the posterior half of a vaginal speculum so that a larger cystocele does not obscure a smaller rectocele.

F. Classification of the severity of a prolapse

1. Grading systems are varied and very subjective. Table 17.1 lists one form of classification.

2. It is best to describe the size of a prolapse in terms of the distance the prolapse descends below or rises above the hymenal ring with the prolapse extended to its fullest (e.g., "The cervix lies 2 cm below the hymenal ring").

3. Describe the diameter of the prolapse to help assist in assessing the severity. The greater the diameter, the more severe the prolapse.

4. Types of prolapse

a. First-degree prolapse is without symptoms and is mildly descended.

b. Second-degree prolapse is halfway into the vagina and is usually asymptomatic.

c. Third-degree prolapse is at the level of the introitus and is usually symptomatic.

d. Fourth-degree prolapse is out of the vagina, even at rest. Symptoms are severe.

G. Evaluating anterior wall support

1. Establishes status of urethral and bladder support

2. Urethra is fused with the lower 3 to 4 cm of the vaginal wall.

3. Urethrocele

a. Diagnosed by descent of the lower anterior vaginal wall to the level of the hymenal ring during straining

b. Seen as a herniation between the urethra and vagina, as the urethra prolapses into the anterior vaginal vault, out of the correct angle with the bladder

  c. Usually associated with stress incontinence and loss of urethral support

  d. Often occurs with a cystocele

  e. Difficult to grade

  f. By itself, it is not usually an indication for use of a pessary.

4. Cystocele

  a. Defective support of the upper portion of the anterior vaginal wall or stretching of the vesicovaginal fascia because the bladder lies adjacent to this portion of the vaginal wall (Figure 17.2)

  b. Herniation occurring between the bladder and the vagina, with descent of a portion of the common wall between these structures

  c. Occurs gradually with stretching, increased bladder capacity, and development of atrophic vulvovaginitis

5. Cystourethrocele—defective support of the entire anterior wall, which is often manifested by descent below the hymenal ring, whether or not stress incontinence is present

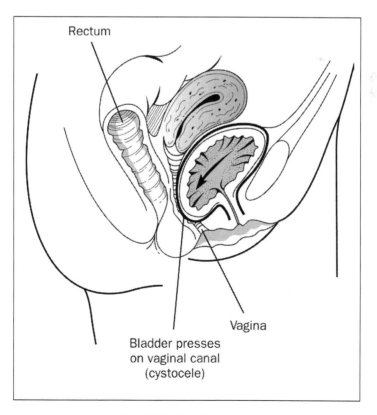

FIGURE 17.2 Cystocele.

    6. Must include direct observation of the urethra while coughing in supine and standing positions

H. Determine the position of the uterus and vagina.

    1. Vagina and cervix are fused with one another.

    2. If the cervix prolapses downward, it brings the upper vagina along with it.

    3. May be caused by

        a. Stretching of the uterosacral and cardinal ligaments

        b. Lacerations or damage to the levator ani and perineal body

    4. Prolapse (or procidentia)

        a. Descent of the uterus below its normal level

        b. As support of ligaments gives way, the uterus moves backward to a retroverted or retroflexed position.

        c. Round ligaments stretch, failing to hold the body of the uterus in the anteverted position.

        d. Uterus next aligns itself with the long axis of the vagina

        e. An increase in intra-abdominal pressure causes the uterus to descend down the vaginal canal (similar to the action of a piston in a cylinder) (Figure 17.3).

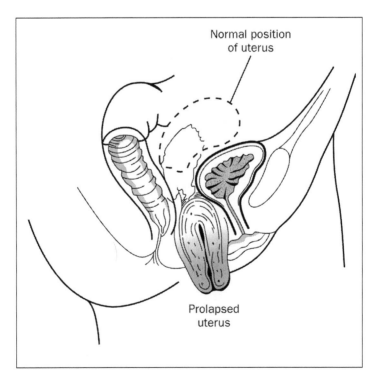

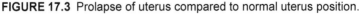

FIGURE 17.3 Prolapse of uterus compared to normal uterus position.

5. Measured by the location of the cervix relative to the hymenal ring
   a. Important: Cervix may not be visible behind a cystocele or rectocele and must be palpated as the patient bears down.
   b. May also test the extent to which the cervix and uterus descend by either of the following methods
      (1) Have the patient stand. Using a mirror placed between her legs, have her observe for descent, while she is asked to bear down.
      (2) Grasp the cervix with a tenaculum to assess, while gently pulling the cervix toward the vaginal opening. (This is certainly the more invasive maneuver.)
   c. If the cervix descends to within 1 cm of the hymenal ring, there is considerable loss of support. Cervical elongation is common in women with a prolapse.
I. Posterior vaginal wall
   1. Rectocele (see Figure 17.4).
      a. Protrusion of the anterior rectal wall and posterior wall of the overlying vagina

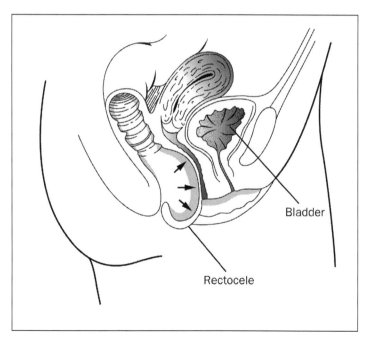

FIGURE 17.4 Rectocele (sagittal section showing relative position of uterus and bladder).

      b. May protrude below the hymenal ring to form a bulging mass originating from the posterior vaginal wall, causing the anterior rectal wall to balloon down through the vaginal ring

      c. Causes

         (1) Disruption of the rectovaginal fascia during childbirth

         (2) Chronic fecal constipation and straining

  2. Enterocele

      a. The cul-de-sac becomes distended with intestine, and bulges the posterior vaginal wall outward.

      b. Hernia of the fascia of the posterior vagina above the rectovaginal septum and below the cervix

      c. Sometimes mistaken for a rectocele

      d. A large enterocele may protrude through the vagina.

      e. Requires correction only if symptomatic

      f. Rarely seen

III. The diagnosis

  A. Assess pelvic muscle tone.

    1. Ask patient to squeeze around your two examining fingers while palpating the levator ani muscle (Table 17.2).

    2. Note the patient's ability to sustain constriction and deflection of finger or fingers upward with a good squeeze. No deflection indicates weaker muscles.

    3. Constriction lasting a few seconds indicates weakening.

    4. Stress incontinence protocol.

  B. Provocative stress test

    1. Ask the patient, when she has a full bladder, to stand and cough.

    2. Observe for small spurts of urine that escape simultaneously with each cough. (May place pad between legs to catch and observe any urine released.)

    3. If urine escapes, place one finger on either side of the urethra.

    4. Ask the patient to cough again.

    5. If there is no loss of urine during the cough, the test is considered positive for stress urinary incontinence.

TABLE 17.2 Assessment of Pelvic Muscle Strength

	0	1	2	3
Pressure	None	Weak	Moderate	Strong—fingers compressed
Duration	None	Less than 1 second	1 to 3 seconds	More than 3 seconds
Displacement	None	Slight incline	Noticeable incline	Fingers drawn in

C. Assess the neuronal support to the sacral dermatone, S2, S3, and S4. These dermatones innervate the micturation reflex.
   1. Lightly stroke the skin area innervated by the dermatones.
      a. Note response to light touch.
      b. Compare contralateral sides.
   2. Bulbocavernosus reflex
      a. Stroke or gently squeeze the clitoris.
      b. Note contraction of the bulbocavernous muscle around the clitoris.
   3. Anal reflex (so-called anal wink)
      a. Lightly stroke the skin lateral to the anus.
      b. Note contraction of the anal sphincter.
D. The cotton-tipped swab (Q-tip) test (see Chapter 18, "Urinary Incontinence")
E. Digital rectal examination
   1. Assess for any fecal impaction.
   2. Note sphincter muscle tone.
F. Assess vulvovaginal area for estrogen status (see Chapter 12, "Atrophic Vaginitis, Vulvovaginal Atrophy").
   1. Observe the vagina for the presence of rugae, degree of moistness, and color.
      a. These features decrease during menopause.
   2. Estrogen status of the vulva and vaginal is important.
      a. The presence of mature squamous epithelium indicates good estrogen nourishment.
      b. Estrogen thickens the layers of the vaginal wall, enhancing support of the bladder and rectum.
G. May refer the patient for a simple cystometrogram or urodynamic techniques (see Chapter 36, "The Simple Cystometrogram")
   1. To assess for detrusor instability before surgery
   2. To evaluate symptoms to determine need for anticholinergic medications
H. Assessment of urinary symptoms
   1. Determine postvoid residual if any retention is suspected.
      a. Should be less than 200 mL
      b. Culture, if pyuria is present
   2. Urinalysis (see Chapter 35, "Urinalysis")
I. Referral as surgical candidates
   1. Based on the particular situation and symptoms of the woman depending on
      a. Size of the prolapse
      b. Degree of symptoms
      c. Any related physiologic complications
      d. Offer the woman a pessary. Explain the conservative approach (see Chapter 46, "Pessary Insertion").
      e. Patient's feelings and attitudes toward surgery

IV. **Symptoms of anterior wall prolapse and uterine prolapse. Note: Symptoms increase with advancing age and tissue atrophy during the postmenopausal years.**
A. Prolapse
1. Dragging sensation
a. Usually occurs in the groin and sacral and lumbar area
b. Caused by downward force on the uterosacral ligaments and fasciae that support the uterus and vagina
c. Discomfort improves when the woman lies flat, relieving the downward pressure.
2. Sensation of peritoneal wetness probably caused by protrusion of moist vaginal walls rather than leakage of urine
3. The patient may complain of a sense of things falling out after prolonged standing.
4. The patient may notice a mass protruding from her vagina, particularly after bearing down, heavy lifting, or prolonged standing.
5. Erosions or ulceration of any mass that has protruded
6. Dyspareunia
B. Cystocele
1. Stress urinary incontinence caused by loss of urethral support of the lower vaginal wall
2. Difficulty emptying the bladder caused by loss of support of the upper anterior vaginal wall and bladder
3. Urinary urgency and frequency probably due to stretching of the bladder base associated with the prolapse, which is often less pronounced when patient is supine
4. Development of recurrent cystitis or a stone from stagnant urine if residual urine occurs
C. Stress incontinence
1. Occurs when intravesical pressure exceeds the maximum urethral closure pressure, in the absence of detrusor muscle contraction
a. Normally, the sphincter at the upper urethra is able to withhold urine.
b. Inability of the sphincter to withstand increased pressure is caused by
(1) Changes in the angle of the bladder
(2) Anatomic descent of the proximal urethra
(3) Failure of the neuromuscular support
(4) Inability of sphincter to resist increased abdominal pressure, resulting in uncontrolled expulsion of urine
2. Loss of support may also cause descent of the bladder neck, with the internal sphincter opening prematurely without voluntary compensation by the muscle surrounding it.

3. Often results from injury to the vesicourethral structure during childbirth
4. The condition is defined as the involuntary loss of urine with a sudden increase in intra-abdominal pressure from physical activity, laughing, lifting, aerobics, coughing, or sneezing.
5. Often leaks only small amounts
6. Need to rule out acute causes such as
   a. Urinary tract infection (usually associated with dysuria, urgency, and frequency)
   b. Atrophic vaginitis (may be present but may not be cause of the incontinence)
   c. Dietary irritants such as coffee, aspartame (Nutrasweet), and alcohol
   d. Medications such as doxazosin (Cardura)
   e. Diabetes (mellitus or insipidus)
   f. Pelvic mass pressing against the bladder or urethra
   g. Chronic urethritis
7. Urgency, frequency, nocturia, and dysuria do not usually occur.
8. Assess for other types of urinary incontinence or mixed disorders.
   D. Rectocele
   1. Feeling of rectal or pelvic pressure
   2. Difficulty in emptying the rectum
   3. Stool fills the rectocele the harder the patient strains.
   4. Must differentiate between true constipation (common in older women) and symptoms of a rectocele
   5. A woman may state that she has to press between the vagina and rectum (to reduce the rectocele) or press in the vagina to help with defecation; further supports the diagnosis.

Bibliography

Culligan, P. J. (2012). Nonsurgical management of pelvic organ prolapse. *Obstetrics & Gynecology, 119*(4), 852–860.

Edwards, S. L., Werkmeister, J. A., Rosamilia, A., Ramshaw, J. A., White, J. F., & Gargett, C. E. (2013). Characterisation of clinical and newly fabricated meshes for pelvic organ prolapse repair. *Journal of the Mechanical Behavior of Biomedical Materials, 23*, 53–61.

Ellington, D. R., & Richter, H. E. (2013). Indications, contraindications, and complications of mesh in surgical treatment of pelvic organ prolapse. *Clinical Obstetrics & Gynecology, 56*(2), 276–288.

Hagen, S., Stark, D., Maher, C., & Adams, E. (2006, October). Conservative management of pelvic organ prolapse in women. *Cochrane Database of Systemic Reviews, 4*, CD003882

Handa, V. L., et al. (2004). Progression and remission of pelvic organ prolapse: A longitudinal study of menopausal women. *American Journal of Obstetrics and Gynecology, 190,* 27–32.

Hawkins, J. W., Roberto-Nichols, D. M., & Stanley-Haney, J. L. (2011). *Guidelines for nurse practitioners in gynecologic settings* (10th ed.). New York, NY: Springer Publishing Company.

Tarnay, C. M. (2007). Pelvic organ prolapse. In A. H. DeCherney et al. (Eds.), *Current diagnosis and treatment obstetrics and gynecology* (10th ed., pp. 720–734). New York, NY: McGraw-Hill.

Urinary Incontinence

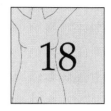

18

Helen A. Carcio

I. **Bladder dysfunction explained**
  A. Statistics
  1. Epidemiological studies suggest that 30% of all adults in the United States have some degree of incontinence.
  2. The actual frequency is probably much higher considering the significant underreporting of the problem because of patients' reluctance (Box 18.1).
  3. An estimated 75% of people affected are women.
  4. Demographic trends are changing the nature of the country and the health care landscape.
     a. The fastest growing segment of the population is the aging baby boomers; those between the ages of 45 and 65 have dramatically increased over the past 10 years.
     b. As the number of elderly increases, so will the need for incontinence services.
  5. Treatment of incontinence is not consumer driven. An astounding 50% of women affected never bring up the subject to their health care provider.
  B. Some thoughts
  1. The most common form of incontinence is mixed incontinence, particularly among older women.
  2. Aging itself does not cause incontinence, but the lower urinary tract does undergo some changes with age. These include
     a. Diminished muscle tone, bladder capacity, and voided volume
     b. The bladder is less compliant and less able to easily stretch with filling.
     c. Uninhibited bladder contractions and postvoid residual volumes increase.
     d. The function of the main pelvic floor muscle, the levator ani, deteriorates.
     e. The above changes are thought to be related to loss of estrogen to the cells and vascular insufficiency.

> **BOX 18.1** *Common Reasons Why Women May Be Reluctant to Discuss Incontinence*
>
> - They believe incontinence is a normal part of aging.
> - They are unaware there are conservative methods of treatment.
> - They erroneously think that surgery is the only treatment option.
> - They don't realize that they are not alone.
> - They are afraid they will be put in a nursing home.
> - They fear it is some form of cancer.
> - They are able to rely on expensive incontinence products.
> - They are not able to find resources to help with their problems.
> - They are ashamed and embarrassed.
> - They feel powerless and are resigned to their situation.

    (1) Symptoms include dysuria, incontinence, urinary frequency, and hematuria

    (2) There is an increased risk of urinary tract infections.

    (3) These symptoms and signs of genitourinary atrophy may develop slowly, over many months or years, or may have a more rapid onset.

    (4) Urogenital atrophy is the most likely consequence of menopause.

  f. The lower urinary tract and pelvic musculature are under the influence of estrogen and share a common embryologic origin with the vagina.

  g. Squamous epithelium of the trigone and urethra thins and blood flow decreases.

II. Pathophysiology of the lower urinary tract system (LUTS)

  A. The bladder and the urethra make up the lower urinary tract (Figure 18.1).

    1. The bladder is both a holding tank and a pump.

      a. Stores urine

      b. Empties when full

    2. Dome: The top of the bladder is the dome and is thin, stretchy, and collapsible.

      a. Extends as the bladder fills, much like a balloon

      b. Collapses when empty

    3. Base: The base of the bladder is the thicker and less distensible portion.

      a. The trigone is the lower portion where the ureters enter the bladder.

      b. The bladder fills from the bottom and rises above the pubic bone when full.

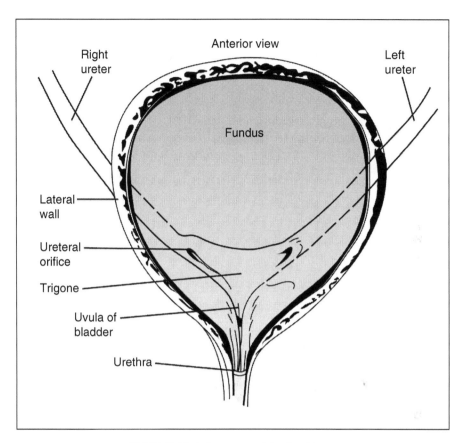

FIGURE 18.1 Anatomy of the bladder.

    c. Bladder fills at a rate of 1 mL per minute.
    d. Has an average capacity of 400 to 500 mL
  B. The bladder wall consists of three layers.
    1. Outer: Adventitial layer of connective tissue
    2. Middle: Contains the main muscle of the detrusor
    3. Inner: Mucous membrane
  C. Urethral sphincter
    1. Passes through the urogenital diaphragm and acts as a purse string to tighten the sphincter
    2. Muscles provide passive compression to keep the urethra closed during filling.
  D. Pelvic floor muscle. The levator ani is an internal diaphragm, which supports and stabilizes the pelvic organs.
    1. Acts as a voluntary sphincter for the urethra
    2. Forms an occlusive layer that closes the lower pelvic floor to resist the downward thrust of an increase in intra-abdominal pressure

   3. Consists of a strong striated long muscle
   4. Figure 18.2 clearly demonstrates a normal and relaxed pelvic floor outlet.
E. Neurophysiology
   1. Distension of the bladder activates stretch receptors at approximately 200 mL of urine.
   2. Sympathetic response facilitates urine storage by inhibiting the bladder contractions and stimulating the urethra to contract.
   3. Afferent impulses travel to the sacral spinal cord and the urge to urinate is felt.

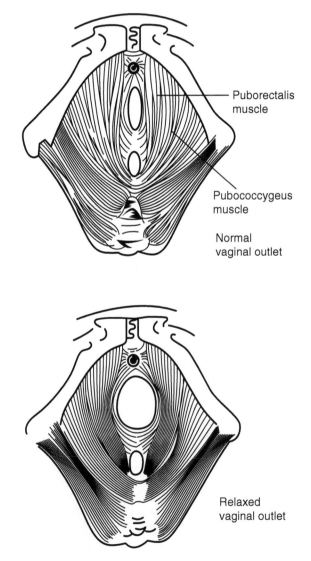

Puborectalis muscle

Pubococcygeus muscle

Normal vaginal outlet

Relaxed vaginal outlet

FIGURE 18.2 Comparison of a normal vaginal outlet to that of a relaxed pelvic outlet.

4. Efferent impulses return via the parasympathetic system.
   a. Detrusor contracts and the bladder empties
   b. The urethral sphincter at the bladder neck simultaneously relaxes to allow the urine to escape.
5. Pudendal nerve causes voluntary relaxation of the external sphincter and levator ani
6. Figure 18.3 provides a schematic diagram of the neurologic innervation of the bladder.

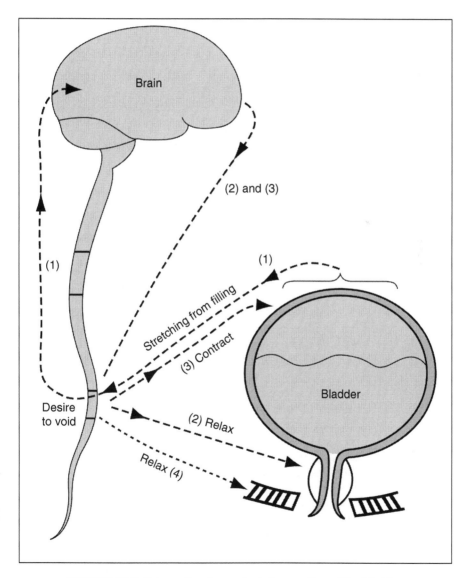

FIGURE 18.3 Schematic of neurologic innervation of the bladder.

III. Urinary incontinence explained
  A. Functional classification
  1. Failure to store
     a. Bladder
        (1) Involuntary muscle contractions
        (2) Low compliance or stretchability
        (3) Hypersensitivity to filling pressures
  2. Failure to empty
     a. Bladder does not contract efficiently
     b. Outlet obstruction due to a stricture or kink in the urethra (cystocele) or the pressure of an enlarged prostate
  3. Incontinence is the ultimate sign of storage failure.
  B. Requirements for urinary continence
  1. Intact intrinsic urethral sphincteric mechanism
  2. Well-supported bladder neck and urethra
  3. Normal bladder storage capacity at low pressure
  4. Good compliance
  5. Competent pelvic floor muscle

IV. Types of urinary incontinence
  A. Stress urinary incontinence (SUI)
  1. Involuntary loss of urine due to increased abdominal pressure on the bladder that exceeds maximal urethral pressure (the ability of the urethra to hold the urine in)
  2. Symptoms
     a. Urine loss, usually occurring at unexpected or inappropriate times
     b. Volume varies and is often described as occurring in spurts or drops.
     c. Precipitated by cough, sneeze, change in position, or other types of impact or exertional activities often related to sports
     d. Rare nighttime occurrence
  3. Cause
     a. Pelvic muscles act as a backboard or spring to absorb any increases in abdominal pressure and prevent overwhelming the urethral sphincter.
     b. When backboard becomes weakened or damaged, the bladder neck becomes displaced and opens the urethra to allow leaking.
     c. Abdominal forces generated to the bladder overcome the closing ability of the urethra and leaking occurs.
  B. Overactive bladder
  1. Symptom
     a. Symptom complex consisting of urgency, frequency, and urge incontinence; may not always be incontinent

    b. Characterized by sudden, strong feeling of urgency caused by uncontrolled (overactive) contractions of the detrusor during filling

    c. The urgency may be very strong or very subtle.

    d. The urge a woman experiences is actually a bladder contraction that creates a false need to empty the bladder before it is full.

    e. If the force of the contractions is too strong or the seal of the urethra is weak, uncontrollable urine leakage can occur.

C. Urge incontinence

    1. The involuntary leakage of urine that is often immediately preceded by an urge to urinate in the absence of physical activity

    2. Frequency associated with "triggers," such as running water or placing the house key in the front door

    3. Urine loss may be substantial since contractions may continue until the bladder is empty.

    4. Must distinguish from a normal strong urge to void, which can be controlled

D. Mixed incontinence

    1. A combination of stress and urge incontinence (Table 18.1)

    2. Probability increases with age

    3. Usually described as being "stress dominant" or "urge dominant" depending on which type of symptoms are more prevalent

    4. It is a combination of symptoms in which each requires special consideration.

    5. Table 18.2 compares the causes of stress and urge incontinence.

TABLE 18.1 Comparison of Presenting Symptoms

SYMPTOM	OAB	STRESS INCONTINENCE	IC
Urgency	X		X
Frequency	X		X
Leaking with physical activity		X	
Leakage volume	Large	Drops to small amounts	Variable
Nighttime urination	X	Rare	X
Inability to reach toilet in time with urgency	X		X
Pelvic pain			X

Mixed is a combination of the symptoms of urge and stress incontinence. OAB, overactive bladder; IC, interstitial cystitis.

TABLE 18.2 Comparison of the Causes of Incontinence

CAUSES OF STRESS INCONTINENCE	CAUSES OF URGE INCONTINENCE/OAB
Pregnancy	Urinary tract infection
Genetic factors	Bladder stones or tumor
Vaginal delivery, particularly if multiple	Lack of vaginal estrogen
Mild to moderate cystocele	Urethritis/urethral diverticulum
Inadequate estrogen levels	Cystocele
Previous pelvic surgeries/radiation	Neurological problems associated with stroke, Parkinson's disease, multiple sclerosis, or spinal cord problems
Obesity, particularly a high waist-to-hip ratio	
High-impact sports	Habitual frequent voiding
Medications (ACE inhibitors, alpha-adrenergic blockers)	Diabetes
	Incomplete emptying of the bladder
Long-term heavy lifting	Smoking
Chronic constipation	
Elevated BMI	
Chronic cough, often related to smoking Vascular changes associated with aging	

BMI, body mass index; OAB, overactive bladder.

E. Transient incontinence: Causes of incontinence that are usually caused by outside forces, which can be controlled or reversed (Box 18.2)
F. Interstitial cystitis (IC)
  1. Symptoms
    a. Complex of symptoms characterized by urinary urgency and frequency, pelvic pain, dysuria, dyspareunia, and nocturia
    b. Bladder is tender and pain increases with filling and is relieved with emptying.
    c. Is often misdiagnosed in the early phases of the condition as overactive bladder or urge incontinence (see Chapter 13, "Assessment of Pelvic Pain")
    d. Pelvic pain increases over the years and is often diagnosed as endometriosis.
    e. Symptoms worsen with intercourse (12–24 hours), menstrual cycle changes, seasonal allergies, and stress.
    f. No underlying cause has been identified.
    g. Diagnosis is difficult and may take up to 7 years of seeing various providers. It is usually made by exclusion.

BOX 18.2 *Causes of Transient Incontinence*

- Delirium/dementia
- Bladder infection
- Atrophic vaginitis/urethritis
- Medications
- Endocrine causes
- Restricted mobility
- Stool impaction/constipation
- Polyuria

V. **Diagnostic testing and differential diagnosis**
   A. Health history
   1. Begin by reassuring the woman that incontinence is a relatively common problem and that effective treatment is available.
   2. History includes the patient's perception of her symptoms, which helps determine the type and extent of urinary incontinence.
   3. Urinary symptoms of frequency, urgency, and incontinence mimic other bladder disorders and require special evaluation.
   4. Assess bowel function and type.
   5. Address the impact that incontinence has on the patient's life, self-esteem, and activities of daily living.
   6. Inquire about prior pelvic surgeries, number of vaginal deliveries, patient motility, medications, and history of urinary tract infection.
   7. Review use and extent of "self-help" measures, such as pad use and fluid reduction.
   8. See Box 18.3 for a sample of a tool used to assess the severity of urinary incontinence.
   B. Bladder voiding diary
   1. Obtain a 3-day recorded history of the woman's day-to-day bladder habits and patterns (see Appendix 18.1 for instructions on how to complete a bladder diary).
   2. Objectively document intake and output and extent of the problem.
   3. The diary allows the woman to focus on her behavior and how it relates to symptoms.
   4. The mere keeping of the diary can be therapeutic, and continence may improve once a causal relationship is established and documented.
   5. See Box 18.4 for a sample recording of the bladder diary.
   6. Review the use of any bladder irritants.
      a. The lining of the bladder is sensitive to certain types of foods and fluids, particularly those with high caffeine and acid content.
      b. It can cause "irritative symptoms" such as urgency and frequency.
      c. Box 18.5 lists the worst offenders in the Carcio "C" list.

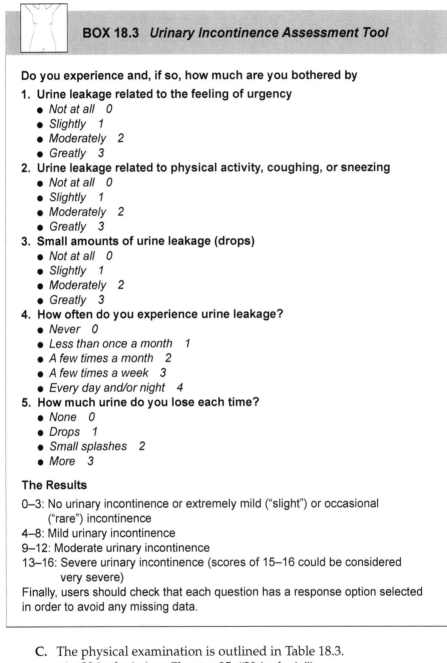

BOX 18.3 *Urinary Incontinence Assessment Tool*

Do you experience and, if so, how much are you bothered by

1. **Urine leakage related to the feeling of urgency**
   - *Not at all   0*
   - *Slightly   1*
   - *Moderately   2*
   - *Greatly   3*
2. **Urine leakage related to physical activity, coughing, or sneezing**
   - *Not at all   0*
   - *Slightly   1*
   - *Moderately   2*
   - *Greatly   3*
3. **Small amounts of urine leakage (drops)**
   - *Not at all   0*
   - *Slightly   1*
   - *Moderately   2*
   - *Greatly   3*
4. **How often do you experience urine leakage?**
   - *Never   0*
   - *Less than once a month   1*
   - *A few times a month   2*
   - *A few times a week   3*
   - *Every day and/or night   4*
5. **How much urine do you lose each time?**
   - *None   0*
   - *Drops   1*
   - *Small splashes   2*
   - *More   3*

The Results

0–3: No urinary incontinence or extremely mild ("slight") or occasional ("rare") incontinence
4–8: Mild urinary incontinence
9–12: Moderate urinary incontinence
13–16: Severe urinary incontinence (scores of 15–16 could be considered very severe)
Finally, users should check that each question has a response option selected in order to avoid any missing data.

C. The physical examination is outlined in Table 18.3.
   1. Urinalysis (see Chapter 35, "Urinalysis")
      a. Rule out infection. Elderly women may not have the characteristic symptoms of a urinary tract infection (UTI), such as burning urination, and may only have frequency and incontinence.

BOX 18.4 Bladder Diary

DATE _____ NAME _____

Complete one page for each of the next 3 days. In order to keep the most accurate diary possible, try to write down events as they happen.
Day: M___ T___ W___ Th___ F___ Sat___ Sun___

	FLUIDS	DID YOU URINATE?				ACCIDENTS		
TIME	What did you drink? How much (in ounces)? 1 cup = 8 oz.	Did you feel a strong, sudden urge to urinate?	What amount each time? (small, moderate, large)	Did you feel any pelvic discomfort?	What activity did this interrupt?	Circle if urine; square if stool	How much urine did you leak? Small: Drops; Med: < 1/4 cup; Lge: > 1/4 cup	What were you doing at the time?
8:45	Coffee 6 oz.	Yes No	S M L	Yes No	Walking	Yes No	Drops	Coughing
		Yes No	S M L	Yes No		Yes No		
		Yes No	S M L	Yes No		Yes No		
		Yes No	S M L	Yes No		Yes No		
		Yes No	S M L	Yes No		Yes No		
		Yes No	S M L	Yes No		Yes No		
		Yes No	S M L	Yes No		Yes No		
		Yes No	S M L	Yes No		Yes No		
		Yes No	S M L	Yes No		Yes No		
		Yes No	S M L	Yes No		Yes No		
		Yes No	S M L	Yes No		Yes No		

> **BOX 18.5 *Common Bladder Irritants***
>
> - Coffee and tea (sometimes even decaffeinated)
> - Chocolate
> - Carbonation
> - Coke and colas (Pepsi)
> - Citrus (whether juice or fresh)
> - Cranberry juice or pills
> - C vitamin
> - Cocktails
> - Crystal Light
> - Candy and other sugars
> - Chili and other tomato-based products
> - Chinese food (spicy or with monosodium gultamate)
> - Cigarette smoking
> - Condiments such as honey and artificial sweeteners—Aspartame (NutraSweet, Equal)
> - Cold remedies

    b. The presence of leukocytes and nitrates on a Multistix Reagent strip is a sensitive and inexpensive indicator.

    c. The presence of glucosuria or proteinuria requires further investigation.

    d. Hematuria may be indicative of bladder cancer and may require referral for cystoscopy.

  2. Postvoid residual

    a. It is the integral result of bladder contractility and urethral resistance.

    b. A high residual may indicate an inability of the bladder to contract against an increase in urethral pressure or a hypotonic bladder.

    c. A measurement of a residual that is 18% or less of the voided volume is acceptable.

  3. Vaginal cultures should be obtained (see Chapter 31, "Vaginal Microscopy").

    a. Urinary frequency may be a symptom of genital herpes.

      (1) Rule out genital herpes with herpes select serology type 2 testing. HSV (herpes simplex virus) 2 may be latent and/or asymptomatic for decades, activating in perimenopause or menopause. Presentations are atypical, further evading easy diagnosis.

  4. Assess for atrophic vaginitis (see Chapter 12, "Atrophic Vaginitis, Vulvovaginal Atrophy").

    a. The maturation index should be assessed in order to determine the presence and extent of atrophic vaginitis (see Chapter 32, "Maturation Index")

TABLE 18.3 The Focused Physical Examination in the Evaluation of Incontinence

Abdominal	Abdominal skin condition Bowel sounds Masses Suprapubic tenderness Bladder distention
Pelvic examination	Perineal skin condition Urethral characteristics Atrophism Vaginal infection Pelvic floor deficits such as cystocele or rectocele Palpation of the strength and symmetry of the levator ani muscle Bladder base tenderness in the anterior vagina Pelvic muscle laxity Pelvic mass Provocative stress test with direct observation of urine loss
Rectal examination	Skin irritation Perineal sensation Sphincter tone Presence and consistency of stool Masses or fecal impaction
Neurological examination	Gait Mental status Knee and ankle reflexes Perineal sensation of S2–S4 dermatones Anal reflex or "wink" (S2–S5) Bulbocavernosus reflex (S2–S4)
Laboratory assessment	Urinalysis for infection, blood, glucose, protein Urine culture for infection Cytology for atypical or malignant cells

  b. The presence of any parabasal cells on a wet mount may be considered documentation of atrophic vaginitis.

  c. Observe for the presence of a urinary caruncle, which can cause symptoms of urgency, frequency, and bleeding.

 D. Assess pelvic muscle tone (see Chapter 17, "Pelvic Organ Prolapse").

  1. Ask patient to squeeze around your two examining fingers while palpating the levator ani muscle.

  2. Note the patient's ability to sustain constriction and deflection of finger or fingers upward with a good squeeze. No deflection indicates weaker muscles.

      3. Constriction lasting a few seconds indicates weakening.

      4. A weakness may be indicative as the cause of SUI.

  E. Provocative stress test

      1. Stress testing has a sensitivity and specificity of more than 90%.

      2. Ask the patient to stand and cough with a moderately full bladder (150 mL).

      3. Observe for small spurts of urine that escape simultaneously with each cough. (May place pad between legs to catch and observe any urine released.)

      4. Delayed or persistant leakage suggests detrusor overactivity (triggered by coughing) rather than outlet incompetence.

      5. If urine escapes, place one finger on either side of the urethra to compress it.

      6. Ask the patient to cough again.

      7. If there is no loss of urine during the cough, the test is considered positive for stress urinary incontinence.

  F. Assess the neuronal support to the sacral dermatone, S2, S3, and S4. These dermatones innervate the micturation reflex (Figure 18.4).

      1. Lightly stroke the skin area innervated by the dermatones in the inner thighs. Note response to light touch. Compare contralateral sides.

      2. Bulbocavernosus reflex

         a. Stroke or gently squeeze the clitoris.

         b. Note contraction of the bulbocavernous muscle around the clitoris.

      3. Anal reflex (so-called anal wink)

         a. Lightly stroke the skin lateral to the anus.

         b. Note contraction of the anal sphincter.

  G. The cotton-tipped swab (Q-tip) test

      1. Determines the degree of the detachment of the proximal urethra (Figure 18.5)

      2. Place cotton-tipped swab through the urethra to the midurethral area.

      3. Ask patient to perform a Valsalva maneuver (hold breath while bearing down).

      4. Note change in the angle of the cotton-tipped swab.

         a. Normally, 10 to 15 degrees from the horizontal position

         b. If there is significant urethral detachment and loss of urethral sphincter muscle, the angle will exceed 30 degrees (Figure 18.5).

  H. Perform a simple cystometrogram (CMG) (see Chapter 36, "The Simple Cystometrogram") to determine the presence of stress incontinence, urge incontinence, or mixes.

VI. Follow-up

  A. Follow-up visits may range from 2 weeks to 3 months based on the patient's problems, response to therapy, and clinician/patient preference.

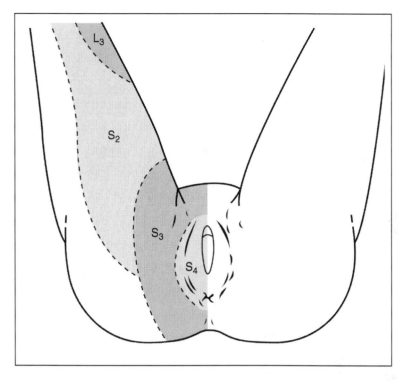

FIGURE 18.4 Sacral neuronal dermatones S2, S3, and S4 that innervate micturition reflex.

  B. Once the diagnosis is established an individualized plan of care is developed with the patient. Options include
    1. Pelvic floor muscle strengthening (see Chapter 37, "Pelvic Floor Electrical Stimulation")
      a. Kegel exercises, which include a rectal tightening and hold for 10 seconds followed by an equal period of relaxation
      b. Exercises should be repeated 30 times a day, 10 reps three times a day.
    2. Biofeedback training
      a. Uses computerized technology to isolate the pelvic floor muscles
      b. Monitors the electrical activity of the muscles through a vaginal or anal sensor and records any unwanted contraction of the accessory muscles using a sensor
      c. Can cure 30% to 70% of motivated patients over a series of six visits.

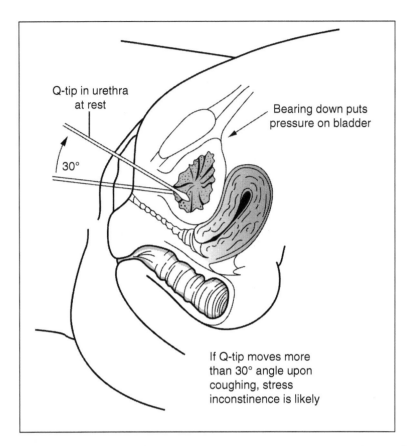

Q-tip in urethra
at rest

30°

Bearing down puts
pressure on bladder

If Q-tip moves more
than 30° angle upon
coughing, stress
inconstinence is likely

FIGURE 18.5 Cotton-tipped (Q-tip) swab test is used to determine the degree of detachment of the proximal urethra.

3. Vaginal support pessary (see Chapter 46, "Pessary Insertion")
   a. Vaginal device that elevates and stabilizes the bladder neck and increases urethral resistance
   b. Takes up redundant vaginal tissue, forming a sling that will support and elevate the uterus, and flatten and support a cystocele
4. Electrical stimulation (see Chapter 37, "Pelvic Floor Electrical Stimulation")
   a. Delivers a weak, painless electrical current to the pelvic floor muscles
   b. Inhibits bladder spasm by affecting the neural pathways between the pudendal nerve and the bladder

BOX 18.6 *Urge Suppression*

PATIENT EDUCATION: Urge

In the following exercises, you will learn to decrease frequency and urgency by calming the bladder. The urgency curve is similar to a labor contraction; you simply have to mentally and physically suppress the urge and ride through the contraction. It is a matter of "mind over bladder." Follow these simple steps. (You may leak a little during this training period.)

The urge strikes!

- Avoid rushing to the toilet. It will make matters worse.
- Sit down and try to relax.
- Do five "quick flicks." This is done by tightening your rectal sphincter for a couple seconds, and releasing for another few seconds. Quickly repeat this sequence five times in a row.
- Next, relax your body totally—try imagery—think of something pleasant and unrelated. (Preferably not the running water of a peaceful waterfall!) The urge should be decreasing by now.
- Do another set of five "quick flicks."
- This may completely make the urge go away, or at least suppress the urge long enough to allow you to squeeze and calmly walk to the bathroom.

5. Urge suppression
   a. Contracting the muscle of the pelvic floor reflexively causes the muscles of the bladder to relax.
   b. Box 18.6 lists the steps to use when teaching urge suppression.
6. Bladder retraining
   a. Bladder training is an important form of behavior therapy that can be effective in treating urinary incontinence.
   b. The goals are to increase the amount of time between emptying your bladder and the amount of fluids your bladder can hold. It also can diminish leakage and the sense of urgency associated with the problem.
   c. Bladder training requires following a fixed voiding schedule, whether or not you feel the urge to urinate.
   d. If you feel an urge to urinate before the assigned interval, you should use urge suppression.
   e. As success is achieved, the interval is lengthened in 15- to 30-minute increments until it is possible to remain comfortable for 3 or 4 hours. This goal can be individualized to suit each woman's needs and desires.

TABLE 18.4 Options in the Treatment of Incontinence

CONTINENCE TREATMENT OPTIONS	STRESS	URGE	MIXED	IC
Pelvic muscle exercises	X	X	X	X
Biofeedback/electromyography (EMG)	X	X	X	X
Reduction in use of bladder irritants		X	X	X
Treatment of vaginal urogenital atrophy	X	X	X	X
Pessary use	X	X	X	
Anticholinergics	Sometimes	X	X	X
Bladder retraining	Sometimes	X	X	X
Urge suppression		X	X	
Weight reduction	X		X	
Vaginal weights	X		X	
Smoking cessation	X	X	X	X

Note how mixed incontinence requires a combination of treatment options for stress and urge incontinence. IC, interstitial cystitis.

7. Table 18.4 summarizes the treatment options in the treatment of urinary incontinence.
C. Certain clinical conditions should be referred to a specialist.
   1. Uncertain diagnosis
   2. Hematuria without urinary tract infection
   3. Urinary retention with persistent symptoms of inadequate bladder emptying
   4. History of previous incontinence surgery, radical pelvic surgery, or pelvic irradiation
   5. Neurological conditions such as MS (muscular sclerosis), spinal cord injury, or neuropathy
   6. Suspicion of fistula or suburethral diverticula

VII. **There are valuable resources for information on urinary incontinence.**
   A. National Association for Continence (NAFC) website (www.nafc.org)
   B. Society for Urologic Nurses and Associates (SUNA)

Bibliography

Abrams, P., Cardozo, L., Fall, M., Griffiths, D., Rosier, P., Ulmsten, U., ... Standardisation Sub-Committee of the International Continence Society. (2003). The standardization of terminology in lower urinary tract function: Report from the standardization subcommittee of the International Continence Society. *Urology, 61*(1), 37–49.

Burgio, K. L. (2004). Behavioral treatment options for urinary incontinence. *Gastroenterology, 126*(1, Suppl. 1), 82S–89S.

Carcio, H. A. (2003). Comprehensive continence care. *ADVANCE for Nurse Practitioners, 12*(10), 26–35.

Carcio, H. A. (2004). Mixed signals: Treating overlapping symptoms of urinary incontinence. *ADVANCE for Nurse Practitioners, 12*(10), 32–36.

Castillo, P. A., Espaillat-Rijo, L. M., & Davila, G. W. (2010). Outcome measures and definition of cure in female stress urinary incontinence surgery: A survey of recent publications. *International Urogynecology Journal and Pelvic Floor Dysfunction, 21*(3), 343–348. [MEDLINE]

Foley, A. L., Loharuka, S., Barrett, J. A., et al. (2012). Association between the geriatric giants of urinary incontinence and falls in older people using data from the Leicestershire MRC Incontinence Study. *Age Ageing, 41*(1), 35–40. [MEDLINE]

Hawkins, J. W., Roberto-Nichols, D. M., & Stanley-Haney, J. L. (2011). *Guidelines for nurse practitioners in gynecologic settings* (10th ed.). New York, NY: Springer Publishing Company.

Kegel, A. H. (1948). Progressive resistance exercise in the functional restoration of the perineal muscle. *American Journal of Obstetrics and Gynecology, 56*, 238–249.

Lucas, M. G., Bosch, R. J., Burkhard, F. C., et al. (2012). EAU guidelines on assessment and nonsurgical management of urinary incontinence. *European Urology, 62*(6), 1130–1142.

Mahoney, C. (2002). Estrogen and recurrent UTI in postmenopausal women. *American Journal of Nursing, 102*(8), 44–52.

Mayo Clinic. (2010). Stress Incontinence. Retrieved June 25, 2012, from http://www .mayoclinic.com/health/stress-incontinence/DS00828

National Kidney and Urologic Diseases Information Clearinghouse. (2010). Urinary incontinence in women. Retrieved June 25, 2012, from http://kidney.niddk.nih. gov/kudiseases/pubs/uiwomen

National Library of Medicine—National Institutes of Health. (2011). Stress Incontinence. Retrieved June 25, 2012, from http://www.nlm.nih.gov/medlineplus/ ency/article/000891.htm

Ouslander, J. G. (2004). Management of overactive bladder. *New England Journal of Medicine, 35*(8), 786–799.

Parsons, C. L. (2002). Interstitial cystitis: Epidemiology and clinical presentation. *Clinical Obstetrics and Gynecology, 45*(1), 242–249.

Resnick, N. M., & Griffiths, D. J. E. (2003). Expanding treatment options for stress urinary incontinence in women. *Journal of the American Medical Association, 290*(3), 395–397.

Samselle, C. M. (2000). Behavioral interventions for urinary incontinence in women: Evidence for practice. *Journal of Midwifery and Women's Health, 45*(2), 94–103.

Sievert, K. D., Amend, B., Toomey, P. A., Robinson, D., Milsom, I., Koelbl, H, ... Newman, D. K. (2012). Can we prevent incontinence? ICI-RS 2011. *Neurourology and Urodynamics, 31*(3), 390–399.

APPENDIX 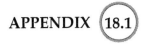 18.1

How to Record a Bladder (Voiding) Diary

Voiding diaries are important to help you understand the functioning of your bladder. It helps you track and know how much and when you drink liquids, how much and when you urinate, when you have that "gotta go" feeling, and how much and when you leak urine.

It describes your day-to-day bladder habits and patterns related to urination. It typically documents the time and amount of fluid intake (great way to look for bladder irritants), the time of each void, each accidental leaking, and a notation of the volume of urine loss.

It is an accurate measure of the urinary frequency, volume, and circumstance surrounding urinary accidents. You should take this chart with you should you decide to talk to your health care provider about your bladder problems. If you leak stool, put a square around the amount; if you leak urine, put a circle around the amount leaked.

How to Complete the Diary

1. Begin your diary when you wake up each day. Take notes throughout the day and continue until you complete 24 hours. For example, if you wake up at 7 a.m. on the first day of your diary, take notes until 7 a.m. the next day.

2. During the day, write down how much liquid you drink. If you do not know exactly how much liquid you are drinking, it's important to take a good guess about the number of ounces every time. Most containers will list the number of ounces they contain. Use these listings to help you make an estimate—for example, an 8-ounce cup of juice, 12-ounce can of soda, or a 20-ounce bottle of water.

3. Take note of how much urine you make during the day. If your health care professional asks you to keep a bladder diary, you will probably get a special collection device to use. It sits under your toilet seat. It is marked with measurements to let you know how much urine you make. Otherwise you can record the amounts in subjective terms of large (more than one-quarter cup), medium (less than one-quarter cup) or small (dribbles).

4. It is best to keep a bladder diary for 3 days in order to get the most accurate picture of your voiding patterns.

The diary is also a method for you to focus on your behavior related to overactive bladder and incontinence. Sometimes the mere fact of keeping the diary is therapeutic in and of itself, and the continence improves once a causal relationship with what you eat and drink and related activities has been established.

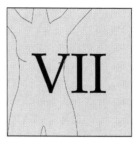

VII

Assessment of Women at Risk

The Sexual-Assault Victim

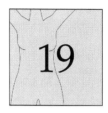

19

Karen Kalmakis

I. **Sexual assault explained**
A. Sexual assault is an invasive, traumatic crime that is accompanied by both legal and health concerns. All women are at risk regardless of age, socioeconomic status, ethnic background, or race.
   1. Twenty-nine percent of female rape victims experience their first rape between the ages of 18 and 24. The Federal Bureau of Investigation (FBI) has identified sexual assault as the most rapidly increasing violent crime in America.
   2. Only one quarter (25%) of rape victims receive medical care post-assault.
B. Many emergency departments are well equipped with a rape crisis team, which often includes sexual-assault nurse examiners (SANEs).
C. The legal definition of rape varies from state to state, but all definitions share similar components.
   1. Nonconsensual sexual penetration involving intimidation or the use or threat of force
   2. Legal definition of penetration: Invasion of the vulva, vagina, mouth, or anus
   3. Legal definition of lack of consent
      a. Assumed when a weapon or brutal force is used
      b. When the victim is a minor
      c. When the victim has physical or mental limitations or is under the influence of alcohol or other substances
D. Certain populations are at higher risk for sexual assault, including the homeless, people who are disabled, and young women.
E. Alcohol and drugs may be used to facilitate sexual assault. Seventy-two percent of sexual assaults among college students involve alcohol consumption by the victim, the assailant or, both.
F. Table 19.1 lists the definition of terms often used with a sexual assault.

TABLE 19.1 Explanation of Terms Used in Sexual Assault

TERM	DEFINITION
Stranger rape	Victim is assaulted by an unknown assailant for unknown purpose
Acquaintance rape	Assaulted by an acquaintance whom the victim has met previously during a nonthreatening social encounter—not considered a friend
Date rape	Occurred during a date or encounter in which the victim agreed to accompany the assailant; may occur after an initial encounter or after many dates of a nonthreatening nature
Intimate or partner rape, or marital rape	Sexual assault perpetrated by an intimate partner
Aggravated assault	Sexual assault of a victim who is disabled (mentally or physically) or elderly; associated with excessive force to cause physical injury
Incest	Sexual assault by a blood relative who is a close family member
Statutory rape	Sexual intercourse with a minor, defined by the state in which the incident occurs; it may be with or without consent

II. **Some reasons why women may not report sexual assault**
   A. Embarrassment
   B. Feelings of self-blame that they are somehow at fault
   C. Fear of retribution, especially if assailant is a known or close acquaintance
   D. Lack of faith in the medical or legal system
   E. Lack of knowledge concerning their legal rights
   F. Lack of access to health care
   G. Concerns about confidentiality
   H. The victim may not believe that date rape constitutes true sexual assault.
   I. The person may have financial constraints.
   J. The person may be unsure where to go for help.

III. **The forensic examination**
   A. Best performed by a specially trained SANE or an emergency department physician
   B. Examinations must be done within 5 days* (120 hours) of the sexual assault. However, the victim may seek health care weeks or months after the assault. (*This time may vary according to the jurisdiction in which the sexual assault occurred.)

C. Once a history of an assault has been identified, the practitioner should follow recommended guidelines.

IV. **Guidelines for the primary care provider following sexual assault**
   A. Facilitate emotional stability and safety of the victim.
   B. Determine time elapsed since the sexual assault and, **if fewer than 5 days and patient consents to forensic evidence collection,** refer to the emergency department for a forensic sexual assault examination.
   C. If **greater than 5 days** since sexual assault **or patient declines forensic exam**
      1. Obtain history of the assault using patient's own words when possible.
      2. Gather information about the victim's prior medical history, particularly her gynecologic history and risk for or presence of pregnancy.
      3. Document any injuries.
      4. If 5 days or less since assault, offer prophylaxis against sexually transmitted infections (STIs) and pregnancy (Box 19.1). If 5 days or more since the assault, offer testing for STIs and pregnancy as indicated. For more information on STI treatment see http://www.cdc.gov/std/default.htm
      5. Recommendations for HIV assessment of adolescent and adult patients 72 hours post–sexual assault.
         a. Assess risk for HIV infection
            (1) Increased risk of contracting HIV is associated with lack of condom use, genital and/or anal trauma, concurrent STIs, and HIV positive or unknown HIV status of assailant(s).
         b. If the patient appears to be at risk for HIV transmission from the assault, discuss antiretroviral prophylaxis options.
         c. Consult with a specialist as needed to discuss nonoccupational postexposure prophylaxis (nPEP) for HIV.
         d. If the patient chooses to start antiretroviral nPEP, give enough medication to last until the next return visit, reevaluate 3 to 7 days after initial assessment, and assess tolerance of medications.
         e. If nPEP is started, perform HIV, CBC (complete blood count), and serum chemistry lab testing at baseline (initiation of nPEP should not be delayed, pending results).
         f. Repeat HIV test at 6 weeks, 3 months, and 6 months.
      6. Arrange mental health counseling as well as physical health follow-up exam.
      7. Complete mandatory report forms as appropriate, for example, provider crime report, weapons report, elder or disabled persons report.

BOX 19.1 *Recommended Prophylactic Medication Regimens*

INFECTION/CONDITION	TREATMENT
Gonorrhea	Ceftriazone 250 mg intramuscularly, **or** cefixime 400 mg orally, **or** (if allergy to penicillin [PCN] or cephlasporines) azithromycin 2 g orally; each is administered in a single dose
Chlamydia	Azithromycin 1 g orally in a single dose, **or** doxucylcline 100 mg orally twice daily for 7 days
Trichomoniasis	Metronidazole 2 g orally in a single dose
Hepatitis B	Hepatitis B vaccination if not already immunized
HIV	Follow nonoccupational postexposure prophylaxis (nPEP) protocol and complete assessment of history, injuries, and risk
Pregnancy	Levonorgesterol (Plan B) l.5 mg **or** ulipristal (Ella) 30 mg orally in a single dose as indicated by history and human chorionic gonadotropin (hCG) testing Alternatively, consider copper-T intrauterine contraception (IUC)

8. Discuss with the patient the possibility of reporting the assault to police.
9. Discharge patient with written instructions to increase adherence to plan of care, including medication regimens.
10. Provide a list of community resources for victim support, for example, sexual assault support centers, women's centers, and rape crisis contact information.
11. Send the victim home in the care of family or friends.

V. Management
   A. Follow-up physical health examinations with health care providers are recommended at 4 to 6 weeks post–sexual assault in cases in which the patient received prophylactic medications immediately after the sexual assault. This follow-up examination should take place in 1 to 2 weeks if no prophylaxis was provided.
      1. Vaginal wet mount for microscopy examination
         a. Trichomoniasis
         b. Bacterial vaginosis

2. Gonorrhea culture from throat, cervix, and rectum as deemed appropriate from patient report of the assault
3. Chlamydia culture
4. HIV antibody screening (complete at 6 weeks, 3 months, and 6 months)
5. Hepatitis B surface antigen with hepatitis B immunizations as needed
6. Other interventions and care as clinically indicated (i.e., herpes lesions)
7. Provide ongoing counseling and support; determine the need for additional mental health counseling and referrals.
8. Pregnancy test if no menses since the sexual assault. If pregnancy test is positive, provide pregnancy-option counseling.
B. Additional follow-up should be scheduled for testing of infections that have a long incubation period before they are discernible in the serum.
1. Test for syphilis at 12 weeks.
2. Test for HIV at 3 and 6 months.
C. Continue mental health counseling as needed.

Bibliography

Brache, V., Cochon, L., Deniaud, M., & Croxatto, H.B. (2013). Ulipristal acetate prevents ovulation more effectively than levonorgestrel: Analysis of pooled date from three randomized trials of emergency contraception regimens. *Contraception, 88*, 611–618. doi:/10.1016/j.contraception.2013.05.010

Draughon, J. E., & Sherican, D. J. (2012). Nonoccupational postexposure prophylaxis following sexual assault in industrialized low-HIV-prelence countries: A review. *Psychology, Health & Medicine, 17*(2), 235–254. doi: 10.1080/13548506.2011.579984

Kalmakis, K. (2010). The cycle of sexual assault and women's alcohol misuse. *Journal of the American Academy of Nurse Practitioners, 22*(12), 661–666. doi: 10.1111/j.1745-7599.2010.00557.x

Linden, J. A. (2011). Care of the adult patient after sexual assault. *New England Journal of Medicine, 365*(9), 834–841. doi: 10.1056/NEJMcp1102869

Tjaden, P., & Thoennes, N. (2006). *Extent, nature, and consequences of rape victimization: Findings from the National Violence Against Women Survey.* Retrieved from fttp://www.ojp.usdoj.gov/nij

Workowski, K. A., & Berman, S. M. (2010). Sexually transmitted diseases treatment guidelines, 2010. *Morbidity and Mortality Weekly Report.* Retrieved from http://www.cdc.gov/mmwr/preview/mmwrhtml/rr5912a1.htm

Intimate Partner Violence

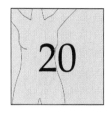

Karen Kalmakis

I. **Violence and abuse explained**
   A. Violence and abuse that is directed at women by their intimate partners is a serious, preventable health problem in the United States.
   B. When responding to the latest national survey, 29% of women reported physical, psychological, or sexual forms of intimate partner violence (IPV).
   C. Definition: Violent, threatening, or controlling behavior that is directed at a woman by a person with whom she has or had an intimate relationship
      1. The overwhelming majority of violence and abuse is perpetrated by men against women.
      2. Violence does occur in same-sex relationships.
      3. There is a small proportion of women who are abusive to men.
   D. There are three main forms of IPV
      1. Physical
         a. Slapping, pushing, punching, biting, burning, kicking, and choking
         b. Use of weapons; stabbing and shooting
      2. Psychological/emotional
         a. Threats of harm to the woman, her family, and pets
         b. Humiliation
         c. Economic control
         d. Isolation and control over activities
         e. Stalking
      3. Sexual
         a. Forced sexual acts
         b. Sexual contact while intoxicated, ill, or disabled
         c. Use of coercion or intimidation for sexual contact

    E. Violence against women interferes with the health of the woman.
      1. Failure to seek routine health care
      2. Delayed health care for injury or illness
      3. Delayed prenatal care
    F. IPV affects
      1. Women of every race, age, sexual orientation, religion
      2. People of all socioeconomic backgrounds and educational levels
      3. Both heterosexual and homosexual relationships
      4. Family members, friends, coworkers, and communities
    G. The relationship with the primary care provider
      1. We are now close to providing careful, sensitive, and safe assessment for violence and abuse in all women in all settings. However, for many reasons, many women in practice settings are still not routinely assessed for IPV. This problem is due more to a lack of knowledge on the part of the provider than to a lack of caring.
      2. Violence and abuse against women are given very little time in curricula; many providers do not understand how severe a health problem this is.
      3. Some providers are afraid women will be offended if they ask about abuse, whereas other providers worry that the woman will disclose violence and the provider will not know how to intervene.

II. **Principles related to assessment of violence and abuse**
    A. In its Clinical Preventive Services for Women report, the Institute of Medicine (IOM) recommended universal screening for IPV.
    B. Many women attempt to conceal the abuse, and any clues to the abuse may be subtle or absent.
    C. Some principles of assessment for abuse are the following
      1. Because abuse may be emotional or sexual, merely observing for signs of physical abuse during a routine visit may not be sufficient to rule out abuse. If there are obvious signs of what might be physical abuse, the provider should address the signs, for example, "Often when I see marks like this on women, it is because someone is hurting them. Is anyone hurting you?"
      2. Always screen for IPV when the woman is alone. She should never be asked questions about violence and abuse in front of anyone else.
      3. Screening questions should be direct and oral (see Box 20.1 for some suggested screening questions).
      4. Screen all women.
      5. The health care provider should be the one to screen for abuse. Do not delegate this task to support staff.
      6. If you do not speak the same language as the woman, you must obtain a professional interpreter to screen for violence and abuse, never use a family member or friend.

BOX 20.1 *Abuse Assessment Screening Questions*

1. Has your partner ever physically hurt you or threatened to hurt you?
2. Are you afraid of your partner?
3. Do you feel that your partner tries to control you?
4. Has your partner ever forced you to have sex when you did not wish to participate?

---

7. Have referral options available to give to women at the time of the visit, including a number she can call 24/7.
8. Make a follow-up appointment with her.
9. If the assessment reveals the woman is not abused, the provider may wish to take advantage of this "teaching moment" to talk about the prevalence of abuse, the seriousness of the problem, and how routine screening is necessary.
10. If the woman is abused, but does not disclose this information to you, your demonstration of concern for her may encourage her to disclose information at a future visit or seek assistance for IPV.
11. During visits in which a pelvic examination is planned, it is very important to ask about past or current sexual abuse since this type of exam may traumatize an abused woman.

D. If a woman discloses IPV, ask her what she wants to do.
   1. The woman herself knows how safe she is and whether she wants to leave the situation.
   2. Leaving the abusive partner may not be the solution, or even an option, for many women.
   3. The time immediately after a woman leaves her abuser is potentially the greatest period of risk for abused women.
   4. Do not encourage the woman to leave her abuser unless she wants to. Instead, listen to the woman, provide her with referrals, tell her how courageous she is, provide her with a safety plan, and have her come back and see you. These actions are interventions.
   5. Pregnant women should be screened for past abuse and abuse during pregnancy. Abuse may begin during pregnancy or may become more severe.

III. **Health consequences of IPV**
   A. Many physical and psychological health problems have been associated with IPV.
      1. In addition to physical injuries as a direct result of physical abuse, chronic health conditions and infections are related to IPV, including headaches, pelvic pain, dyspareunia, gastrointestinal reflux, sexually transmitted infections, and urinary tract infections.

2. Psychological conditions, such as anxiety, depression, eating disorders, and sleep disturbances, have also been associated with IPV.

3. Children who witness IPV in the household have poorer health throughout their lives.

IV. **Some concluding comments**

A. There now exists a solid body of literature about the health consequences of violence and abuse of women.

B. Most states have some type of protective orders to protect women from their abusers; some are good, and some are not. The courts in most states try to prosecute perpetrators.

C. Violence and abuse against women by their partners continues to be a public health problem that deserves the attention of all health care providers.

D. The goal it to provide sensitive, kind, well-informed, universal screening with appropriate referrals to all women who suffer from IPV.

Bibliography

Black M. C., Basile K. C., Breiding M. J., Smith, S. G., Walters, M. L., Merrick, M. T., … Stevens, M. R. (2011). *The National Intimate Partner and Sexual Violence Survey (NISVS): 2010 summary report.* Atlanta, GA: National Center for Injury Prevention and Control, Centers for Disease Control and Prevention. http://www.cdc.gov/violenceprevention/pdf/nisvs_executive_summary-a.pdf

Centers for Disease Control and Prevention. (2008). Adverse health conditions and health risk behaviors associated with intimate partner violence–United States, 2005. *Morbidity and Mortality Weekly Report, 57*(9), 113–117. http://www.cdc.gov/mmwr/preview/mmwrhtml/mm5705a1.htm

Decker, M. R., Frattaroli, S., McCaw, B., Coker, A., Miller, E., Sharps, P., … Gielen, A. (2012). Transforming the healthcare response to intimate partner violence and taking best practices to scale. *Journal of Women's Health, 21*(12), 1222–1229. doi: 10.1089/jwh.2012.4058

Domesticviolence.org

Dube, S. R., Anda, R. F., & Felitte, V. J. (2002). Exposure to abuse, neglect, and household dysfunction among adults who witnessed intimate partner violence as children: Implications for health and social services. *Violence, (17)*1, 3–17.

Institute of Medicine. (2011). *Clinical preventive services for women: Closing the gaps.* Washington, DC: The National Academies Press.

Weil, A. (2013). Intimate partner violence: Epidemiology and health consequences. In S. W. Fletcher & H. N. Sokol (Eds.), *UpToDate.* Retrieved from http://www.uptodate.com.silk.library.umass.edu/contents/intimate-partner-violence-epidemiology-and-health-consequences?source=see_link

Sexually Transmitted Infections

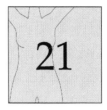

21

R. Mimi Secor

I. **Sexually transmitted infections (STIs) explained**
    A. Statistics and trends
        1. Previously known as sexually transmitted diseases, now referred to as STIs
        2. Approximately 20 million new infections occur each year (incidence) in the United States per the Centers for Disease Control and Prevention (CDC). The CDC also estimated there are more than 110 million total STIs (prevalence) among men and women in the United States.
        3. Nearly 50% affect 15- to 24-year-olds
        4. One in four teens has one or more STIs
        5. One in two African American teens has one or more STIs
        6. STIs are twice as common in African American populations.
        7. Significant physical and psychological consequences resulting from STIs
        8. The total for direct medical costs of managing STIs is estimated to be $16 billion (in 2010 dollars). These current estimates are based on CDC's analyses of eight common STIs: chlamydia, gonorrhea, hepatitis B virus (HBV), herpes simplex virus type 2 (HSV-2), human immunodeficiency virus (HIV), human papillomavirus (HPV), syphilis, and trichomoniasis.
        9. Reportable STIs include gonorrhea, chlamydia, and syphilis.
        10. STIs not reportable include HPV, HSV (herpes simplex virus), and *trichomoniasis*.
        11. Biological factors place women at greater risk than men for acquiring STIs and suffering from more severe health consequences associated with STIs.

B. Epidemiology. See Table 21.1 for a summary of STI assessment of the female.

  1. Chlamydia is the most common reportable STI
     a. With an estimated 1.3 million (in 2010) new cases each year
     b. More than half of the new cases remain undiagnosed and unreported.
     c. Leading cause of PID (pelvic inflammatory disease) and infertility in United States; also associated with chronic pelvic pain
  2. Gonorrhea is the second most common reportable STI
     a. An estimated 309,341 (in 2010) new cases each year; gonorrhea is also underdiagnosed and underreported
     b. Likely twice as common as reported numbers
     c. More common in southern and western United States
     d. More common in MSM (men having sex with men)
     e. Increases susceptibility to HIV threefold to fivefold
     f. Widespread fluoroquinolone-resistance among MSM and heterosexual populations
  3. Genital herpes is the most prevalent STI.
     a. Affecting one in five Americans, 25% of women, one out of three women over 30 years old, and over 50% of non-Hispanic Blacks are seropositive for HSV-2
     b. Most transmission occurs when patients are asymptomatic.
     c. Most symptoms are atypical.
     d. When signs do occur, they typically appear as one or more painful blisters in the urogenital area or rectum. The fluid-filled blisters soon break, leaving tender ulcers (sores) that may take 2 to 4 weeks to heal if it is the primary outbreak. Blisters infrequently appear on mucous membranes and are of very short duration when they do occur.
     e. HSV type 1 accounts for up to 35% of primary genital infections but rarely causes recurrences after first year.
     f. HSV type 2 is associated with the highest shedding and recurrence rate the first year with up to 1 in 3 days associated with asymptomatic or symptomatic shedding. Recurrences and/or asymptomatic shedding may continue over a lifetime, waxing and waning in variable ways per individual.
  4. HPV is the most common STI with the highest incidence among young populations
     a. Ubiquitous exposure among the sexually active young population
     b. Usually transient infection, clearing within 9 to 12 months
     c. HPV is the cause of cervical cancer, and this is a rare complication associated with persistent HPV infection with high-risk subtypes, including 16, 18, 31, and others.

    d. More than 100 different strains or subtypes exist, 30 of which are sexually transmitted.

    e. HPV can infect the genital area of men and women, including the skin of the penis, vulva, anus, and the vagina, cervix, and rectal mucosa.

  5. Syphilis rates have increased in recent years, especially among women

    a. Rates are six times higher in MSM than among heterosexual women.

    b. This is a decade-long trend.

      (1) Ten years ago, rates were equal among men and women.

    c. Recent 11% increase in women, reason unclear

    d. Known as "the great imitator" because the signs and symptoms are indistinguishable from those associated with other STIs and nonvenereal skin problems

C. Complications associated with STIs

  1. Chlamydia and gonorrhea, often asymptomatic and undiagnosed, if untreated, may lead to pelvic inflammatory disease (PID), ectopic pregnancy, chronic pelvic pain, and infertility.

  2. Long-term complications of chlamydia are much more serious in women.

  3. Many STIs increase risk of acquiring HIV, including gonorrhea, herpes, bacterial vaginosis, and syphilis.

  4. Several STIs are associated with preterm labor, including trichomoniasis and bacterial vaginosis.

  5. Cervical cancer is a rare complication from persistent HPV infection.

    a. HPV is the cause of cervical cancer.

D. Female considerations

  1. Women are more susceptible to STIs due to the extensive mucous membrane tissue lining the female genital area.

  2. Many STIs in women are asymptomatic, and most cases go undiagnosed.

  3. Chlamydia is three times more common in women than in men.

  4. HIV is increasing more rapidly in heterosexual women than in other groups.

  5. Women may be reinfected with STIs if their partners are not diagnosed and appropriately treated.

II. Clinical evaluation of female

  A. History

    1. Symptoms

      a. Onset, duration, severity, course

      b. Past history of same problem, symptoms, diagnosis, management

c. Self-care to present
d. Associated symptoms with review of symptoms (ROS)
  (1) Constitutional: malaise, fatigue, myalgia, chills, fever, weight loss, anorexia
  (2) HEENT (head, eye, ear, nose, and throat) (HSV-1, HSV-2, gonorrhea, syphilis)
    • Sores, lesions, oropharnygeal erythema, exudate, tenderness
  (3) Respiratory tuberculosis (TB)
    • Wheezing/rhonchi, rales, reduced breath sounds, pain with breathing
  (4) Cardiac (syphilis, gonorrhea associated endocarditis)
    • Murmurs, irregularity, other abnormal findings
  (5) Gastrointestinal (GI) (hepatitis, PID, HIV)
    • Abdominal, PID, back pain (pyelonephritis), upper right quadrant pain (liver), bloating, indigestion, nausea, vomiting, diarrhea, anorexia, weight loss
  (6) Genital/urinary (GU) (HSV-1, HSV 2, gonorrhea, chlamydia, trichomoniasis, bacterial vaginosis, candidiasis)
    • Urinary symptoms of frequency, urgency, dysuria, hematuria, odor, abnormal color to urine, back pain
    • Genital itching, sores, tears, lesions, burning, pain, discharge, odor, dyspareunia
  (7) Neurological (syphilis)
    • Mental status changes
  (8) Skin (syphilis, gonorrhea, HSV)
    • Sores, lesions, blisters, rashes, tattoos, branding, body piercings, icterus (hepatitis)
  (9) Extremities (gonorrhea, syphilis, lymphogranuloma venereum [LGV])
    • Arthralgias, joint stiffness, pain, swelling
2. Gynecologic history
  a. Pregnancy history summary including gravida, parous
    (1) Abortions: spontaneous, medical, surgical, miscarriage
  b. Menstrual history
    (1) Last menstrual period: Was it normal, late, lighter than normal?
    (2) Age of first period or menarche: How often, how many days; dysmenorrhea, new onset or worsening of dysmenorrhea; abnormal bleeding; bleeding after intercourse; type of protection used (tampons and/or pads)
  c. STI history
    (1) Record all STIs, including vaginal infections; dates of infections, how previously diagnosed and treated, inquire about any incomplete treatments; record

follow-ups, partner notification, and subsequent treatments

(2) Date last tested, what tests done, and results

d. Sexual history

(1) Record sexual partner, partners, gender, date of most recent sexual encounter, behaviors involved, frequency of sexual activity; daily, weekly, weekends only; dates of first penile/vaginal intercourse or coitarche, total number of sex partners, male, female, history of new partner in past 1 to 2 months, stated sexual orientation/preference

(2) Risky behaviors
- Unprotected vaginal, anal, oral (receptive, expressive); use of condoms (percentage); sex with money exchange; intravenous (IV) drug use; tattooing; body piercing; branding; violence; rape; abuse including violent sex play; using dirty sex toys
- High-risk partner(s)
  - Exposure to HIV, hepatitis B, hepatitis C, chlamydia, gonorrhea, IV drug use, sex worker, MSM, bisexual, group sex, abusive controlling partner with unknown history or suspected high-risk history

(3) Contraceptive history
- History of unprotected intercourse, consenting, rape, reluctant consent, access to emergency contraception (Plan B, ulipristal [Ella], or intrauterine contraception [IUC])
- Current contraceptive method, methods used in past, dates, problems, satisfaction with current method, complaints, and compliance with method of choice

(4) Pregnancy history

(5) Infertililty

e. Gynecologic surgery, procedures, problems

f. Personal hygiene

(1) Douching may increase risk of recurrent vaginal infections (e.g., BV [bacterial vaginosis]) and PID

(2) Tampon or pad use; deodorant tampons, synthetic, or cotton, note brand, use of panty liners; frequency of wear (daily versus with menses only)

(3) Type of underwear (i.e., thong underwear associated with vaginal infections)

(4) Hygiene practices
- Including poor hygiene, not wiping front to back, not washing after anal intercourse, not washing sex toys, poor oral hygiene, not washing hands or genitals before sex

- Use of soap, type, amount used, bubble baths, feminine hygiene sprays, other chemicals
  - Baths versus showers; source of water in bath or shower
  - **(5)** Clothing: tight clothing, workout clothing, pantyhose, bathing suit, duration of wear; particularly extended hours
  - **(6)** Genital and oral piercings
- **3.** Social history
  - **a.** History of sexual, physical, and verbal abuse
  - **b.** Lifestyle history; diet, exercise, sleep, stressors, occupation, recreation
- **4.** Medical history
  - **a.** Medical conditions: past and present, stable or unstable
  - **b.** Immunization status including TB, hepatitis A, hepatitis B
  - **c.** Date of last tuberculosis test and results
- **5.** Medications
  - **a.** Prescription: Borrowed or self-medication
  - **b.** Medication allergies
  - **c.** Over-the-counter medications
- **6.** Family history
- **B.** Examination
  - **1.** Vital signs
  - **2.** Skin
    - **a.** Lesions, rashes, ulcers, palmar or foot sole rash (syphilis), tattoos, piercings, brandings
  - **3.** Oral
    - **a.** Erythema, tenderness, sores, lesions; warts, exudate, plaques, thrush, Kaposi's sarcoma (KS)
    - **b.** Foul odor, gum disease, plaque, dental caries, poor hygiene
  - **4.** Respiratory
    - **a.** Determine whether there has been exposure to TB or if there are symptoms.
  - **5.** Cardiac
    - **a.** Tertiary syphilis
  - **6.** Abdominal
    - **a.** Absence of bowel sounds or increased bowel sounds
    - **b.** Masses, enlargement
      - **(1)** Lower abdominal mass consider PID with tubo–ovarian abscess (TOA)
      - **(2)** Right upper abdominal mass, consider hepatitis
      - **(3)** Inguinal nodes swelling and/or tenderness, consider HIV, pelvic, genital infection
    - **c.** Tenderness
      - **(1)** Cardiovascular accident (CVA) tenderness with pyelonephritis
      - **(2)** Right upper quadrant, consider hepatitis
      - **(3)** Lower abdominal, consider PID, cystitis

7. Pelvic examination
  a. External genitalia
    (1) Inguinal node tenderness or enlargement
    (2) Erythema, lesions, urethral discharge, fissures, tears, tenderness
    (3) Bartholin gland areas at 5 and 7 o'clock of vaginal introitus
    (4) Skene's glands at 3 and 9 o'clock of urethral meatus
    (5) Urethral caruncle, discharge
  b. Vagina
    (1) Introital erythema (focal or diffuse), lesions, tenderness, particularly between labial folds (displace tissue to fully visualize tissues)
    (2) Erythema, lesions
    (3) Discharge
      • Color, quality; flocular, creamy, coaty, clumpy, frothy; amount
    (4) Vaginal pH, amine potassium hydroxide (KOH) test; foul-fishy odor is positive
    (5) Vaginal microscopy/wet mount (see Chapter 10, "Assessment of Menopausal Status")
  c. Cervix
    (1) Redness, cervical erosion, ectropion, mucopus, friability, bleeding
    (2) Cervical os, size, shape, mucopus from os, quantity
    (3) Cervical motion tenderness; mild, moderate, severe, or positive chandelier test suggestive of PID
  d. Bimanual exam of uterus and adnexae
    (1) Tenderness; mild, moderate, severe, rebound, localized, masses, mobility
    (2) Uterus size, shape, mobility, firmness, tenderness
    (3) Ovaries
      • Palpable or nonpalpable
      • Tenderness; mild, moderate, severe
      • Fullness or masses
  e. Rectal
    (1) Lesions; sores, blisters, warts, tags, fissures, tears, hemorrhoids
    (2) Erythema, hemorrhoids, lesions, tenderness, discharge
8. Extremities
  a. Joint swelling, tenderness, increased heat, reduced range of motion
C. Diagnostic testing per the CDC STI Guidelines
  1. Chlamydia testing
    a. Yearly screening of all sexually active women under the age of 25 years

       b. Screen women 25 years old and older if new or multiple sexual partners or history of high-risk behaviors

       c. Retesting 3 months after treatment to prevent reinfection

       d. If retesting in 3 months doesn't occur, then retesting within 12 months following initial treatment is recommended.

  2. Gonorrhea testing

       a. Men having sex with men, bisexual, heterosexual females with sex partners of unknown risk, or who have high-risk partners, females not using condoms, new partner

       b. History of STIs

       c. Women with previous gonorrhea infection; those who engage in commercial sex work and drug use; women in certain demographic groups; and those living in communities with a high prevalence of disease

       d. The U.S. Preventive Services Task Force (USPSTF) does not recommend screening for gonorrhea in men and women who are at low risk.

  3. Genital herpes

       a. Cultures if fluid-filled blisters or very moist lesions

       b. Polymerase chain-reaction (PCR) culturing is four times more accurate than non-PCR; therefore, nonblistering lesions may be tested with greater accuracy.

       c. HSV type 1- and type 2-specific IgG (immunoglobulin G) antibody testing are the gold standard diagnostic tests for nonprimary HSV testing.

         (1) Nearly 100% seroconversion within 4 months of infection

         (2) Initial negative test indicates probable primary infection with recent acquisition of infection

         (3) There is no type-specific Immunoglobulin M (IgM) antibody test and therefore IgM should not be ordered.

  4. HIV

       a. MSM, bisexual, IV drug use, high-risk partner

       b. Possible false-positive rate with point-of-care salivary testing (orasure); confirmatory serology testing should be done

       c. CDC recommends universal screening unless at very low risk. Of the 50,000 new cases each year in the United States, 25% report no risk factors.

  5. Hepatitis B

       a. MSM, bisexual, IV drug use, high-risk partner

  6. Hepatitis C

       a. MSM, bisexual, IV drug use, high-risk partner

       b. CDC recommends one-time screening of all adults. This is because 1 out of 30 adults in the United States is positive for hepatitis C, and most are unaware they are infected.

  7. Syphilis

       a. MSM, bisexual, IV drug use, high-risk partner

       b. On the increase among heterosexual women

TABLE 21.1 Sexually Transmitted Infection Assessment of the Female

INFECTION	CAUSE	PREVALENCE	SYMPTOMS	DIAGNOSIS
Chancroid	Hemophilus ducreyi, gram-negative bacillus	More common in populations exchanging sex for money	Women are often asymptomatic, single painful genital ulcer in men; usually fewer than 4 lesions	Culture + or polymerase chain reaction (PCR) + for *H. ducreyi*, rule out more common HSV, also HIV, syphilis by rapid plasma reagin (RPR)
Chlamydia	Obligate intracellular parasite susceptible to antibiotics	Most common reported STI, 3 million new cases a year; leading cause of preventable infertility	Often asymptomatic in women, so need for widespread screening < 26 years old	Universal screening if < 26 years old urine, cervico-vaginal, or cervical NAAT/PCR (nucleic acid amplification test/polymerase chain reaction) testing
Genital herpes	Type 1 or 2 herpes virus; both can infect genitals	Estimated 55 million Americans infected	Most asymptomatic, most transmission when asymptomatic; symptoms may include painful genital lesions; first infection most severe, recurrences most common with HSV-2, widely variable symptoms	Classic symptoms suspect HSV culture if lesions PCR culture more sensitive, expensive; type-specific serology IgG/herpes select; 98% seroconversion 4 months post-HSV acquisition
Genital warts	Nononcogenic HPV, 6, 11	1 million visits yearly; HPV affecting up to 80% of sexually active young women in the United States	Single or multiple, soft, fleshy, nontender, cauliflower-like lesions in genital area including vulvovaginal, anal, or cervix	By exam, HPV DNA testing not recommended; RPR to rule out condylomata lata of syphilis; colposcopy and/or biopsy of atypical lesions

(continued)

TABLE 21.1 Sexually Transmitted Infection Assessment of the Female *(continued)*

INFECTION	CAUSE	PREVALENCE	SYMPTOMS	DIAGNOSIS
Gonorrhea	*Neisseria gonorrhoeae*, gram-negative diplococcus bacteria	Second most common STI in the United States, especially among MSM	Women commonly asymptomatic, or abnormal vaginal discharge, dysuria, abnormal menses	Gram stain, (50% sensitivity) culture, NAAT of cervical or vaginal secretions; urine NAAT an option too
Pelvic inflammatory disease (PID)	Polymicrobial, various combinations, *N. gonorrhoeae*, *C. trachomatis*, anaerobes, and others	1 million new cases yearly; leading cause of female infertility	Many have no symptoms or atypical symptoms; symptoms include pain/tenderness lower abdomen, uterus, ovaries, fever, chills, elevated WBCs/ESR (erythrocyte sedimentation rate), associated with menses	High index of suspicion, low threshold for diagnosis, + cultures, CDC criteria, pelvic exam tenderness, mucopus, WBCs on vaginal microscopy
Syphilis	*Treponema pallidum* spirochete	Increasing among MSM, unusual in women unless risk factors: higher rates in the Southwest	Primary: Classic chancre is painless indurated ulcer in genital area at site of exposure, may evade diagnosis if vaginal Secondary: Variable skin rash, may involve palmar hands, soles of feet Latent: No signs or symptoms, positive serology, negative spinal tap	Primary: Darkfield exam of chancre, with RPR serology Secondary: Latent; RPR serology
Trichomoniasis	Motile protozoan	Most common curable STI in the United States and worldwide, 3 million U.S. women infected yearly may be asymptomatic for years	Excessive, frothy, yellow-green vaginal discharge, exam findings variable, sometimes with genital erythema, swelling, and pruritus	Vaginal microscopy for typical motile trichomonads and WBCs; Pap should be verified with culture or microscopy Various vaginal cultures may also be used PCR

Acknowledgment

Thanks to Dr. Jeffrey Gilbert for his review of this chapter.

Bibliography

American Academy of Pediatrics. (2013). Diagnostic testing for sexually transmitted infections. Healthy Children. Retrieved from http://www.healthychildren.org/ English/health-ssues/conditions/sexually-transmitted/pages/Diagnostic-Testing-for-Sexually-Transmitted-Infections.aspx

American Cancer Society. (2014). Testing for HPV. American Cancer Society. Retrieved from http://www.cancer.org/cancer/cancercauses/othercarcinogens/ infectiousents/hpv/humanpapillomavirusandhpvvaccinesfaq/hpv-faq-h-p-v-testing

American Sexual Health Association. (2013). Getting tested for STDS/STIS. American Sexual Health Association. Retrieved from http://www.ashasexualhealth.org/ std-sti/get-tested.html

Batteiger, B. E. (2014). Screening for chlamydia trachomatis. UpToDate. Retrieved from http://www.uptodate.com/contents/screening-for-chlamydia-trachomatis

CDC. (2010). 2010 STD treatment guidelines. Retrieved from http://www.cdc.gov/ std/treatment/2010/default.htm

CDC. (2011). Sexually transmitted disease surveillance, 2011. Retrieved from http:// www.cdc.gov/std/stats

CDC. (2013). Public health grand rounds: Reducing the burden of HPV-associated cancer and disease through vaccination in the US. Retrieved from http://www. cdc.gov/about/grand-rounds/archives/2013/February2013.htm

Handsfield, H. H. (2013). Real-world strategies to maximize guideline-driven serology screening for HIV and syphilis. *Sexually Transmitted Diseases, 40*(4), 275–347.

Minichiello, V., Rahman, S., Hawkes, G., & Pitts, M. (2012). STI epidemiology in the global older population: Emerging challenges. *Perspectives in Public Health, 132*(4), 178–181.

Office on Womens Health. (2012). Sexually transmitted infections fact sheet. Office on Womens Health. Retrieved from http://www.womenshealth.gov/publications/ our-publications/factsheet/sexually-transmitted-infections.html

Owusu-Edusei, K., Chesson, H, W., Gift, T. L., Tao, G., Mahajan, R., Ocfemia, M. B., & Kent, C. K. L. (2013). The estimated direct medical cost of selected sexually transmitted infections in the United States. *Sexually Transmitted Diseases, 40*(3), 197–201.

Planned Parenthood. (2014). Sexually transmitted diseases. Planned Parenthood. Retrieved from http://www.plannedparenthood.org/health-topics/stds-hivsafer-sex-101.htm

Satterwhite, C. L., Torrone, E., Meites, E., Dunne, E. F., Mahajan, R., Ocfemia, M. C. B., & Weinstock, H. (2013). Sexually transmitted infections among women and men: Prevalence and incidence estimates. *Sexually Transmitted Diseases, 40*(3), 187–205.

Swygard, H., & Cohen, M. C. (2013). Screening for sexually transmitted infections. *UpToDate*. Retrieved from http://www.uptodate.com/contents/screening-for-sexually-transmitted-infections

Torrone, E. A., Johnson, R. E., Tian, L. H., Papp, J. R., Datta, S. D., & Weinstock, H. S. L. (2013). Prevalence of neisseria gonorrhoeae among persons 14 to 39 years of age, United States, 1999 to 2008. *Sexually Transmitted Diseases, 40*(3), 202–205.

World Health Organization. (2014). Sexually transmitted infections. World Health Organization. Retrieved from http://www.who.int/topics/sexually_transmitted_ infections/en

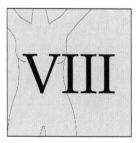

VIII

Infertility and Subfertility Assessment

Initial Evaluation of Infertility

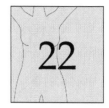

22

Carol Lesser

I. Infertility explained

A. Infertility affects the ability to conceive and carry a pregnancy to term.

1. Infertility affects approximately 7.3 million women and their partners or approximately 15% to 20% of the reproductive age population in the United States.

2. Infertility affects both females and males. Both should be evaluated.

3. Most patients are not infertile, but instead, subfertile. Choice of words can affect patient self-perception.

4. Primary infertility refers to trying to conceive with no prior history of pregnancy.
   a. Trying to conceive for 12 months or more younger than 35 years
   b. Trying to conceive 6 months or more 35 years and older
   c. Also includes those with known problems that prevent pregnancy, such as blocked tubes, anovulation, or male factor problems

5. Secondary infertility refers to women who have trouble conceiving a child after prior success.
   a. Bureau for Health Statistics estimates more than 3 million women of reproductive age in the United States have secondary infertility
   b. Age is most often a factor.

6. The number of infertility clinics in the United States is more than 400.
   a. Since the birth of the first IVF baby in 1978, in vitro fertilization (IVF) centers have offered comprehensive evaluation and treatments with significant advances in the field of reproductive medicine.
   b. Worldwide, more than 3 million babies have been born as a result of IVF.

7. Assisted reproductive technology (ART) is the term used for fertility-related treatments.

8. Physicians who offer these services work in the field of reproductive endocrinology and infertility and are called REIs (reproductive endocrinology and infertility).

   a. Advanced practice clinicians can play a key role in the assessment and treatment of the fertility patient.

   b. Advanced practice clinicians can facilitate prompt referral to assisted reproductive technology services when appropriate.

9. Most individuals with a fertility-related problem never seek evaluation or treatment. IVF and its associated technologies remain an underutilized mode of treatment, often due to misconceptions that clinicians can help redress.

10. The clinician's goal is to help diagnose, treat, and resolve infertility. Find the best resources to assist them in moving forward. These include

    a. Helping those who prefer adoption

    b. Third-party reproduction

    c. Child-free living

B. More women than ever before are seeking diagnosis and treatment of fertility-related problems. Several factors have contributed to this increase.

1. Delayed childbearing has become the norm for increasing numbers of women who start trying to conceive after 35 when natural fertility rates have already declined.

2. Infertility centers are increasingly taking care of women who are past their reproductive prime and as a result may require more intensive treatments.

3. Availability of third-party reproduction, including donor egg and gestational carriers, is available in most centers.

4. The development of egg banks similar to sperm banks has made donor egg treatment more affordable and attractive to more individuals.

5. Singles and same-sex couples are increasingly requesting fertility-related services as our societal acceptance of alternative ways for family building increases.

6. Availability of adoptable babies remains a challenge as costs, screening requirements, and numbers of healthy infants limit access for many. This has contributed to the popularity of ART treatments.

7. Infertility causes significant stress and affects every aspect of a woman's life and relationship. Increasingly fertility centers offer a range of services to address these needs.

C. Causes of infertility

1. The cause may be due to female or male factors and often is a combination of both. Counsel patients to avoid blame.

⌐ **BOX 22.1** *Causes of Infertility and Subfertility*

- Advanced maternal age
- Ovulatory factor
- Tubal factor
- Uterine factor
- Male factor
- Cervical factor
- Combined
- Unexplained

Infertility is a "couples" issue except in the case of those using donor gametes.

2. Female factors include advanced age, ovulation disorders, tubal and uterine factors. Female age is a prime contributor, often causing subfertility or premature ovarian insufficiency (POI).

3. Male factor includes obstructive and nonobstructive causes of absent sperm (azoospermia).

   a. Males are evaluated for potential anatomic and or endocrine issues; prior infection or trauma; genetics; lifestyle; and environmental/occupational exposure as causes of subfertility, infertility, or sterility.

   b. The initial female workup (for those who present with a partner) always includes a semen analysis.

4. The single most important factor that influences the ability to conceive is maternal age. Remember, fertility starts to measurably decline in a woman's 20s.

5. Monthly fecundity in the general population has been estimated between 15% to 20%, decreasing exponentially with advanced age. Most individuals overestimate their monthly chances to conceive and equate ovulation with fertility.

6. Unexplained infertility accounts for a small percentage of cases. In general, unexplained infertility can be attributed to age.

7. Box 22.1 contains a summary of the causes of infertility.

II. **Health assessment of the infertile woman/couple**

A. Initiate a workup for anyone trying to conceive if there is a known fertility problem such as anovulation or blocked tubes, recurrent miscarriage, or any reason to question the ability to conceive. There is no good reason to turn a patient away who wants reassurance regarding her fertility potential.

B. Increasingly, younger women present for fertility preservation if they are diagnosed with cancer requiring gonadotoxic treatments during their reproductive years.
   1. Learn where to refer these patients. Fertility preservation programs are often regional.
   2. The national organization, Fertile Hope, can assist with patient support and referrals.
C. Take a thorough history of both parties.
   1. Be sensitive to issues of confidentiality.
   2. Women may not want partners to know about a previous therapeutic termination.
D. When treatment is started, informed consent involves both parties. If couples disagree on treatment, counseling is strongly recommended.
E. Identify risk factors
   1. Gynecologic factors including prior intrauterine device (IUD) use, loop electrosurgical excision procedure (LEEP) or coninization of the cervix, pelvic inflammatory disease (PID), irregular cycles, menorrhagia, severe dysmenorrhea or dyspareunia, which might suggest endometriosis.
   2. Reassure patient that cervical polyps will not adversely affect fertility. If they are annoying and friable, they may be removed for those reasons.
   3. Smoking is the most deleterious habit to screen for but check for any substance abuse.
   4. Occupational exposures such as nitrous oxide are associated with reduced fertility and spontaneous abortions. Dry-cleaning chemicals and mercury have also been associated with decreased fecundity.
F. Be aware that the level of stress associated with infertility is similar to what is experienced in a terminal illness.
   1. Anger, depression, frustration, and anxiety are commonly reported. Try to remain nonreactive and offer timely support and appropriate referrals as needed.
   2. A well-informed patient who understands her treatment options and prognosis will be easier to care for. Support groups or individual counseling resources are available.
   3. Accommodating patient requests for appointments in a timely manner is important. Patients feel that time is running out. Tests are often cycle-day dependent and patients are very sensitive to "losing a month" while waiting to be seen.
G. A thorough history and physical should be performed initially.
H. See Appendix 22.1 for assessment forms for female and male.

BOX 22.2 *Ferriman–Galwey Tool to Assess Hirsuitism*

- Hair growth is rated from 0 (no growth of terminal hair) to 4 (complete and heavy cover)
- Nine locations: upper lip, chin, chest, upper back, lower back, upper abdomen, lower abdomen, the upper arms and the thighs
- Maximum score of 36
- In White women, a score of 8 or higher is regarded as indicative of androgen excess
- With other ethnic groups, the amount of hair expected for that race should be considered.

III. **Physical examination of the infertile woman**
A. A complete physical is recommended before treatment is initiated.
  1. Check height, weight, and body mass index (BMI) or another method of evaluating body-fat composition.
     a. Women of very short stature may need evaluation for Turner's (XO) syndrome. Check karyotype.
     b. Extremes in weight (BMI) are associated with health risks as well as infertility or subfertility.
     c. Extremely low BMI may be associated with anovulation secondary to hypothalamic hypogonadism, which baseline hormones can usually detect.
     d. Elevated BMI is often associated with polycystic ovarian syndrome (PCOS), hyperinsulinemia and, in severe cases, metabolic syndrome, requiring a multidisciplinary approach.
  2. Check for hirsutisim.
     a. The Ferriman–Gallwey grading system can be helpful. Many women seek electrolysis or laser treatment so ask whether they have had these procedures done (Box 22.2).
     b. Hyperandrogenic states are often associated with PCOS and less often with congenital adrenal hyperplasia (CAH), which can affect ovulation.
     c. Excessive hair growth on the upper torso and back can suggest more significant hyperandrogenism.
     d. If acanthosis nigricans (leathery brown discoloration of skin at back of neck, axilla, or other skin folds) is found, this also suggests the severe hyperandrogenism associated with hyperinsulinemia and metabolic syndrome.

    e. These sequelae are seen in more severe cases of PCOS. Similarly, facial acne or more extensive acne on the upper torso and back are associated with PCOS or other hyperandrogenic states.

3. Thyroid examination should be performed.

    a. Thyroid nodules or enlargement may provide an explanation for difficulty in conceiving.

    b. Thyroid function tests should always be performed, including thyroid antibodies, if patient is hypothyroid or has a strong family history since the presence of thyroid antibodies may be more significant than the finding of subclinical hypothyroidism.

4. Breast examination with attention to nipple discharge (galactorrhea), either spontaneous or expressive

    a. May be associated with hyperprolactinemia, which can block ovulation, thus preventing pregnancy

    b. If appropriate, a mammogram should be ordered. Always check a prolactin level.

5. A pelvic exam should be performed.

    a. If cervical motion tenderness or unusual discharge are noted, then sexually transmitted infection (STI) testing should be performed.

    b. Chlamydia affects 4 to 5 million women annually in the United States. If untreated, it can cause tubal factor infertility.

    c. If a Pap smear has not been done, then either perform one or arrange for this to be done.

6. Blood pressure, cardiac, and lung auscultation should be performed. Abdominal exam and skin evaluation are also required.

7. The time of the exam can be an optimal opportunity to check for smoking or drug use. Often the smell of cigarettes will be noted on the serious smoker.

    a. Fertility is adversely affected for both males and females, and this issue should be addressed at the outset.

    b. Women who smoke are at risk for earlier menopause and embryo quality is negatively affected by nicotine.

    c. Miscarriage rates are higher for smokers.

    d. Signs of drug abuse may prompt permission for toxicology tests and counseling.

8. Women of advanced age, usually described as older than 45, are often required to have a more thorough initial exam, including mammogram, EKG, and oral glucose tolerance testing, as well as a request for clearance from her ob/gyn for pregnancy-related treatments and ability to carry a pregnancy.

9. Ensure that vaccinations are up to date, including rubella and varicella, as well as seasonal flu vaccination. It is always best to address preconception.

IV. **The initial workup**
A. The infertility evaluation begins with a visit with both parties ideally, if a couple is involved. Allotting a full hour is reasonable. This allows for history, exam, discussion, and ordering of appropriate tests.
   1. Evaluative tests should be accomplished within 1 to 2 months.
   2. Patients often present with unnecessary fears of tests and treatments. A thorough review of the basic tests, including blood, ultrasound, and x-ray for females and semen analysis and blood tests for men, can help patients feel less anxious.
   3. Make yourself accessible to answer patient questions and concerns promptly.
   4. Education regarding sexual intercourse
      a. Inform patients that only sperm-safe lubricants are acceptable and that many over-the-counter lubricants are not recommended. Sperm safe pH-balanced lubricants mimic midcycle secretions. When in doubt, natural oils work well, without interfering with sperm.
      b. Do not tell patients how often to have intercourse. There is no data to suggest that too frequent ejaculations will have a negative effect on conception.
      c. No need for women to remain on their backs or with raised hips or in bed after intercourse
      d. Douching after intercourse is not permitted.
   5. A menstrual cycle history will suggest if a woman is ovulatory.
      a. Regular cycles are highly correlated with ovulation. For those with regular cycles, midcycle secretions suggest preovulation.
      b. Instructing the couple to have intercourse twice a week should be adequate to cover her ovulation.
      c. Telling a woman that too much sex is harmful is not evidence based. Only one properly timed exposure can be adequate.
      d. It is stressful to give overly restrictive advice that is not based in fact.
   6. Taking a thorough history will reveal particular risk factors. Query for
      a. Prior and current medical, surgical, gynecologic, infectious, and genetic problems for the patient, her partner, and immediate family
      b. Previous cervical conization or LEEP may have affected cervical mucus secretory glands or caused stenosis.

    c. Significant dysmenorrhea and/or dyspareunia might be associated with endometriosis.

    d. Menstrual history including age at menarche and interruptions to normal cyclicity and for how long

    e. Ask about normal pubertal milestones.

    f. Check for history of irregular or dysfunctional bleeding, eating disorder, excessive athleticism, or obesity.

    g. Prior methods of birth control

       (1) IUD use and positive STI history may have caused tubal damage.

       (2) Hydrosalpinges reduce implantation most likely due to the adverse affect of backflow of the intratubal fluid on the endometrium.

    h. Previous obstetrical history including parity, miscarriages, ectopics, terminations, premature deliveries

    i. Gynecologic procedures such as laparoscopy, laparotomy, or hysteroscopy with surgical findings

    j. Fibroids, endometriosis, and adenomyosis

       (1) Submucosal fibroids can have the greatest impact on fertility.

       (2) Fibroids that impinge on the cavity and measure greater than 5 cm may need to be removed.

    k. Endometriosis should be staged. No clear evidence that medical or surgical treatment enhances fertility. IVF is generally recommended to best address this issue.

    l. Screen for over-the-counter (OTC), prescription, or recreational drug use or abuse that might impact fertility. For example, non-steroidal anti-inflammatory drugs (NSAIDs) are not recommended when trying to conceive.

7. Preconception counseling includes explaining to patients the importance of carrier testing prior to conception.

    a. The American College of Obstetricians and Gynecologists (ACOG) and other professional organizations recommend screening every patient for cystic fibrosis prior to conception.

    b. Increasingly, clinicians are screening for the spinal muscular atrophy (SMN 1) gene.

    c. Check Tay-Sachs for those of Ashkenazi, French Canadian, and Cajun descent.

    d. Check a hemoglobin electrophoresis to rule out thalessemias for those of Mediterranean descent and sickle cell trait for those of African descent.

    e. Patients are increasingly unsure of their ethnicity, so consider pan screening to be on the safe side.

BOX 22.3 *Summary of Basic Fertility Evaluation*

- Ovarian reserve testing: "Day 3" follicle-stimulating hormone (FSH), estradiol, anti-Müllerian hormone (AMH) level
- If anovulatory: Complete hormonal workup
- Hysterosalpingogram
- Semen analysis
- Preconception blood work: Thyroid-stimulating hormone (TSH), prolactin, complete blood count (CBC), STI panel, rubella, varicella, blood type, and antibody screen
- Genetic screening: Cystic fibrosis (CF), spinal muscular atrophy (SMA), and Fragile X, Ashkenazi panel, and hemoglobin (Hgb) electrophoresis as indicated by ethnicity.

Consider broader screening if patient is uncertain of ethnicity.

---

    f. For those with premature ovarian failure and insufficiency, check for Fragile X as premutation carrier status can affect ovarian reserve.

  8. If BMI is greater than 30 to 35, refer to nutritionist or primary care for further evaluation and intervention. Elevated BMI is associated with hyperinsulinemia in PCOS patients and adversely affects ability to conceive and carry pregnancy to term.

  9. Couple should leave their first visit aware of what tests they need and why. Speaking with a financial counselor will help them address any financial or insurance-based concerns.

  10. Give patients reading materials or online links, as the first visit is usually overwhelming due to information overload.

  11. Box 22.3 summarizes the basic infertility evaluation.

V. Male assessment

  A. Semen analysis (SA)

    1. Checks for volume, count, motility, and morphology

    2. Better results if specimen is produced at home under more relaxed circumstances than a medical office or bathroom

    3. Use a nontoxic specimen container for the collection.

    4. Transportation of semen

      a. Keep out of direct sunlight while transporting.

      b. Avoid extreme temperatures.

      c. Best to keep warm next to body

      d. Do not refrigerate the specimen.

      e. Do not use lubricants when producing the specimen.

    5. If the specimen was partially lost, report this, as it will affect the findings.

6. If abnormal, repeat, as sperm parameters can vary widely in the same individual. A single abnormal test is not conclusive.
7. If two abnormal semen analyses are reported, refer to a reproductive urologist.

B. History and screening
1. Take a thorough male history including undescended testes (bilateral cryptochordism), mumps orchitis, urologic infections, prior urologic surgeries including hernia repair, sports injuries, endocrine disorders such as diabetes mellitus, diethylstilbestrol (DES) exposure of his mother, epilepsy, obesity.
2. Screen for use of recreational drugs including nicotine and alcohol as well as testosterone supplements, which can stop sperm production, including anabolic steroids and performance-enhancing substances that may contain testosterone or its derivatives.
3. Ask if he has close male relatives with infertility or males who have never fathered children.
4. A full sexual history including ejaculatory problems and whether he has fathered a child or been involved in any prior pregnancies
5. Certain prescription drugs are detrimental to sperm production such as calcium channel blockers, cimetidine, Dilantin, sulfasalazine, allopurinol, colchicine, nitrofurantoin. and certain chemotherapy agents.
6. STI testing as there is still significant STI transmission due to lack of detection and awareness
7. Screen for varicoceles, or varices of the testes, more common on the left side
   a. Controversial as they are common and also found in fertile men
   b. In some cases they are large and cause pain.
   c. They should be evaluated by a reproductive urologist to determine if they are clinically significant.
8. If male is unable to produce a specimen for semen analysis, he may require a collection condom available from specialty pharmacies or online. These condoms are not toxic to sperm and allow intercourse to take place for collection.
9. Refer males for a complete exam with primary care physician or urologist to check for normal virilization, testes size and consistency (including presence of varicioceles), presence or absence of the vas deferens, and phimosis.
10. Box 22.4 lists organizations that offer support for infertility and subfertility.

BOX 22.4 *National Advocacy Groups*

Resolve: The National Infertility Association
703-556-7172
www.rrsolve.org

American Fertility Association (AFA)
888-917-3777
wwwtheafa.org

The American Society for Reproductive Medicine (ASRM)
205-978-5000
ww.asrm.org

National Council for Adoption
703-299-6633
www.adoptioncouncil.org

Fertile Hope
855-220-7777
www.fertilehope.org

Bibliography

Bayer, S. R., Alper, M. M., & Penzias, A. S. (Eds.). (2012). *The Boston IVF handbook of infertility: A practical guide for practitioners who care for infertile couples* (3rd ed.). Boca Raton, FL: Taylor & Francis.

Brinsden, P. R. (Ed.). (2005). *Textbook of in vitro fertilization and assisted reproduction: The Bourn Hall guide to clinical and laboratory practice* (3rd ed.). Boca Raton, FL: Taylor & Francis.

Burns, L. H., & Covington, S. N. (Eds.). (2000). *Infertility counseling: A comprehensive handbook for clinicians*. New York, NY: Parthenon.

Campbell, L. (2013). *Single infertile female: Adventures in love, life, and infertility*. CreateSpace Independent Publishing.

Carcio, H. A., & Secor, M. C. (2010). *Advanced health assessment of women: Clinical skills and procedures* (2nd ed.). New York, NY: Springer Publishing Company.

Carr, S. C. (2011). Ultrasound for nurses in reproductive medicine. *Journal of Obstetrics, Gynecologic, & Neonatal Nursing, 40*(5), 638–653. doi: 10.1111/j.1552-6909.2011.01286.x

Cedars, M. I. (2005). *Infertility: Practical pathways in obstetrics & gynecology*. New York, NY: McGraw-Hill.

Committee on Gynecologic Practice of the American College of Obstetricians and Gynecologists and The Practice Committee of the American Society for Reproductive Medicine. (2008). Age-related fertility decline: A committee opinion. *Fertility and Sterility, 90*(3), 486–487. doi: 10.1016/j.fertnstert.2008.08.006)

Crawshaw, M., & Balen, R. (Eds.). (2010). *Adopting after infertility: Messages from practice, research and personal experience*. Philadelphia, PA: Jessica Kingsley Publishers.

Cronister, A., Teicher, J., Rohlfs, E. M., Donnenfeld, A., & Hallam, S. (2008). Prevalence and instability of fragile X alleles: Implications for offering fragile X prenatal diagnosis. *Obstetrics & Gynecology, 111*(3), 596–601.

DeCherney, A., Nathan, L., Goodwin, T. M., Laufer, N., & Roman, A. (2013). *Obstetrics & gynecology* (11th ed.). Current diagnosis and treatment. New York, NY: McGraw-Hill.

Domar, A. D., & Kelly, A. L. (2004). *Conquering infertility: Dr. Alice Domar's mind/body guide to enhancing fertility and coping with infertility.* New York, NY: Penguin Books.

Fritz, M. A., & Speroff, L. (2011). *Clinical gynecologic endocrinology and infertility* (8th ed.). Philadelphia, PA: Lippincott Williams & Wilkins.

Goldstein, M., & Schlegel, P. N. (Eds.). (2013). *Surgical and medical management of male infertility.* New York, NY: Cambridge University Press.

Gordon, J. D., Rydfors, J. T., & Druzin, M. L. (2001). *Obstetrics, gynecology and infertility: Handbook for clinicians-resident survival guide* (5th ed.). Arlington, VA: Scrub Hill Press.

Lebovic, D., Gordon, J. D., & Taylor, R. (2013). *Reproductive endocrinology and infertility, handbook for clinicians* (2nd ed.). Arlington, VA: Scrub Hill Press.

Lipshultz, L. I., Howards, S. S., & Niederberger, C. S. (Eds.). (2009). *Infertility in the male* (4th ed.). New York, NY: Cambridge University Press.

Marrs, R., Bloch, L. F., & Silverman, K. K. (2011). *Dr. Richard Marrs' fertility book: America's leading infertility expert tells you everything you need to know about getting pregnant.* New York, NY: Dell Publishing.

Practice Committee of American Society for Reproductive Medicine. (2008). Vaccination guidelines for female infertility patients. *Fertility and Sterility, 90*(5), S169–S171. doi: 10.1016/j.fertnstert.2008.08.056

Practice Committee of the American Society for Reproductive Medicine. (2012). Diagnostic evaluation of the infertile female: A committee opinion. *Fertility and Sterility, 98*(2), 302–307. doi: 10.1016/j.fertnstert.2012.05.032)

Practice Committee of the American Society for Reproductive Medicine. (2012). Diagnostic evaluation of the infertile male: A committee opinion. *Fertility and Sterility, 98*(2), 294–301. doi: 10.1016/j.fertnstert.2012.05.033)

Practice Committee of the American Society for Reproductive Medicine. (2012). Smoking and infertility: A committee opinion. *Fertility and Sterility, 98*(6), 1400–1406. doi: 10.1016/j.fertnstert.2012.07.1146

Practice Committee of the American Society for Reproductive Medicine. (2012). Testing and interpreting measures of ovarian reserve: A committee opinion. *Fertility and Sterility, 98*(6), 1407–1415. doi: 10.1016/j.fertnstert.2012.09.036

Practice Committee of the American Society for Reproductive Medicine. (2012). The clinical relevance of luteal phase deficiency: A committee opinion. *Fertility and Sterility, 98*(5), 1112–1117. doi: 10.1016/j.fertnstert.2012.06.050

Racowsky, C., Schlegel, P. N., Fauser, B. C., & Carrell, D. T. (Eds.). (2011). *Biennial review of infertility (volume 2).* New York, NY: Springer Publishing Company.

Schoolcraft, W. (2010). *If at first you don't conceive: A complete guide to infertility from one of the nation's leading clinics.* New York, NY: Rodale Press.

Sedaka, M., & Rosen, G. (2011). *What he can expect when she's not expecting: How to support your wife, save your marriage, and conquer infertility.* New York, NY: Skyhorse Publishing.

Speroff, L., Glass, R. H., Kase, N. G., & Seifer, D. B. (2001). *Clinical gynecologic endocrinology & infertility: text, self-assessment and study guide* (6th ed.). [CD-ROM]. Philadelphia, PA: Lippincott Williams & Wilkins.

Stadtmauer, L., & Tur-Kaspa, I. (Eds.). (2013). *Ultrasound imaging in reproductive medicine: Advances in infertility work-up, treatment, and ART.* New York, NY: Springer Publishing Company.

Wardell, H. (2003). *Childfree after infertility: Moving from childlessness to a joyous life.* Lincoln, NE: iUniverse, Inc.

Wilcox, A. J, Dunson, D., & Baird, D. D. (2000). The timing of the "fertile window" in the menstrual cycle: Day specific estimates from a prospective study. *British Medical Journal, 321*(7271), 1259–1262. doi: http://dx.doi.org/10.1136/British Medical Journal.321.7271.1259

Wright, H. (2010). *The PCOS diet plan: A natural approach to health for women with polycystic ovary syndrome.* New York, NY: Celestial Arts.

APPENDIX 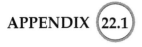 22.1

Health History

Female Fertility Evaluation
Please complete the following:
Name:_____
Member #: _____
Date of birth: _____ Age: _____
Partner's name:_____ Member #:_____
Date of birth: _____ Age: _____
Primary care provider: _____
OB/GYN provider: _____
How long have you been trying to get pregnant?_____
Weight:_____ Height: _____ Current medications: _____
Allergies: _____ Reaction:_____

Menstrual History
Date of last menses:
Age at onset of your menstrual period:
Average length between cycles:
Any history of irregular menses, spotting, or missed menses? If yes, please
    explain (include dates):
Painful menses?

List any medications you take for cramps.

Ovulation

Do you experience:

Premenstrual cramps?   Yes ❐   No ❐

Clear discharge midcycle?   Yes ❐   No ❐

Monthly cycles?   Yes ❐   No ❐

Pain at midcycle?   Yes ❐   No ❐

Have you ever used the following?
Basal body temperature: _____ months. Temperature shift: _____
Day of shift:_____
Ovulation predictor kit:
Name of kit:_____
Number of cycles: _____
Day of surge:_____
LH surge seen?   Yes ❐   No ❐

Birth Control
Have you ever used any of the following?
Birth control pills, IUD, diaphragm, condoms, Norplant, Depo-Provera, foam, sponge, other
(please describe)

METHOD	DATES	HOW LONG	WHY STOPPED	COMPLICATIONS

Obstetric History

PREGNANCY NUMBER	YEAR	TIME TO CONCEIVE	TYPE OF FERTILITY TREATMENT? (IF ANY) WEEKS CARRIED	OUTCOME	TYPE OF DELIVERY (VAGINAL/ C-SECTION)	COMPLICATIONS	CURRENT PARTNER

Gynecologic History
Please include dates and treatment if you ever had

Mother who took DES

Pelvic infection

Chlamydia/gonorrhea

Herpes

Vaginitis

Endometriosis

Ovarian cysts

Genital warts

Ectopic pregnancy

Miscarriage

Abortion

List date and nature of any pelvic surgery: Have you had a tubal ligation? If so, when was it reversed? Were you ever treated for an abnormal Pap smear? If yes, list date and nature of treatment.

Sexual History

Please describe any positive responses.

Do you have painful intercourse?

Do you use vaginal lubricants or douches?

Hormonal Assessment

Have you experienced any of the following?

Weight gain/loss of 10+ lb

Discharge from nipples

Change in vision

Unusual sensitivity to hot or cold

Excessive change in hair growth/loss

Thyroid disease, diabetes, or other hormonal abnormalities

Medical History
Please list any medical or psychiatric conditions that you have or had in the past and any medications used in treatment. List dates.

Surgical/Hospitalization History
Please list any surgeries or hospitalizations you have had. List dates.

Family History
Please list any family history of infertility, genetic problems, thyroid disease, diabetes, cancer, or any other major medical problems.

Social History
Occupation: Travel for work?   Frequency?
Caffeine intake:
Do you smoke cigarettes?   _____ packs per day
Alcohol consumption: _____ drinks/week   Type:
Medications
    Prescription:
    Over the counter:
    Recreational (marijuana, hallucinogens, crack/cocaine, other addictive drugs; if yes, explain):

List the form and frequency of any regular exercise. Have you ever been told you have or suspected you have an eating disorder?

Previous Infertility Treatment
Describe results. Include dates.
Name of physician/practice:
Has your partner ever had a semen analysis?
Have you had any hormonal blood tests?
Have you ever had an endometrial biopsy?
Have you ever had an x-ray of your tubes and uterus (hysterosalpingogram [HSG])?
Have you ever had a laparoscopy?
Have you ever taken medications to stimulate ovulation?
Have you ever had intrauterine insemination?
Have you ever had advanced reproductive technology procedures performed (IVF, gamete intrafallopian transfer [GIFT], intracytoplasmic sperm injection [ICSI])?
Why do you think you are not getting pregnant?

FEMALE PARTNER FERTILITY EVALUATION
Please complete the following:
Name:_____ Member #: _____
Date of birth: _____ Age: _____
Partner's name:_____ Member #: _____

Gynecologic History

Please include dates and treatment if you ever had

Pelvic infection
Chlamydia/gonorrhea
Herpes
Vaginitis
Genital warts
Were you ever treated for an abnormal Pap smear? If yes, list date and nature of treatment.

Methods to Detect Ovulation

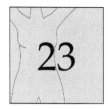

23

Carol Lesser

I. **Methods to detect ovulation**
   A. Key concepts
      1. Take a menstrual history.
         a. Determine if there is a history of amenorrhea or long cycles, greater than 35 to 40 days or short cycles less than 25 days.
         b. A sign of perimenopause is the shortening of cycle length, so determine if short cycles are chronic or a new occurrence.
      2. Previously, women were instructed to check their basal body temperature (BBT) using a digital thermometer to record their early-morning temperature before food or drink, every day of the menstrual cycle.
         a. The BBT rises 0.4° to 0.8°F after ovulation and a biphasic pattern emerges due to a thermal shift.
         b. After ovulation the temperature remains elevated until the corpus luteum recedes and stops making progesterone. Menses ensues, accompanied by a BBT drop.
         c. If pregnancy occurs, the BBT remains elevated for the duration of pregnancy.
      3. Checking for spinnbarkeit (clear, stretchy secretions) is difficult for many women to grasp and is highly subjective. However, this information can be useful if other testing is not available.
      4. These older methods have been replaced by other more reliable methods of determining midcycle (see Box 23.1) for fertility patients.
         a. Most clinicians no longer recommend BBT charting as it is time-consuming and confusing.
         b. It gives better information retrospectively than prospectively.
      5. Mobile applications are available to help women track their cycles and symptoms. One free app is Period Tracker Lite.

BOX 23.1 *Basic Fertility Evaluation*

- Ovarian reserve testing: "day 3" follicle-stimulating hormone (FSH), estradiol, anti-Müllerian hormone (AMH) level
- If anovulatory: Complete hormonal workup
- Hysterosalpingogram
- Semen analysis
- Preconception blood work: Thyroid-stimulating hormone (TSH), prolactin, complete blood count (CBC), sexually transmitted infection (STI) panel, rubella, varicella, blood type and antibody screen
- Genetic screening: Cystic fibrosis (CF), spinal muscular atrophy (SMA), and Fragile X, Ashkenazi panel, and hemoglobin (Hgb) electrophoresis as indicated by ethnicity. Consider broader screening if patient uncertain of ethnicity.

   B. Ovulation predictor kits (OPK)

      1. OPK or ovulation predictor kits and monitors are widely used.

      2. No home-based method is completely reliable so care must be taken to educate the patient in their proper use. Urine strips and fertility monitors are available. Some kits work better for individuals than others requiring a trial-and-error approach. Women frequently complain that their kits are hard to read and interpret.

      3. Cost varies and often affects decision on which to use.

      4. All kits detect the luteinizing hormone (LH)

      5. The LH surge precedes ovulation.

         a. A color change or positive indicator indicates that ovulation is approaching, usually in 12 to 36 hours.

         b. Must follow instructions for the kit or monitor being used. Some are daily and others focus on a more limited window of testing.

         c. Most urine-testing kits instruct that the first morning void be discarded, as it may be too concentrated.

         d. Read instructions carefully and familiarize yourself with the kits you recommend.

      6. Testing too late in the cycle will miss the surge and chance to conceive. This is the most common error. Remaining sexually active is a safeguard against this for those who have a partner and can do so.

      7. If a woman has regular cycles and knows when she is ovulating, then kits are not necessary.

      8. Timing of intercourse does not have to be so precise.

         a. Pregnancy occurs if exposure to sperm takes place in a 6-day window leading up to and including ovulation.

BOX 23.2 *Presumptive Signs That Ovulation Is Occurring (Moliminal)*

Molimina (Premenstrual Signs) That Signify Ovulation

Menstrual characteristics
- Predictable bleeding pattern every 21 to 35 days
- Bleeding that lasts 3 to 5 days
- Breast tenderness that resolves with menses
- Mild to moderate cramps

Periovulatory characteristics
- Spinnbarkeit, mid-cycle stretchy cervical secretions resembling clear egg white
- Mild cramping (Mittelschmerz)
- Occasional mid-cycle spotting (Hartman's sign)
- Increase in sexual desire

  b. Wilcox et al. confirmed greatest chance of pregnancy occurred with intercourse beginning 2 days prior to ovulation. No pregnancies occurred if intercourse took place after ovulation.

  c. Sperm can live for up to 5 days in the reproductive tract while the oocyte lives for less than 24 hours.

  d. This is why intercourse or exposure to sperm postovulation is ineffective.

II. Hormonal evaluation of ovulation

 A. Estradiol rises as the follicle matures. At ovulation the estradiol level is usually between 150 to 250 pg/mL per follicle. Estradiol is checked with a blood test. Newer saliva tests are being developed and hold promise for the future.

 B. As the follicle reaches maturity, LH rises. At its peak a surge occurs.

 C. A rise in progesterone is diagnostic for postovulation.

  1. Labs use different assays and cutoffs so it is important to know what the periovulatory levels are for your lab.

  2. Generally, progesterone greater than 1.5 ng/mL is diagnostic for postovulation.

  3. Progesterone levels dip right before menses. A low progesterone level can mean menses is approaching, or is suggestive of anovulation or preovulation.

  4. Progesterone is released in pulses every 2 to 3 hours. Levels can vary widely, making a single level less diagnostic.

 D. Moliminal premenstrual symptoms (Box 23.2) are highly diagnostic for ovulation.

E. Luteal-phase defect is a concept now considered controversial and outdated.
  1. Infertility centers rarely check for this anymore.
  2. An exception is a patient who has failed multiple in vitro fertilization (IVF) cycles despite the creation of high-quality embryos. Specialized tests can be ordered that go far beyond the endometrial dating assessed during a routine endometrial biopsy.

III. The endometrial biopsy
  A. The issues
  1. In the past, endometrial biopsy was routinely performed to rule out a luteal-phase deficiency (LPD).
  2. It was theorized that some ovulatory women had inadequate progesterone production in the luteal phase, negatively impacting endometrium maturation and receptivity for implantation and ongoing pregnancy.
  3. The luteal phase can be between 13 to 16 days long but the tests were interpreted in light of a 14-day luteal phase, leading to overdiagnosis.
  4. For these reasons, it is no longer routinely offered in fertility centers.
  5. See Chapter 40, "Endometrial Biopsy" regarding gynecologic indications for this test.
  6. Can still be used to rule out endometritis and hyperplasia or atypia (see Chapter 44, "Intrauterine Insemination").

IV. Uterine cavity and fallopian tube assessment
  A. The basics
  1. Pregnancy depends on normal uterine and fallopian tube anatomy.
  2. Pregnancy can occur if only one fallopian tube is present or open.
  3. Advanced practice practitioners can perform these tests.
  4. Check for Müllerian defects such as unicornuate, bicornuate, or didelphys uterus; fibroids, polyps, or Asherman syndrome; as well as tubal disease, most notably hydrosalpinges.
  5. In the case of fibroids, the cavity evaluations are looking for impingement on the cavity that would interfere with implantation or pregnancy advancement.
  B. Tests include
  1. Pelvic ultrasound to rule out any obvious pathology including fibroids, ovarian cysts or dermoids, or obvious structural defects. Evidence of polycystic ovarian syndrome (PCOS) like ovaries with their characteristic "string of pearls" appearance ringing the perimeter should be noted.

2. Hysterosalpingogram to assess tubal patency and assess the internal uterine cavity for fibroid impingement, polyps, Müllerian defects or Asherman syndrome. Done in a radiology-equipped room or facility after menstrual flow but before ovulation if trying to conceive that cycle.
3. Sonohysterogram is a procedure done in the office in which a small amount of saline is inserted into the uterus through the cervix.
   a. Often used to assess abnormal bleeding or recurrent miscarriage. Done after menstrual flow but before ovulation if trying to conceive that cycle (see Chapter 33, "Sonohysterography [Fluid Contrast Ultrasound]").
4. Office hysteroscopy when defects need further evaluation and possible treatment such as polypectomy or lysis of adhesions from Asherman syndrome
5. Operative hysteroscopy may be indicated based on findings if more extensive surgery is needed.
6. Laparoscopy may be indicated if the patiente has significant pelvic pain or a history of endometriosis or large fibroids that need intervention.

V. **Ovarian reserve (OR) testing**
   A. Background
      1. Integral part of the infertility evaluation. Commonly refers to oocyte quantity, quality, and reproductive potential.
      2. Offers valuable information to help determine appropriate diagnosis and treatment
      3. Can be assessed by blood and ultrasound, often interpreted together in the context of patient history (e.g., age, how long trying to conceive, obstetrical history, etc.)
      4. Chronologic age affects oocyte quality and quantity and younger patients tend to have more and better quality eggs.
         a. The highest number of eggs is present in the ovaries at 20 weeks gestational age with a steady decline until menopause and a precipitous drop in the later reproductive years.
         b. Fertility measurably declines in a woman's 20s but is usually not of concern.
      5. OR tests measure the relative quantity of eggs remaining but chronologic age is still an excellent predictor of success. Therefore, younger patients whose levels suggest decreased ovarian reserve tend to fare better than older patients, even if their levels look good.

B. The tests

1. Anti-Müllerian hormone (AMH)

   a. The newest OR test that many find to be the most helpful predictor of ovarian reserve. Expressed by the granulosa cells of the ovary.

   b. Can be done on any cycle day including while on oral contraceptives, when anovulatory, breastfeeding, or postpartum

   c. Often used when screening potential oocyte donors

   d. Generally, higher numbers are reassuring and are seen with PCOS. Lower numbers are associated with perimenopause and premature ovarian insufficiency and failure (Table 23.1).

   e. Earliest known marker for detecting ovarian aging and decline

   f. Some studies suggest that results from younger women can be predictive of age at onset of menopause.

2. Follicle-stimulating hormone (FSH) and estradiol

   a. Basal FSH concentrations increase with advancing age until their peak at menopause.

   b. An elevated FSH is associated with decreased ovarian reserve or premature ovarian insufficiency. Menopausal FSH levels in a younger woman indicate premature ovarian failure (POF) (Table 23.2).

      (1) Younger patients with FSH elevations should be counseled to seek reproductive treatments as soon as possible if childbearing is desired.

      (2) If ovulatory, check in the early follicular phase, typically on days 1, 2, 3, or 4. This is when basal FSH levels should be at their lowest, before follicle recruitment.

      (3) If anovulatory, basal FSH levels can be drawn on any day since follicle recruitment is not taking place.

   c. Estradiol suppresses FSH. Best to interpret the FSH level with an estradiol level drawn at the same time.

TABLE 23.1 Interpretation of AMH Levels

AMH	LEVEL	OVARIAN RESERVE
1–3	ng/mL	Normal
< 1	ng/mL	Reduced
< 0.83	ng/mL	Further reduced
< 0.1	ng/mL	Poor prognosis

Note: AMH level reflects the remaining follicular pool.

TABLE 23.2 Interpretation of Cycle Day 3 Hormone Levels

FSH (MIU/ML)	ESTRADIOL (PG/ML)	OVARIAN RESERVE
> 10	< 70	Reduced
> 10	> 70	Reduced
2-10	> 70	Reduced
2-10	< 70	Normal

Notes: An ovulatory younger woman with elevated FSH has a significantly higher chance of pregnancy than an older woman with the same level. Provide general guidelines: No level can predict pregnancy. Ovarian reserve tests are quantitative not qualitative assessment tools.

    d. If the estradiol is significantly elevated, this can be associated with perimenopause.
        (1) Levels greater than 70 pg/mL are considered elevated and lower the FSH level.
        (2) FSH would need to be repeated on a future cycle when the estradiol was within the normal range.
    e. Elevations in estradiol are common in perimenopause and can happen intermittently or frequently.
    f. OR testing from a specialty lab can be arranged by the patient.
  3. Basal antral follicle (BAF) count
    a. Technician dependent and must be done by trained personnel
    b. A simple test that measures antral follicles, which are small follicles (2 to 8 mm in size) that are visible on the ovaries via ultrasound. They are also known as resting follicles and give a representation of the pool of primordial follicles that remain.
    c. The higher the number of antral follicles, the greater the ovarian reserve potential. Lower counts are associated with decreased ovarian reserve or ovarian insufficiency.

VI. Baseline hormone testing
  A. What to test and when
    1. Hormones are best checked in the early follicular phase if including OR tests. Otherwise, any cycle day will suffice.
    2. Check FSH, estradiol, and AMH as described previously.
    3. Check LH. Although it was previously taught that LH and the FSH:LH ratio are increased in PCOS, this is not always the case. A normal LH does not preclude the diagnosis of PCOS.

4. Check prolactin if there is menstrual irregularity or anovulation or galactorrhea.
5. Check TSH for all patients with infertility. If the TSH is elevated, check for thyroid antibodies as they are associated with infertility and miscarriage.
6. If oligo or anovulatory, screen for hyperandrogenism. Check LH, testosterone, and consider sex hormone binding globulin and adrenal hormones such as 17Ohydroxyprogesterone (17OH-P) and dehydroepiandrosterone sulfate (DHEA-S).
7. If congenital adrenal hyperplasia (CAH) is suspected, further testing will be indicated. Consider a 24-hour urinary cortisol or congenital adrenal hyperplasia (adrenocorticotropic hormone [ACTH]) challenge test.
8. Most patients with oligo or anovulation have PCOS. They often have elevated basal estradiol levels produced by their active ovaries.

VII. Postcoital test
1. Microscopically tests the survival of sperm postcoitus in cervical mucus at midcycle.
2. Cervical mucus would be examined under microscope and graded for its degree of ferning, which peaks at midcycle as estradiol levels rise.
   a. A small amount of cervical mucus is allowed to air dry on a clean, saline-free glass slide.
   b. In the presence of high levels of estrogen, just prior to ovulation, the cervical mucus forms fern-like patterns due to crystallization of sodium chloride on mucus fibers.
3. The number and degree of motility of living sperm per high-power field (HPF) would be recorded.
4. No longer considered part of the routine infertility evaluation.
5. Test was not found to be reliable or predictive so has been dropped.

VIII. Ovulation induction
A. Define the cause.
1. If oligo or anovulatory due to PCOS, offer ovulation induction medication.
   a. Most popular oral agent is clomiphene citrate, a selective estrogen receptor modulator (SERM).
      (1) Prescribed for those with open tube(s) and normal semen parameters or using donor sperm
      (2) Dose: 50 to 150 mg for 5 days. This can start on day 2, 3, 4, or 5 of the menstrual cycle. Lowest effective dose is typically prescribed. For severe PCOS with impaired glucose tolerance (IGT), metformin is often also prescribed.

    b. If anovulatory, assess the uterine lining to rule out hyperplasia. If normal, can prescribe with or without a withdrawal bleed. Clomiphene citrate can thin the endometrium due to its hypoestrogenic effect. Some studies suggest better implantation without a prior induced bleed that can further diminish lining.

    c. Efficacy can be assessed by waiting for a menstrual cycle to occur within 35 days, highly correlated with ovulation. If the patient experiences molimina for the first time, this too is reassuring.

    d. A progesterone level can be obtained after day 21 to see if it is in the postovulatory level, generally greater than 1.5 ng/mL, but check your lab cutoff.

    e. An OPK checks for an LH surge. If a woman's baseline LH is always elevated, then the kit may always test positive and is not the best way to assess clomiphene's efficacy or her ovulatory status.

    f. Fertility centers can offer serum monitoring of estradiol, LH, and progesterone as well as pelvic ultrasound to track mature follicle(s) if necessary.

    g. Clomiphene citrate has approximately a 10% to 15% success rate per cycle and a 10% chance of twins.

        (1) Side effects including hypoestrogenic complaints such as hot flashes, moodiness, and thinning of endometrium and cervical secretions have been described.

        (2) Alternative to clomiphene citrate and equally effective but an off-label use is letrozole, an aromatase inhibitor (AI). The off-label aspect is the chief factor limiting its broader use. Patients prefer it to clomiphene citrate.

        (3) Prescribed in the same way as clomiphene citrate for 5 days starting on days 2, 3, 4, or 5. Dose is 2.5 to 7.5 mg daily. Lowest effective dose is typically prescribed.

    h. Advantage of AI is lack of hypoestrogenic side effects and slightly lower risk of twins.

  2. Hypothalamic amenorrhea

    a. Hypogonadotropic hypogonadism, although not common, is most often self-inflicted and associated with eating disorders, low body mass index (BMI), and excessive athleticism now or in the past. Rarely, Kallmann syndrome will be the cause, characterized by anosmia and gonadotropin-releasing hormone (GnRH).

    b. Psychological counseling is often indicated for eating disorders but can be a very difficult disorder to treat.

    c. Hormonal assays reveal depressed FSH, LH, and estradiol. Panhypopituitarism is sometimes seen with lowered TSH and prolactin as well.

    d. Treatment is usually injectable gonadotropin therapy, which patient can self-administer subcutaneously, delivering a combination of FSH and LH in a 1:1 ratio. A trigger shot of human chorionic gonadotropin (hCG) acting as an LH surrogate is also needed to complete final follicle maturation and ovulation.

        (1) Main risks are hyperstimulation syndrome and multiple births. Offering IVF with single embryo transfer ameliorates these concerns.

        (2) Requires careful monitoring and extremely low dose to decrease these risks. Patients with low BMI can become ovulatory with modest weight gain.

Bibliography

Bayer, S. R., Alper, M. M., & Penzias, A. S. (Eds.). (2012). *The Boston IVF handbook of infertility: A practical guide for practitioners who care for infertile couples* (3rd ed.). Boca Raton, FL: Taylor & Francis.

Brinsden, P. R. (Ed.). (2005). *Textbook of in vitro fertilization and assisted reproduction: The Bourn Hall guide to clinical and laboratory practice* (3rd ed.). Boca Raton, FL: Taylor & Francis.

Burns, L. H., & Covington, S. N. (Eds.). (2000). *Infertility counseling: A comprehensive handbook for clinicians.* New York, NY: Parthenon Publishing Group Inc.

Campbell, L. (2013). *Single infertile female: Adventures in love, life, and infertility.* CreateSpace Independent Publishing.

Carcio, H. A., & Secor, M. C. (2010). *Advanced health assessment of women: Clinical skills and procedures* (2nd ed.). New York, NY: Springer Publishing Company.

Carr, S. C. (2011). Ultrasound for nurses in reproductive medicine. *Journal of Obstetrics, Gynecologic, & Neonatal Nursing, 40*(5), 638–653. doi: 10.1111/j.1552-6909.2011.01286.x

Cedars, M. I. (2005). *Infertility: Practical pathways in obstetrics & gynecology.* New York, NY: McGraw-Hill.

Committee on Gynecologic Practice of the American College of Obstetricians and Gynecologists and The Practice Committee of the American Society for Reproductive Medicine. (2008). Age-related fertility decline: A committee opinion. *Fertility and Sterility, 90*(3), 486–487. doi: 10.1016/j.fertnstert.2008.08.006

Crawshaw, M., & Balen, R. (Eds.). (2010). *Adopting after infertility: Messages from practice, research and personal experience.* Philadelphia, PA: Jessica Kingsley Publishers.

Cronister, A., Teicher, J., Rohlfs, E. M., Donnenfeld, A., & Hallam, S. (2008). Prevalence and instability of fragile X alleles: Implications for offering fragile X prenatal diagnosis. *Obstetrics & Gynecology, 111*(3), 596–601.

DeCherney, A., Nathan, L., Goodwin, T. M., Laufer, N., & Roman, A. (2013). *Obstetrics & gynecology* (11th ed.). Current diagnosis and treatment. New York, NY: McGraw-Hill.

Domar, A. D., & Kelly, A. L. (2004). *Conquering infertility: Dr. Alice Domar's mind/body guide to enhancing fertility and coping with infertility.* New York, NY: Penguin Books.

Fritz, M. A., & Speroff, L. (2011). *Clinical gynecologic endocrinology and infertility* (8th ed.). Philadelphia, PA: Lippincott Williams & Wilkins.

Goldstein, M., & Schlegel, P. N. (Eds.). (2013). *Surgical and medical management of male infertility.* New York, NY: Cambridge University Press.

Gordon, J. D., Rydfors, J. T., & Druzin, M. L. (2001). *Obstetrics, gynecology and infertility: Handbook for clinicians–resident survival guide* (5th ed.). Arlington, VA: Scrub Hill Press.

Lebovic, D., Gordon, J. D., & Taylor, R. (2013). *Reproductive endocrinology and infertility, handbook for clinicians* (2nd ed.). Arlington, VA: Scrub Hill Press.

Lipshultz, L. I., Howards, S. S., & Niederberger, C. S. (Eds.). (2009). *Infertility in the male* (4th ed.). New York, NY: Cambridge University Press.

Marrs, R., Bloch, L. F., & Silverman, K. K. (2011). *Dr. Richard Marrs' fertility book: America's leading infertility expert tells you everything you need to know about getting pregnant.* New York, NY: Dell Publishing.

Practice Committee of American Society for Reproductive Medicine. (2008). Vaccination guidelines for female infertility patients. *Fertility and Sterility, 90*(5), S169–S171. doi: 10.1016/j.fertnstert.2008.08.056

Practice Committee of the American Society for Reproductive Medicine. (2012). Diagnostic evaluation of the infertile female: A committee opinion. *Fertility and Sterility, 98*(2), 302–307. doi: 10.1016/j.fertnstert.2012.05.032

Practice Committee of the American Society for Reproductive Medicine. (2012). Diagnostic evaluation of the infertile male: a committee opinion. *Fertility and Sterility, 98*(2), 294–301. doi: 10.1016/j.fertnstert.2012.05.033

Practice Committee of the American Society for Reproductive Medicine. (2012). Smoking and infertility: A committee opinion. *Fertility and Sterility, 98*(6), 1400–1406. doi: 10.1016/j.fertnstert.2012.07.1146

Practice Committee of the American Society for Reproductive Medicine. (2012). Testing and interpreting measures of ovarian reserve: A committee opinion. *Fertility and Sterility, 98*(6), 1407–1415. doi: 10.1016/j.fertnstert.2012.09.036

Practice Committee of the American Society for Reproductive Medicine. (2012). The clinical relevance of luteal phase deficiency: A committee opinion. *Fertility and Sterility, 98*(5), 1112–1117. doi: 10.1016/j.fertnstert.2012.06.050

Racowsky, C., Schlegel, P. N., Fauser, B. C., & Carrell, D. T. (Eds.). (2011). *Biennial review of infertility (vol. 2).* New York, NY: Springer Publishing Company.

Schoolcraft, W. (2010). *If at first you don't conceive: A complete guide to infertility from one of the nation's leading clinics.* New York, NY: Rodale Press.

Sedaka, M., & Rosen, G. (2011). *What he can expect when she's not expecting: How to support your wife, save your marriage, and conquer infertility.* New York, NY: Skyhorse Publishing.

Speroff, L., Glass, R. H., Kase, N. G., & Seifer, D. B. (2001). *Clinical gynecologic endocrinology & infertility: text, self-assessment and study guide* (6th ed.). [CD-ROM]. Philadelphia, PA: Lippincott Williams & Wilkins.

Stadtmauer, L., & Tur-Kaspa, I. (Eds.). (2013). *Ultrasound imaging in reproductive medicine: Advances in infertility work-up, treatment, and ART.* New York, NY: Springer Publishing Company.

Wardell, H. (2003). *Childfree after infertility: Moving from childlessness to a joyous life.* Lincoln, NE: iUniverse, Inc.

Wilcox, A. J, Dunson, D., & Baird, D. D. (2000). The timing of the "fertile window" in the menstrual cycle: Day specific estimates from a prospective study. *British Medical Journal, 321*(7271), 1259–1262. doi: http://dx.doi.org/10.1136/bmj.321.7271.1259

Wright, H. (2010). *The PCOS diet plan: A natural approach to health for women with polycystic ovary syndrome.* New York, NY: Celestial Arts.

Donor Insemination

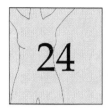

24

Carol Lesser

I. **Donor insemination explained**
  A. More than 80,000 donor inseminations are performed annually.
  B. More than 5,000 babies are born by donor insemination in the United States each year.
  C. Legal issues vary from state to state. Familiarize yourself with the laws of your state.
  D. Increase in number of single women and lesbian couples interested in having a biological child with increased societal acceptance
  E. Reduced availability of adoptable babies has increased its use.
  F. Psychological, social, and ethical questions should be addressed before proceeding. Specific attention should be given to donor identification for a child who is 18 or older.
  G. Equally important is counseling to help individual or couple determine disclosure to a child.
  H. If pregnancy with a specific donor is requested, additional vials from the same donor may be purchased and reserved for future pregnancies. This offers the possibility for a full sibling.
  I. No increase in pregnancy complications or birth defects in babies born with donor sperm
  J. Provide woman or couple with a list of available cryogenic banks that your office has had good experience working with in terms of quality and reliability.
  K. As soon as your patient has been cleared to proceed, obtain informed consent from the individual or couple and help her chose the method to predict ovulation.

II. **Indications**
  A. Donor insemination may be recommended when the male partner has the following
    1. Azoospermia
      a. Prior vasectomy (not reversed)
      b. Congenital or surgical absence of either testes or vas deferens

    2. Severe male factor not resolved with assisted reproductive technologies (ART) intervention (or couple refuses ART)

    3. Male or female sexual dysfunction making intercourse impossible at midcycle

B. Women without male partners

    1. Same-sex couples

    2. Single women

C. Genetic disorders

    1. Autosomal dominant disorder in male (e.g., Huntington's disease)

    2. Recessive genetic trait in both partners (e.g., Tay-Sachs or cystic fibrosis) if preimplantation genetic diagnosis is not feasible (with in vitro fertilization [IVF]).

D. Women with history of fetal loss caused by Rh sensitization. (These patients could opt to choose an Rh-negative donor.)

III. Success rates

A. Success rates with frozen sperm are comparable to fresh sperm when a sperm bank is used. They may be lower when partner sperm is used if sperm parameters are reduced.

B. Success rates are cumulative and age related. Younger patients tend to conceive faster than patients with decreased ovarian reserve.

IV. Source of donor

A. Counseling is recommended to make sure that all parties accept this form of third-party reproduction.

    1. Decisions regarding disclosure to close family members and a child should be made prior to conception.

B. All donor sperm is frozen and quarantined for 6 months before release, after it has been determined that the person has remained free of any sexually transmitted diseases.

C. Known donors

    1. Although less common, identified or known donors may be selected if they undergo Food and Drug Administration (FDA) screening and appropriate counseling, including legal advice.

    2. Patients may opt to use a local cryogenic bank or request this service from an IVF center.

D. Anonymous donors

    1. Most popular option

    2. Sperm banks have both open and closed donors. Open donors who allow for contact when the child turns 18 are becoming more popular and available, but may incur an extra fee.

    3. Sperm banks do not reveal the identity of the donor if there is no prior agreement to do so.

    4. Most sperm banks do not inform the donor if a conception has occurred.

BOX 24.1 *FDA-Required Testing for Communicable Diseases for Sperm Donors*

- HIV 1, 2
- HBV (hepatitis B virus)
- HCV (hepatitis C virus)
- RPR (rapid plasma reagin)
- *Chlamydia trachomatis*
- *Neisseria gonorrhoeae*
- Human T-lymphotropic virus, type 1, 2
- Cytomegalovirus

5. Sperm banks "retire" a donor once he has achieved a certain number of pregnancies, but this policy varies depending on the sperm bank.
6. A very small percentage of men who present to a sperm bank will be accepted into the donor program. Semen analysis and medical, family, and social history must be optimal in order to be accepted.
7. The issue of cytomegalovirus (CMV), immunoglobulin G (IgG) status causes confusion.
   a. Donors are routinely tested and some programs routinely test their patients.
   b. Sperm banks accept men with a prior history of CMV (IgG positive).
   c. Sperm banks never accept a man who is immunoglobulin M (IgM) positive, which would suggest current infection.
   d. The decision to choose an IgG-positive donor if the woman is CMV negative is a personal one to be determined between her and her clinician.
   e. Patients who have been counseled may opt to choose a CMV-positive donor, as many clinicians do not feel that this will put them at increased risk for CMV.

V. Shipping of frozen specimens
   A. No change, except it may be cost-effective to ship multiple vials at one time. One to 10 vials cost the same amount.

VI. Preparation of the donor
   A. The Centers for Disease Control and Prevention (CDC) and the FDA have imposed restrictions on the use of donor specimens by mandating that only guaranteed frozen specimens be used, as described below (Box 24.1 contains a list of FDA-required testing).

B. Testing
  1. The donor is tested for HIV. The specimen is quarantined for 60 to 180 days and released only after a second HIV antibody titer is negative.
C. Additional tests required of donors
  1. Blood type and Rh
  2. Complete blood count
  3. Blood chemistry
  4. Antihepatitis B core antibody
  5. Gonorrhea and chlamydia
  6. Rapid plasma reagin (RPR) test for syphilis
  7. Herpes simplex virus
  8. Antihepatitis
  9. Hepatitis B surface antigen
  10. HIV-1 and HIV-2
  11. Fluid culture on semen
D. Carrier testing for donors. Most sperm banks screen for 23 more common genetic disorders, including cystic fibrosis (CF), spinal muscular atrophy (SMA), and thalassemias with hemoglobin electrophoresis.
E. Additional testing may be necessary if the woman is a carrier for a rare disorder. There is an extra cost for this.
F. Donors are generally young; between 18 and 35 years.
G. Donors need a full evaluation.
  1. FDA questionnaire must be completed.
  2. Health and family history covering three generations
  3. Complete physical exam, including urologic exam
  4. Semen analysis: Men with suboptimal parameters will not be accepted.
H. Description of donor includes
  1. Ethnicity
  2. Level of education
  3. Hair and eye color
  4. Height and weight
  5. Blood type
  6. Religion
  7. Occupation
  8. Special interests
  9. Some sperm banks provide photographs, including baby pictures, audiotapes, videotapes, and/or essays or letters that could be later shared with a child. Check with each sperm bank for the different options and associated fees.
I. Choosing a donor
  1. Short forms give basic information.
  2. Long forms provide more in-depth information for an additional fee.

3. When a donor is selected, it is recommended to reserve multiple vials since popular donors tend to be depleted due to increased demand.

VII. Specimen quality
A. Intracervical insemination (ICI) specimens are less expensive than intrauterine insemination (IUI) specimens. For couples pursuing IVF, IUI specimens are generally preferred. IUI-prepared sperm offers higher success rates. If ICI sperm is purchased, it performs better if IUI prepared. This generally is not cost-effective.

VIII. Home insemination using frozen sperm
A. After discussing the various alternatives, a woman may decide on home insemination.
B. It is the clinician's responsibility to offer support, education, and guidance.
C. Review timing of procedure
   1. Using ovulation predictor kits
      a. Day of color change or day after if using frozen sperm
      b. Day after color change if using sperm from a known donor
D. Thawing of specimen
E. Procedure for deposition of sperm in the vagina
   1. Intravaginal: May use syringe and catheter to simply deposit sperm in the vagina.
   2. Purchase sperm cup.
      a. The entire specimen of semen is placed in the cup and placed against the cervix, thus protecting the semen from a hostile vaginal environment.
      b. The sperm cup should be left in place for approximately 8 hours.
   3. The advantage of the home-insemination option is that it eliminates the necessity of transporting the specimen to the provider's office, electing for the quieter, more natural environment of the home; this seems to be less invasive.
   4. Disadvantage of home inseminations
      a. Technique is not monitored
      b. No check of adequacy of sperm specimen
      c. IUI specimens are not recommended for home insemination.

Bibliography

American Fertility Society. (1993). Guidelines for therapeutic donor insemination: Sperm. *Fertility and Sterility, 59*, 1S–4S.

Bordson, B. L., Ricci, E., Dickey, R. P., Dunaway, H., Taylor, S. N., & Curole, D. N. (1986). Comparison of intracervical, intrauterine, and intratubal techniques for donor insemination. *Fertility and Sterility, 59*, 339–342.

Carcio, H. A. (1998) *Management of the infertile woman*. Philadelphia, PA: Lippincott-Raven.

Carrell, D. T., Cartmill, D., Jones, K. P., Hatasaka, H. H., & Peterson, C. M. (2002). Prospective, randomized, blinded evaluation of donor semen quality provided by seven commercial sperm banks. *Fertility and Sterility, 78*(1), 16–21. doi: 10.1016/S0015-0282(02)03179-5

Degl'innocenti, S., Filimberti, E., Magini, A., Krausz, C., Lombardi, G., Fino, M. G., Rastrelli, G., ... Baldi, E. (2013). Semen cryopreservation for men banking for oligospermia, cancers, and other pathologies: Prediction of post-thaw outcome using basal semen quality. *Fertility and Sterility, 100*(6), 1555–1563. doi: 10.1016/j.fertnstert.2013.08.005

Goldstein, M., & Schlegel, P. N. (Eds.). (2013). *Surgical and medical management of male infertility*. New York, NY: Cambridge University Press.

Gordon, J. D., Rydfors, J. T., & Druzin, M. L. (2001). *Obstetrics, gynecology and infertility: Handbook for clinicians–resident survival guide* (5th ed.). Arlington, VA: Scrub Hill Press.

Kang, B. M., & Wu, T. C. (2006). Effect of age on intrauterine insemination with frozen donor sperm. *Obstetrics and Gynecology, 88*, 93–98.

Klock, S. C. (1993). Psychological aspects of donor insemination. *Infertility and Reproductive Medicine Clinics of North America, 4*, 455–469.

Lebovic, D., Gordon, J. D., & Taylor, R. (2013). *Reproductive endocrinology and infertility: Handbook for clinicians* (2nd ed.). Arlington, VA: Scrub Hill Press.

Lipshultz, L. I., Howards, S. S., & Niederberger, C. S. (Eds.). (2009). *Infertility in the male* (4th ed.). New York, NY: Cambridge University Press.

Speroff, L., & Fitz, M. (2005). *Clinical gynecologic endocrinology and infertility* (7th ed., pp. 435–437). Philadelphia, PA: Lippincott Williams & Wilkins.

Stenchever, A. (2001). *Comprehensive gynecology* (4th ed., pp. 1204–1206). St. Louis, MO: Mosby.

Wainer, R., Bailly, M., Merlet, F., Tribalat, S., Ducat, B., & Lombroso, A. (1995). Prospective randomized comparison of intrauterine and intracervical insemination with donor spermatozoa. *Human Reproduction, 10*, 2919–2922.

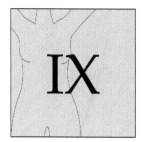

Contraception

Medical Eligibility Criteria for Contraceptive Use

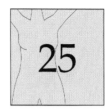

25

R. Mimi Secor

I. **The Centers for Disease Control and Prevention (CDC) medical eligibility criteria explained: In 2010 the issued the first ever U.S. Medical Eligibility Criteria (MEC) for contraceptive use.**
   A. These guidelines were issued in response to the 2009 WHO contraceptive guidelines.
   B. The CDC MEC guidelines provide evidence-based guidance on whether women and men with particular medical conditions or physical characteristics can safely use certain methods of contraception.
   C. Two-page summary charts are available and can be printed double-sided, laminated, and used by health care providers as a reference and also when counseling women.
   D. The categories of risk are based on a scale of 1 to 4 and these categories are summarized in Table 25.1.

II. **In 2011 the CDC updated the 2010 MEC guidelines for combined hormonal contraceptive use among postpartum women, on the basis of new scientific evidence.**
   A. Due to the persistence of the pregnancy-associated hypercoagulopathy state, women should not use combination contraceptive methods for the first 21 days postpartum.

III. **Recommendations for hormonal contraceptive use among women at high risk for HIV or infected with HIV were revised and updated by the CDC in 2012 based on new scientific evidence.**
   A. HIV-positive women may now use intrauterine contraceptives (IUC) as they have not been found to be associated with increased shedding or transmission of HIV.

TABLE 25.1 Categories for Medical Eligibility Criteria (MEC) for Contraceptive Use

RATING	DEFINITION
1	A condition for which there is no restriction for the use of the contraceptive method.
2	A condition for which the advantages of using the method generally outweigh the theoretical or proven risks.
3	A condition for which the theoretical or proven risks usually outweigh the advantages of using the method.
4	A condition that represents an unacceptable health risk if the contraceptive method is used.

Source: CDC (2010).

    B. Progestin-only methods are also considered acceptable; however, the risk of HIV transmission is unclear with the use of progestin-only medroxyprogesterone acetate (depot medroxyprogesterone acetate [DMPA]) injectable contraceptives.

IV. Issued in 2013, U.S. Selected Practice Recommendations (US SPR) for Contraceptive Use is a companion document to the CDC MEC, and addresses how to use contraceptive methods.
    A. Although the CDC MEC provides guidance on who can use various methods of contraception, the US SPR provides guidance on how contraceptive methods can be used and how to remove unnecessary barriers for patients in accessing and successfully using contraceptive methods.

Bibliography

American Congress of Obstetricians and Gynecologists (ACOG). (2011). Understanding and using the U.S. medical eligibility criteria for contraceptive use. *Obstetrics and Gynecology, 118*(3), 754–760. Retrieved from http://www.acog.org/Resources_And_Publications/Committee_Opinions/Committee_on_Gynecologic_Practice/Understanding_and_Using_the_US_Medical_Eligibility_Criteria_for_Contraceptive_Use_2010

CDC. (2010). United States medical eligibility criteria for contraceptive use. Retrieved from http://www.cdc.gov/reproductivehealth/UnintendedPregnancy/USMEC.htm

CDC. (2010). U.S. medical eligibility criteria for contraceptive use, 2010. *Morbidity and Mortality Weekly Report, 59*(RR04), 1–85. Retrieved from http://www.cdc.gov/reproductivehealth/unintendedpregnancy/USMEC.htm

CDC. (2011). Update to CDC's U.S. medical eligibility criteria for contraceptive use, 2010. Revised recommendations for the use of contraceptive methods during the postpartum period. *Morbidity and Mortality Weekly Report, 60*(26), 878–883. Retrieved July 7, 2011 from http://www.cdc.gov/mmwr/pdf/wk/mm6026.pdf

CDC. (2012). Update to CDC's U.S. medical eligibility criteria for contraceptive use, 2010. Revised recommendations for the use of hormonal contraception among women at high risk for HIV or infected with HIV. *Morbidity and Mortality Weekly Report, 61*(24), 449–452. Retrieved from http://www.cdc.gov/mmwr/preview/ mmwrhtml/mm6124a4.htm?s_cid=mm6124a4_e%0d%0a

CDC. (2013). U.S. selected practice recommendations for contraceptive use (US SPR). Centers for Disease Control and Prevention. Retrieved from http://www.cdc. gov/reproductivehealth/UnintendedPregnancy/USMEC.htm

World Health Organization. (2009). *Medical eligibility criteria for contraceptive use* (4th ed.). Geneva, Switzerland: WHO. Available at http://whqlibdoc.who.int/ publications/2010/9789241563888_eng.pdf

The FemCap

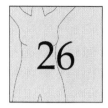

26

Rebecca Koeniger-Donohue

I. **The FemCap explained:** The FemCap is ideal for women of childbearing age who cannot or do not want to use hormonal contraceptives or an intrauterine device (IUD) and may be interested in using a female barrier contraceptive, especially one that requires no involvement by the male partner.

    A. The FemCap is a nonhormonal, latex-free female-controlled barrier contraceptive.

    B. Available by prescription with no side effects (unlike hormonal methods)

    C. Comes in three sizes. Proper size selection based on a woman's obstetric history based on the fact that pregnancy and delivery are the two major factors that have the greatest impact on the elasticity of the vagina and the size of the cervix.

    D. Approved by the U.S. Food and Drug Administration (FDA) in March 2003.

    E. Unique design: Brim designed to flare outward like an inverted funnel—flaring of the brim is met by the physiological inward concentric contraction of the vagina. Unlike the former Prentif cervical cap, which had to be snug over the cervix, the FemCap is held in place by the vaginal contraction, which allows the vagina to hold and support the FemCap in place without causing any pressure over the cervix.

    F. Reusable for longer than 1 year

    G. Does not interfere with the menstrual cycle, libido, or sexual pleasure for either partner

    H. Easy to insert and remove

    I. Designed to cover the cervix completely, delivers spermicide on the cervical—and most important—on the vaginal side, to meet the sperm head on

    J. It is effective in preventing pregnancy when used as directed and is safe to use, with no systemic side effects.

    K. May potentially prevent sexually transmitted infections (STIs)

    L. Advantages and disadvantages are summarized in Box 26.1.

II. **Overview of cervical caps**

    A. The cervical cap dates back more than 150 years, with a longer history of contraceptive use than the diaphragm.

    B. Before FDA approval of the FemCap, the only cervical cap available to women in the United States was the Prentif cavity rim cervical cap, which was manufactured by Lamberts Ltd. of London and is now off the market.

    C. Cervical caps differ from diaphragms in that they are designed to cover the cervix only; they are not designed to fit in the entire vagina.

    D. Cervical caps have been touted as one of the "best-kept secrets" of the Modern Age. However, they have never been used on a large scale in North America because of lack of clinician interest and lack of access.

III. **Description of the FemCap**

    A. Made of soft, durable, hypoallergenic, silicone rubber

    B. Its shape resembles a sailor's hat with an upturned brim that lies against the vaginal walls around the cervix.

    C. The design conforms to the anatomy of the cervix and the physiologic changes of the vagina that occur during sexual arousal. The dome of the FemCap fits over the cervix "like a glove," covering it completely.

    D. Complete cervical coverage prevents sperm from entering the cervix and the uterus.

        1. The rim of the cervical cap provides a snug fit into the vaginal fornices and covers the vaginal vault, and the brim covers the vaginal walls surrounding the cervix.

        2. The brim is longer posteriorly to conform to the unique anatomy of the vaginal walls.

        3. The out-flaring of the brim facing the vaginal opening has a unique groove that acts as a trap for sperm and a reservoir for any spermicide, or any microbicidal/spermicide that will soon be developed in the future, to reinforce the mechanical barrier of the FemCap.

        4. The FemCap is held in place by the muscular walls of the vagina and does not have to be snug around the cervix or hinge behind the pubic bone.

    E. The FemCap has a strap over the dome to facilitate removal of the device and provide added protection to the vaginal walls and cervix from possible fingernail abrasions during removal.

    F. When the FemCap is placed correctly, users should rarely, if ever, be aware of its presence. During the several clinical trials, fewer than 2% of women and 22% of men reported a sense of awareness of the FemCap and it did not interfere with their sexual pleasure.

BOX 26.1 *Advantages and Disadvantages of the FemCap*

Advantages
- Easy to use
- No systemic side effects or local effects
- Silicone rubber has a longer shelf life than latex rubber
- Safe for latex-allergic women or partners with a latex allergy
- Can be left in place for up to 48 hours
- Cannot be punctured by fingernails
- Does not break down with petroleum-based products
- Does not absorb odors; easy to clean
- Immediately reversible if and when pregnancy is desired
- Compared with diaphragm—Associated with fewer UTIs, needs less spermicide, more comfortable
- Compared with IUD—Less invasive
- Compared with hormonal contraceptives—Does not have systemic or serious side effects, does not change the menstrual cycle, does not decrease libido
- Compared with male condom—Does not interrupt spontaneity or reduce sexual pleasure for either partner; is under the woman's control

Disadvantages
- Requires a prescription and a pelvic exam
- Necessitates that a woman touch her genitalia, which may be culturally or personally unacceptable
- Theoretical risk of toxic shock syndrome

STI, sexually transmitted infection; UTI, urinary tract infection; IUD, intrauterine device

---

G. The anatomical design and the nonallergenic material of the FemCap offers an additional benefit when compared with the latex diaphragm. Unlike the diaphragm, the FemCap reduces the likelihood of contracting a urinary tract infection (UTI). It is occlusive for the cervix, and yet, unobtrusive to the vagina and urethra.

H. The FemCap can be cleansed easily with hand soap and water.

I. It does not deteriorate from exposure to heat, body fluids, or petroleum-based products. It is reusable for about 1 year without any deterioration.

J. To avoid the theoretical risk of toxic shock syndrome, it must not be used during menstruation.

IV. **Size selection**

A. Selecting the correct size is based on obstetric history and pelvic exam.

> ### BOX 26.2 *FemCap: Contraindications*
>
> - Adhesions between the cervix and the vaginal walls
> - Third-degree uterine prolapse
> - Flat cervix
> - Acute cervicitis
> - Cancer of the cervix
> - Active pelvic inflammatory disease
> - History of toxic shock syndrome
> - Cut or tear in the vagina or cervix visualized on pelvic exam
> - Allergy to spermicide
> - Women who are adverse to touching their genitals (cultural norms or personal preference)

  B. The pelvic exam is essential to estimate the size of the cervix and to exclude women who have contraindications such as cancer, laceration, infection, or a flat cervix. Box 26.2 summarizes contraindications to the FemCap.

  C. Available in three sizes
    1. Small (22 mm internal diameter) for nulligravida women
    2. Medium (26 mm) for women who have been pregnant but have had a miscarriage, therapeutic abortion, or delivered by Caesarian section.
    3. Large (30 mm) for women who have had at least one full-term vaginal delivery.
    4. If the woman denies ever having been pregnant, but the cervix looks bigger on pelvic exam than a nulligavida cervix, then provide her with the 26-mm FemCap. If in doubt about the fit it is safest to use the 26-mm size.

  D. Cost: The retail price for a single FemCap kit is $89. For added preparation and convenience, a 2-pack FemCap kit is available for $130.00. Each kit comes with an instructional videotape, which is also available online in many languages; illustrated color brochure; and FDA package insert.

  E. It is recommended that the FemCap be replaced every year (or sooner if it shows signs of deterioration).

  F. For information and orders please visit www.femcap.com.

  V. Protection against STIs and HIV/AIDS
    A. Using the FemCap with spermicide, the diaphragm with spermicide, or Lea's shield with spermicide have *not* been shown to protect against STIs.

B. No studies have yet demonstrated a protective effect against HIV by limiting access to cells in the cervix. These studies are still in the research stages.

C. Nonoxynol-9 spermicide alone does not provide protection against HIV, chlamydia, and gonorrhea.

D. Frequent use of large doses of spermicide alone can cause disruption of the single-layer endocervical columnar epithelium. This disruption creates microabrasions or ulcerations that, at least in theory, could *increase* susceptibility to HIV transmission.

VI. **Efficacy and acceptability**

A. The typical failure rate (Pearl index) of the second-generation FemCap was estimated to be 7.6 per hundred women per year.

B. Effectiveness of the FemCap varies, depending on the motivation of the user and on whether she uses the device correctly and consistently.

C. Labeling recommends the use of an emergency contraceptive pill if a woman uses the FemCap incorrectly or fails to use it during an act of intercourse.

D. Seven requirements for perfect use of the FemCap are listed in Box 26.3.

VII. **Candidate selection and counseling**

A. Clinicians can enhance correct and consistent use of the FemCap by discussing the following key points
   1. Emphasizing motivational and lifestyle factors
   2. Establishing a habit or routine of FemCap contraceptive use
   3. Keeping two FemCaps on hand (one for home and one for travel)

BOX 26.3 *Seven Requirements for Perfect Use of the FemCap*

1. Motivation for consistent and correct use of the FemCap
2. Viewing of the instructional video provided with the FemCap prior to use
3. Use of backup method of contraception during the learning phase
4. Insertion of the FemCap before any sexual arousal
5. Application of a small amount of spermicide; checking the FemCap's position before each use
6. Leaving the FemCap in place for at least 6 hours after the last act of intercourse
7. Use of emergency contraception (morning-after pill) if the FemCap was not used or if it was used incorrectly

4. Inserting the FemCap *before* any sexual arousal to ensure proper fit and to avoid interruption of spontaneity
5. Maintaining a diary to record dates of insertion, removal, and menstrual cycles
6. Strongly advising emergency contraception, as soon as possible, if the woman had unprotected intercourse or used the FemCap incorrectly

VIII. **FemCap protocol for clinicians: One can request information on the FemCap, as well as request a kit, by logging on to www.femcap.com.**
   A. The clinician should
      1. Schedule a 30- to 45-minute visit for cap fitting and instructions.
      2. Perform a pelvic examination to exclude any anatomical or pathological contraindications.
      3. Discuss the advantages and disadvantages and reinforce the importance of adherence with its use.
      4. Provide the woman with her FemCap size, according to obstetrical history (one of three sizes).
      5. Provide her with the package insert and videotape.
      6. Allow her privacy and time to practice inserting and removing the FemCap, making sure she can identify and cover her cervix with the FemCap.
      7. Encourage her to practice insertion and removal several times.
      8. Practice should be continued until she can successfully insert, remove, and recognize proper placement of the FemCap.
      9. Have the woman leave the FemCap in place for clinician to recheck for proper fit by digital examination.
      10. Speculum examination (if needed for further confirmation)
      11. Use only a plastic disposable speculum as it has blunt tips and allows good lighting.
      12. Insert the speculum halfway into the vagina and open it enough at this point to be able to see the FemCap covering the cervix without dislodging it.
      13. Some comments
         a. Unlike the diaphragm, the bulk of the spermicide is stored in the grooved area between the dome and brim of the FemCap, facing the vaginal opening, to expose sperm to the spermicide on deposition into the vagina.
         b. The FemCap does not require measurement for custom fitting like the diaphragm.
         c. The woman can insert and remove the FemCap in a squatting position on her own much easier and faster than any clinician can insert it for her, no matter how skillful.

IX. **Directions for use**
  A. Insertion
    1. Place ½ teaspoon of spermicide in the groove between the dome and the brim of the FemCap and ¼ teaspoon of the spermicide over the rim and in the bowl of the device.
    2. Spread a thin layer all over the brim of the FemCap except for the spots where the finger and the thumb are holding the device.
    3. Squeeze and flatten the device, insert it into the vagina with the bowl facing upward and the long brim entering first.
    4. The FemCap is inserted downward toward the rectum and then downward and back as far as possible in the vagina to be sure the cervix is covered.
    5. It is important to ensure that the FemCap is not partway between the vaginal opening and the cervix.
    6. With repeated acts of intercourse, check the position of the FemCap and insert ½ teaspoon of spermicide (without removing the device).
    7. If the FemCap is placed correctly, the woman should not be aware of its presence during intercourse or daily activities. It should fit comfortably over the cervix, with the rim fitting snugly to the vaginal fornices and the brim adhering to the vaginal walls.
    8. It *must* be placed in the vagina *before* any sexual stimulation and may be worn for up to 48 hours maximum. The device should remain in place for at least 6 hours after sexual intercourse, but no longer than 48 hours altogether.
  B. Removal
    1. The woman should squat and bear down, which will bring the removal strap closer to the fingers, facilitating removal of the device.
    2. The device can then be rotated and removed comfortably by pushing the tip of the finger against the dome of the FemCap to dimple it. This will break the suction and allow room for the finger to be inserted between the dome and the removal strap and then it can be pulled out gently by hooking a finger into the removal strap.
    3. The woman should develop a routine for insertion and removal, such as after her daily shower.
  C. Detailed instructions are provided by the manufacturer on the DVD and in written materials included in the FemCap kit.

X. **Care of the FemCap**
  A. The FemCap should be washed with antibacterial soap and rinsed thoroughly with tepid tap water and air dried or patted dry with a clean soft towel.

B. It should be stored in the plastic container supplied with it and kept in a cool, dry place. Do not use powder.

C. It should never be placed in a microwave or cleaned by synthetic detergents, organic solvents, or sharp objects.

D. This process is 99.9% effective in eliminating all bacteria and viruses from the FemCap.

Bibliography

Karim, Q. A., Karim, S. S., Frohlich, J. A. Grobler, A. C., Baxter, C., Mansoor, L. E., ... CAPRISA 004 Trial Group. (2010). Effectiveness and safety of tenofovir gel, an antiretroviral microbicide for the prevention of HIV infection in women. *Science, 329*(5996), 1168–1174.

Koeniger-Donohue, R. (2006). The FemCap: A non-hormonal contraceptive. *Women's Health Care: A Practical Journal for Nurse Practitioners* (Primary Care Edition), *5*(4), 79–91.

Shihata, A. (n.d.). FemCap. Retrieved from http://www.femcap.com

Shihata, A., & Brody, S. (2011). HIV/STIs and pregnancy prevention: Using a cervical barrier and microbicide. *World Journal of AIDS, 1*, 131–135. doi:10.4236/wja.2011.14018

The Diaphragm

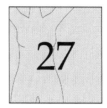

Helen A. Carcio

I. **The diaphragm explained**
  A. The diaphragm is an effective form of contraception.
    1. It is considered a barrier method, which means that it provides a barrier between the ejaculated sperm and its entrance into the uterus.
    2. The anterior rim fits securely behind the pubic bone, and the posterior rim fits behind and below the cervix, covering the cervix with the spermicidal jelly-filled cup.
    3. Correct fitting, consistent use, and proper insertion are critical to the success of the use of the diaphragm.
  B. Mechanism of action
    1. The diaphragm prevents contraception by eliminating the possibility of the sperm fertilizing the egg.
    2. It forms a mechanical barrier to prevent sperm from entering the cervical canal.
    3. It acts as a receptacle for the spermicide, which immobilizes the sperm.
  C. Historical perspective
    1. The diaphragm has been used ever since the beginning of recorded history.
    2. There are early references to use of honey, spice, oils, sticky plugs, and other substances for birth control.
    3. The actual diaphragm was invented in the late 1800s, although it was not well promoted.
  D. Use today
    1. Has fallen in and out of vogue over the past 10 to 20 years
    2. Has been replaced by the more effective and easier-to-use cervical cap (see Chapter 26, "The FemCap")
  E. Advantages
    1. It offers the woman a large degree of control over her body, which women are seeking.

2. Acts as a barrier to many sexually transmitted diseases when used with contraceptive jelly, foam, or cream (This feature is under investigation.)
3. Provides a local contraceptive effect, rather than a systemic effect, such as that provided by oral contraceptives or Depo-Provera
4. It is inexpensive.
5. The diaphragm is durable, easy to care for.
6. Serious side effects are rare.
7. No data as yet regarding effect on transmission of human immunodeficiency virus (HIV)

F. Disadvantages
1. User dependent: Depends on the motivation of the user
2. It cannot be bought over the counter, such as contraceptive foam.
3. Requires that the woman see her practitioner for proper sizing and prescribing
4. May interfere with the spontaneity of lovemaking because spermicide must be added after each act of intercourse (The woman may teach her partner to insert the diaphragm as part of the ritual.)
5. Spermicidal cream or jelly is perceived as being messy.
6. The partner may feel the diaphragm. A different size or type of diaphragm might help.
7. The diaphragm may be uncomfortable if it is fitted improperly.
8. It is difficult to conceal its use.
9. The woman's partner may object to the taste of spermicide. Suggest the diaphragm be inserted after oral sex.
10. There is expense related to the use of spermicide if intercourse is frequent.
11. Women need to feel comfortable with touching their own bodies.
12. One needs time and privacy for insertion and removal of the diaphragm.
13. Prolonged retention can cause vaginal irritation.
14. Possibility of toxic shock syndrome. Most research today states that the incidence of this syndrome is rare.
15. Not all women can use the diaphragm. See Box 27.1 for a list of contraindications.

G. Effectiveness
1. The diaphragm is 97% effective.
2. It is nearly as good as the birth control pill, but not as effective as Depo-Provera and the intrauterine device (IUD).
3. A major factor that increases the effectiveness of the diaphragm is the ability of the user to use it consistently.

BOX 27.1 *Contraindications to Diaphragm Use*

- Allergy to rubber, spermicide, or both—may try changing brands
- Inability of patient or partner to learn insertion technique
- Inability to physically hold diaphragm and insert into vagina
- Prolapsed uterus
- Large cystocele
- Markedly shallow pubic arch
- Vesicovaginal fistula
- Full-term delivery in past 12 weeks
- Acute pelvic inflammatory disease or cervicitis
- Undiagnosed vaginal bleeding
- Abnormal Pap smear
- Recent cervical procedure

II. Description
  A. The diaphragm is a small rubber cup, with a firm rim stabilized by a rubber-covered steel spring.
    1. The diaphragm fits behind the pubic bone within the vaginal vault.
    2. Saucer-like disc made of latex with a flexible rim
  B. Types: There are many different types of diaphragms, the choice of which depends on the woman's pelvic muscle tone, as well as the anatomic shape of the vagina and the pubic bone, which holds the diaphragm tightly in place (see Table 27.1 for comparison of various types).
  C. Sizes
    1. Sizes range from 50 to 105 mm in diameter, in increments of 2.5 to 5 mm.
    2. Most women use between size 65 and 80 mm.

TABLE 27 .1 Comparison of Types of Diaphragms

DIAPHRAGM TYPE	STRENGTH	INDICATIONS	CONTRAINDICATIONS
Flat spring	Thin rim with gentle strength	Normal vaginal tone	Shallow pubic arch
Coil spring	Intermediate strength	Good muscle tone	Deep recess behind pubic arch
Arcing spring	Strong, firm double spring	Vaginal delivery	Poor vaginal muscle tone

D. Use of spermicide
1. Diaphragms must always be used with spermicide.
2. Spreading the cream on the edge of the diaphragm may ease insertion but may also make the diaphragm more slippery, thus possibly making insertion more difficult.
3. Spermicide is usually effective for 6 hours.
   a. Some clinicians believe that 2 hours should be the cutoff point for intercourse after spermicide application.
   b. Probably best to err on the side of caution; therefore, their recommendation is that if more than 2 hours have elapsed since insertion, additional spermicide should be added vaginally with subsequent intercourse.
4. Warn the woman never to substitute petroleum jelly or other lubricants for spermicide.
   a. Other lubricants lack spermicidal effects.
   b. Petroleum jelly can deteriorate the latex in the diaphragm.

III. Indications for use
A. The diaphragm is well liked by many women, but not every woman can use a diaphragm.
B. It is an appropriate method for a couple in a monogamous relationship who are motivated to work together to prevent pregnancy.
1. The failure rate decreases with increasing age and duration of use.
2. The failure rate increases with single status and increased coital frequency.
C. The diaphragm is an excellent choice for the woman who is comfortable with touching her genitals and who is committed to using the device every time she has intercourse.

IV. The fitting procedure
A. Timing of fitting
1. Fitting of the diaphragm can occur at any time of the month.
2. It is best to wait until at least 6 weeks after delivery of a child.
3. Menses makes the fitting more uncomfortable for the patient.
4. If any infection is present or there are abnormal findings on the woman's Pap smear, wait until condition resolves.
B. Fitting kits
1. Fitting kits can be obtained from the companies that produce the diaphragm.
2. The kit should be available in the examining room.
3. Fitting diaphragms are better to use than fitting rings.
C. Health history
1. Inquire about contraindications listed in Box 27.1.
2. Ask about the woman's success with other methods of contraception.

3. Assess comfort with and use of tampons.
    a. Address woman's comfort with touching her genital area.
    b. Help in learning how to use the diaphragm if the woman has prior experience with tampons.
D. Before insertion, review
    1. Printed instructions
    2. Effectiveness
    3. Insertion and removal technique
    4. Discuss when to insert and remove.
    5. Explain that the diaphragm comes in many sizes and that the woman may have to try two or three different ones to get the right fit.
    6. Explain that she will be allowed time to practice in the examination room, taking the diaphragm in and out a few times.
E. Perform the pelvic examination.
    1. Note the size and position of the uterus.
    2. Check for irritation or infection.
        a. Observe the cervix for any signs of infection.
        b. Perform a wet mount, if indicated, and treat any diagnosed infection.
    3. Have the woman bear down to determine whether a cystocele is present. Measure depth of the pubic arch.
        a. Normal pubic arch: Choose coil spring.
        b. Shallow pubic arch: Choose flat spring.
        c. Markedly shallow pubic arch: Consider an alternate method.
F. Fitting the diaphragm
    1. Explain each step of the procedure, eliciting feedback from the patient.
    2. Move the tips of the examining fingers into the posterior fornix of the vagina.
    3. Make note of where the hand comes in contact with the pubic bone.
    4. The rim of the fitting diaphragm should extend from the tip of the middle examining finger to just in front of the point noted on the examining hand.
    5. The average sizes used are 70, 75, and 80. Start with one of those three sizes and adjust up or down as needed.
    6. Grasp the edges of the diaphragm, and squeeze the edges together rim to rim.
    7. While holding labia apart, insert diaphragm deep into the vagina, sliding it posteriorly under the cervix and tucking the anterior rim behind pubic bone (see Figure 27.1).
    8. Checking for proper fit
        a. If the woman can feel the diaphragm, it may be too big or improperly placed.

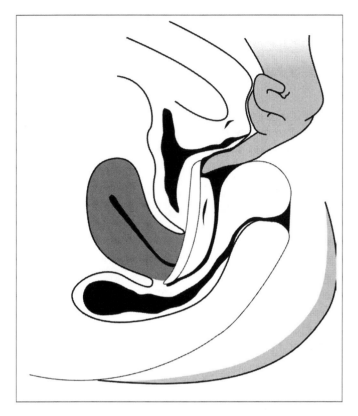

FIGURE 27.1 Tucking the rim behind the pubic bone for a proper fit.

    b. The diaphragm should not be able to move from side to side or from front to back.
    c. The rim should not be buckled.
    d. One should only be able to get the tip of one finger between the rim of the diaphragm and the pubic bone.
    e. The fit should be on the snug side because the vagina expands with sexual excitement.
  9. Once the diaphragm is inserted
    a. Have woman cough or bear down.
    b. Allow time for the woman to walk around the room, sit down, and stand up a few times.
    c. Give the woman privacy to practice insertion and removal two or three times.
    d. Ask her to leave the diaphragm in place.
  10. Recheck position and proper size.
    a. Evaluate whether the diaphragm still covers the cervix and is tucked behind the pubic bone.
  11. Remove the diaphragm and check for any tears.

G. Document
  1. Size and type of diaphragm
  2. Perceived patient comprehension
  3. Fit
  4. Demonstration and redemonstration

V. Patient education

A. Review causes of method failure.
  1. Dislodgment during coitus particularly with
     a. Change in coital position
     b. Use of the female superior position
     c. Expansion of the vagina with sexual excitement
  2. If the diaphragm is too large, the woman will experience
     a. Lower back and/or rectal pain
     b. Lower abdominal pain
     c. Difficulty voiding
     d. Cramps in thighs
  3. If the diaphragm is too small, it moves out of proper position.
  4. Failure to insert before every occasion of coitus
  5. Failure to tuck the rim of the diaphragm behind the pubic bone, allowing the penis to override the diaphragm
  6. Failure to check coverage of cervix
B. Discuss adjustment period
  1. It does take a period of time to become adjusted to using the diaphragm.
  2. Use of the diaphragm soon becomes much easier once it becomes more habitual.
C. The woman should call the health center or return to the office if
  1. Pain or discomfort occur with the diaphragm in place
  2. A change in vaginal discharge occurs

VI. Instructions to the woman for use at home

A. Initial trial
  1. Practice insertion and removal every night.
  2. Use backup method until return visit.
  3. Return in 2 to 4 weeks with the diaphragm in place.
B. Before insertion
  1. Hold diaphragm up to the light and observe for any holes or cracks, especially near the rim.
  2. Rinse off any powder.
  3. Make sure your fingernails are short so that there is no possibility of tearing the diaphragm.
  4. Box 27.2 summarizes the insertion and removal techniques.
  5. If the diaphragm is left in for more than 24 hours, be alert for signs and symptoms of toxic shock syndrome (Box 27.3).

BOX 27.2 *Inserting and Removing a Diaphragm*

Insertion

- The diaphragm is inserted up to 2 hours before intercourse.
- Apply spermicidal jelly or cream to rim and inside of dorne.
- Holding dorne down, squeeze rim until sides touch.
- Stand with one foot propped, squat, or lie down.
- Spread labia, insert folded diaphragm deep into vagina.
- Push diaphragm back as far as possible, then tuck front rim up behind the pubic bone inside the vagina.
- Check for placement; feel for cervix covered with rubber dorne.
- For repeated intercourse, add more spermicide without removing diaphragm.
- Leave diaphragm in place for 6 to 8 hours after last intercourse.

Removal

- To remove diaphragm, place index finger behind front rim; pull down.
- If suction is tight, insert finger between pubic bone and rim to break suction, then pull down.
- Clean diaphragm with soap and water, rinse, and dry. Dust with cornstarch or unscented powder; perfumed powders can damage rubber or irritate tissue.
- Store diaphragm in plastic container in cool, dry place.
- Check diaphragm before and after every use for tears and holes.
- Do not use petroleum jelly because it causes deterioration of rubber.

C. Care of the diaphragm

1. The diaphragm can last for years, as long as it has been carefully maintained.
2. After use, the diaphragm should be washed with warm water, using a mild soap, and allowed to air dry.
3. The diaphragm should be powdered with cornstarch, which will help absorb excess moisture and odors. (Talc should not be used because its use has been linked to cervical cancer.)
4. Cornstarch should be washed off before the next use.
5. Always be sure to hold the device up to the light to observe for any tiny cracks and holes, particularly around the rim.
6. A diaphragm that has been tucked away in a drawer should be checked carefully.
7. Store in a plastic container in cool, dry location.
8. Do not
   a. Store in alcohol, because it will ruin the diaphragm.
   b. Put the device in the microwave for sterilization. The metal ring will ruin the microwave.

BOX 27.3 *Reducing the Risk of Toxic Shock Syndrome*

Toxic shock syndrome (TSS) can occur with the use of the diaphragm and cervical cap.

To reduce the risk of TSS with these contraceptives, you should do the following:

- Wash your hands thoroughly with soap and water before insertion or removal.
- Never leave in place for more than 24 hours.
- Never use during your menstrual period or if you have any vaginal bleeding or spotting.
- Wait 12 weeks before using a contraceptive after a full-term pregnancy.
- Watch for TSS danger signs
  - Fever (temperature 101°F or more)
  - Diarrhea
  - Vomiting
  - Muscle aches
  - Rash (similar to sunburn)
- Remove the contraceptive right away if you develop these signs, and see your health care provider.
- Choose a different type of contraceptive if you have ever had TSS.

    D. Common errors
        1. Inserting diaphragm into the anterior fornix, above the cervix
        2. Failing to tuck the diaphragm behind the pubic bone, which allows the penis to override the diaphragm during penetration
    E. The follow-up visit
        1. Return in 2 to 4 weeks.
        2. Have the diaphragm in place.
        3. Use an alternate form of birth control (i.e., condoms) until you become comfortable with the diaphragm.

VII. The return visit
    A. Inquire about any difficulty with
        1. Insertion technique: Checking fit over the cervix
            a. A critical aspect
            b. Some women do not check because they feel uncomfortable touching their own genitals.
        2. Removal
        3. Cleaning
        4. Use of spermicide
        5. Partner satisfaction

    B. Perform the pelvic examination
        1. Check for proper position of the diaphragm over the cervix.
        2. Recheck for proper size.
        3. Remove the diaphragm. Check for any tears.
        4. Observe the cervix for any signs of infection.
        5. Check for vaginal irritation.
    C. Educate the woman as to when the diaphragm must be refitted.
        1. With change in weight of plus or minus 20 pounds
        2. Postpartum
        3. After any pelvic surgery
        4. If it has been more than a year since it was used
        5. If another form of contraception is desired
        6. Occurrence of stress incontinence
        7. If the diaphragm is damaged or deteriorating
    D. Call or return with any concerns listed previously.

Bibliography

American College of Obstetricians and Gynecologists. (n.d.).*Barrier methods of contraception.* Retrieved November 16, 2011 from http://www.acog.org/publications/faq/faq022.cfm

Association of Reproductive Health Professionals. (n.d.). *Choosing a method of birth control.* Retrieved November 14, 2011, from http://www.arhp.org/Publications-and-Resources/Quick-Reference-Guide-for-Clinicians/choosing/Cervical-Cap

Barbieri, R. L. (n.d.). *How to fit and use a diaphragm for contraception.* Retrieved November 16, 2011, from http://www.uptodate.com/home/index.html

Cates, W., Holmes, K.K., & Stone, K.M. (2011). Vaginal barriers and spermicides. In R. A. Hatcher et al. *Contraceptive technology* (20th ed., p. 391). New York, NY: Ardent Media.

Office of Population Affairs. (n.d.). *Diaphragm fact sheet.* Retrieved November 16, 2011 from http://www.hhs.gov/opa/reproductive-health/contraception/diaphragm

Trussell, J. (2007). Choosing a contraceptive: Efficacy, safety, and personal considerations. In R. A. Hatcher et al. (Eds.), *Contraceptive technology* (19th ed., pp. 19–47). New York, NY: Ardent Media.

Zieman, M., Guillebaud, J., & Weisberg, E. (2010). Female-controlled barrier methods. *A pocket guide to managing contraception* (p. 63). Tiger, GA: Bridging the Gap Communications.

Intrauterine Contraception

28

R. Mimi Secor, Marcia Denine, and Linda Pettit

I. **The intrauterine contraceptive (IUC) explained**
  A. Definition: The IUC is a plastic contraceptive device that is inserted into the uterine cavity through the cervical canal.
    1. There are three kinds of intrauterine contraceptives available in the United States. All types have a two-strand, polyethylene monofilament string that protrudes from the cervical os.
      a. Copper IUC (ParaGard) (www.paragard.com) with white strings
      b. Levonorgestrel (LNG) containing IUC (Mirena) (www.mirena.com) with brown strings
      c. Levonorgestrel containing IUC (Skyla) (www.skyla-us.com) with blue strings
    2. IUC is for contraceptive use only. No intrauterine contraceptive is intended to offer any protection against STI (sexually transmitted infection) transmission. If STI risk, encourage consistent use of condoms.
    3. Efficacy equivalent to sterilization yet reversible
    4. Cost-effective
  B. The ParaGard T380A is a copper-releasing intrauterine contraceptive (Cu-IUC).
    1. Manufactured by Teva Pharmaceuticals
    2. One size; fine-copper wire wound around vertical limb of T
    3. Releasing free copper and copper salts, affecting the endometrium
    4. Advantages
      a. Is the longest acting contraceptive method available
      b. Metabolically neutral
      c. Can remain in place for 10 years; off-label for 12 years
      d. Has the lowest expulsion rates
      e. Can be inserted into nulliparous women

    f. Safety and efficacy have been established in women older than 16 years of age.

    g. Ideas about how ParaGard works include preventing sperm from reaching the egg, preventing sperm from fertilizing the egg, and possibly preventing the egg from attaching (implanting) in the uterus. ParaGard does not stop your ovaries from releasing an egg (ovulating) each month. ParaGard is not an abortifacient.

  5. Contraindicated in women with known allergy to copper or a diagnosis of Wilson's disease

  6. Disadvantage: May alter bleeding pattern and increase menstrual flow, as well as increase cramping associated with menses

C. The Mirena IUC is a levonorgestrel-containing intrauterine contraceptive (LNG-IUC).

  1. Manufactured by Bayer HealthCare

  2. Progestin-only hormone-releasing device with initial release of 20 mcg time-released every day that diminishes by 50% after 5 years (per package insert)

  3. The progestin is contained in a vertical limb that releases low-dose progestin locally into the endometrial cavity.

  4. Offers continuous contraceptive protection for 5 years

  5. Cumulative 5-year failure rate is 0.5 to 0.7 per 100 women

  6. Thins endometrial lining

  7. Thickens cervical secretions

  8. Decreases menstrual flow

  9. Reduces dysmenorrheal and menstrual blood loss. After 8 months 50% of women have no menstrual bleeding, only monthly spotting. Twenty percent of women have amenorrhea in the first year.

  10. Food and Drug Administration (FDA)-approved indications include contraception and treatment of heavy menstrual bleeding for women who choose to use intrauterine contraception as their method of contraception (package insert, 2013).

  11. Recommended for women who have had at least one child (package insert, 2013).

  12. Appropriate for parous women or nulliparous women with dysmenorrhea or menorrhagia

D. Skyla IUC is a progestin-releasing LNG-IUC.

  1. Manufactured by Bayer HealthCare

  2. Releases levonorgestrel at a rate of 14 mcg/day after 24 days and declines to 5 mcg/day after 3 years

  3. Provides continuous contraceptive protection for 3 years

  4. Actions are the same as the Mirena LNG-IUC (see above)

  5. Cannot be used for postcoital contraception

    6. Appropriate for parous or nulliparous women

    7. Skyla is a smaller device (28 mm horizontally) than the Mirena and is the preferred LNG-IUC for a nulliparous woman.

E. Contraindications for IUC use

    1. Both Cu-INCs and LNG-IUCs

        a. Pregnancy or suspicion of pregnancy

        b. Congenital or acquired uterine anomaly if it distorts the uterine cavity

        c. Acute pelvic inflammatory disease (PID) (initiation only is category 4). Past history of PID is not a contraindication if no known current risk factors for STIs. Increased risk of STIs is category 3 for both IUCs for initiation only.

        d. Immediate post–septic abortion and puerperal sepsis

        e. Known or suspected uterine or cervical neoplasia (while awaiting treatment)

        f. Unexplained vaginal bleeding (initiation only is category 4)

        g. Current untreated acute cervicitis or chlamydia or gonorrhea infection (initiation only is category 4). Vaginitis including *Trichomonas vaginalis* and bacterial vaginosis are not a contraindication (category 2).

        h. Severe cirrhosis, benign hepatocellular adenoma, malignant hepatoma (LNG-IUC only are category 3). Cu-IUC is category 1 for these conditions.

        i. A previously inserted IUC that has not been removed (per package insert).

        j. Breast cancer (LNG-IUC only), current is category 4, past history, and no evidence of current disease for 5 years is category 3.

        k. Systemic lupus erythematosus (SLE) with positive or unknown antiphospholipid antibodies (category 3 for LNG-IUC only)

        l. Solid organ transplantation; complicated graft failure (initiation only for both is category 3)

        m. Pelvic tuberculosis (initiation only is category 4 for both IUCs)

        n. HIV is *not* a contraindication for either IUC. These guidelines were updated in 2012.

    2. Mirena should be used with caution in patients who have

        a. Coagulopathy or are receiving anticoagulants

        b. Migraine, focal migraine with asymmetrical visual loss, or other symptoms indicating

        c. Transient cerebral ischemia

        d. Exceptionally severe headaches

        e. Marked increase of blood pressure

        f. Severe arterial disease, such as stroke or myocardial infarction

F. Historical perspective (listed in chronologic order)
   1. The first intrauterine device was a ring-shaped device described in 1909 by a German gynecologist, Ernest Grafenberg.
   2. During the 1960s and 1970s, 10% of women in the United States who used contraception chose the IUC.
   3. The Dalkon Shield was introduced in 1970.
      a. Within 3 years, a high incidence of pelvic inflammatory disease (PID) was recognized.
      b. It was documented that the braided multifilament tail of the Dalkon Shield provided a pathway for bacteria to pass through the protective cervical mucus and ascend into the uterus.
      c. A large number of women sued the manufacturer.
      d. The number of IUCs used decreased in proportion to the increase in IUC litigation.
   4. The controversy and litigation surrounding the Dalkon Shield tainted the image of all IUCs.
   5. Additionally, two studies in the mid-1980s reported that the use of IUCs was associated with infertility, this further frightened women.
   6. Many IUCs were removed from the market in 1986 because of the concern regarding medical liability, giving the message that IUCs are unsafe.
   7. Women become distrustful because they remember the Dalkon Shield.
   8. The number of women using IUCs in the United States declined by two thirds from 1981 to 1989.
   9. Today, manufacturers have made great strides to protect the product.
      a. Package materials include an informed consent.
      b. Strict patient-selection criteria are listed.
      c. Appropriate clinician–patient dialogue is strongly encouraged.
      d. Label comes with extensive warnings
   10. Despite the above-mentioned measures, IUCs now account for less than 1% of the contraception used in the United States.
   11. Worldwide, IUC is the most popular method of reversible contraception.
G. Some comments and considerations regarding selection of contraception
   1. The prescription of any contraception needs to be individually tailored.
   2. Patient selection and proper insertion technique are vital.
      a. Group A streptococcal infection has been reported following IUC insertion. Strict aseptic technique is essential during insertion (per package insert).

3. Factors influencing a woman's choice of contraceptive
    a. Sexual lifestyle
    b. Number of partners and frequency of coitus
    c. Status of marriage or relationship
    d. Cultural or religious beliefs
    e. Motivation of the woman and her partner
    f. Degree of comfort with one's body
    g. Lactation status
    h. Confidence in the method
    i. Effectiveness
    j. Safety
    k. Access to health care
    l. Convenience
    m. Temporary or permanent nature of the method
    n. Previous experience or experience of others
    o. Educational and cognitive status
    p. Cost
    q. Health concerns
G. Advantages of the IUC in general
    1. It is safe, highly effective, and economical.
    2. Offers long-term contraceptive protection with few compliance issues

II. **The insertion**
A. Timing of insertion; controversial
    1. Can occur at any time as long as contraindications and potential pregnancy have been ruled out
    2. Insertion during menses
        a. Insertion may be easier—cervical canal is lubricated with menstrual blood
        b. Relatively sure that the patient is not pregnant
        c. Os is slightly dilated
        d. The disadvantage is that menstrual blood may provide a medium for bacterial growth. The infection rate and expulsion rate are higher when the IUC is inserted during menses.
    3. Insertion at mid-cycle
        a. Cervical os is dilated
        b. Must have used protection the previous week
    4. Insertion immediately on the removal of another IUC
    5. Following delivery or abortion. May be inserted following these procedures. Expulsion rate is lower if the clinician waits until 4 to 8 weeks postpartum visit.
B. Preinsertion visit, with IUC insertion at next visit
    1. Complete history
        a. Emphasize contraindications (Box 28.1).
        b. Inquire about previous episode of syncope.

BOX 28.1 *Sample Patient Consent Form*

I have read this brochure in its entirety and discussed its contents with my clinician. My clinician has answered all my questions and has advised me of the risks and benefits associated with the use of ParaGard T380A, with other forms of contraception, and with no contraception at all.

    I have considered all these factors and voluntarily choose to have the ParaGard T380A inserted by _____ on _____

Clinician _____

Patient Signature _____

The patient has signed this brochure in my presence after I counseled her and answered all her questions.

Clinician_____Date_____

This ParaGard T380A is scheduled for removal on _____

Distributed courtesy of Teva Pharmaceutics.

---

    c. Focus on the patient's history of heart disease.
    d. Note date of last menses, length, flow, and any associated pain.
    e. Ask whether any odor or change in vaginal discharge is present.
    f. Inquire about any signs of pregnancy.
    g. Determine past and present sexual partners.
    h. Assess behavioral risk of STIs.
  2. Pelvic examination, including bimanual examination
    a. Inspect vulva, vagina, and cervix, noting any signs of infection or cervical stenosis.
    b. Note size, shape, contour, and position of uterus or any tenderness or masses on palpation.
    c. Establish absence of infection, pregnancy, or neoplasia.
  3. Use the 2010 Centers for Disease Control (CDC) STI Treatment Guidelines to assess for STIs and consider a wet mount to assess for vaginitis, if indicated.
    a. If WBCs (white blood cells) are present, culture for gonorrhea and chlamydia. Delay insertion of the IUC until after treatment if culture is positive. Explain the risks.
    b. If bacterial vaginosis is present, the IUC may still be inserted and bacterial vaginosis (BV) treated, preferably with oral metronidazole or oral clindamycin per the 2010 CDC STI Treatment Guidelines.
  4. Counseling regarding disadvantages and advantages
  5. Encourage questions.
  6. Explain procedure.

7. The patient may read and sign informed consent, or she may bring to next visit (Box 28.1).
8. Explain the necessity of proper protection against pregnancy until insertion visit.
9. Laboratory tests
   a. Hemoglobin and hematocrit measurement recommended, particularly if the patient has a history of heavy menses.
   b. Pap smear, per the 2012 American Cancer Society (ACS) Pap HPV screening guidelines, the American Society for Colposcopy and Cervical Pathology (ASCCP), and the American Society for Clinical Pathology (ASCP) Consensus Guidelines.
   c. Sedimentation rate, STI testing per the 2010 CDC STI Treatment Guidelines, and vaginal microscopy if PID suspected
   d. Routine urinalysis and urine pregnancy test as needed
   e. Chlamydia and gonorrhea screening per 2010 CDC STI Treatment Guidelines according to age and risk
10. Discuss analgesia. Prostaglandin inhibitor such as ibuprofen for discomfort
    a. Take nonsteroidal anti-inflammatory drugs (NSAIDs) one-half hour before appointment.
11. Discuss use of antibiotics.
    a. No consensus as to effectiveness of use of antibiotics in reducing postinsertion infection
    b. If subacute endocarditis is present, most clinicians do not recommend use of IUC.
C. Insertion visit
   1. If irregular or absent menses are noted, perform sensitive (within 10 days postovulation) pregnancy test.
   2. Review laboratory results.
   3. Obtain signed consent if this was not done at the previous visit.
   4. Allow time for any questions.
D. Some comments and considerations
   1. Move slowly and gently during all phases of IUC insertion to minimize chance of perforation and vasovagal reaction.
   2. Use strictest sterile technique.
   3. Always read the manufacturer's instructions included in the IUC package because they vary slightly.
   4. The withdrawal technique may minimize risk of uterine perforation.
   5. Explain the procedure carefully to help the patient relax.
   6. Show the IUC, and review the insertion technique.
   7. Vasovagal reactions are more common in women who
      a. Have not been pregnant for many years
      b. Are nulliparous
      c. Are very nervous and fearful
      d. Have an empty stomach

e. Have a history of previous episodes of fainting
f. Reactions are usually transient and spontaneously subside.
8. Slow manipulation with the instruments decreases occurrence of syncope.
9. Patient discomfort
   a. The woman may feel menstrual-type cramps during the sounding of the uterus and the actual insertion of the IUC.
   b. The tenaculum may cause a pinching sensation.
E. Equipment
   1. Sterile gloves
   2. Bivalve speculum
   3. Ring forceps
   4. Six to eight cotton balls
   5. Single-toothed tenaculum
   6. Uterine sound
   7. Antiseptic solution
   8. Rectal swab (four)
   9. Sterile IUC in unopened package
   10. Scissors to trim string after insertion
   11. Optional: Paracervical block tray
F. Technique of the examination
   1. Perform a bimanual examination to reassess the position of the uterus (although this was done previously). Perforations occur most often in an ante flexed or retroflexed uterus that was not diagnosed before the IUC was inserted.
   2. Visualize the cervix, and wash the cervix with an antiseptic solution. If iodine is present in the antiseptic solution, rule out an allergy to iodine.
   3. A topical local anesthetic (Hurricane) may be used at this point during the insertion process, over the area where the tenaculum is to be placed.
   4. Grasp the anterior lip of the cervix with a tenaculum about 1.5 to 2.0 cm from the os. Close the single-toothed tenaculum slowly, one notch at a time. (Use of a tenaculum is not always necessary, although it is generally recommended.) Apply gentle traction to stabilize the uterus and straighten the canal.
      a. Warn that the woman may feel a pinching sensation.
      b. The tenaculum should avoid areas of blood vessels on the cervix.
         (1) If the cervix is anteverted, apply tenaculum at the 10 o'clock and 2 o'clock positions.
         (2) If the cervix is retroverted, apply the tenaculum to the cervix at the 4 o'clock and 8 o'clock positions.
   5. Sound the uterus slowly and gently until the resistance of the fundus is felt, to determine depth, direction, and configuration of uterus.

6. Measure the depth of the fundus by sounding.
    a. Place a cotton swab at the cervix when the sound is all the way in.
    b. Remove sound and swab while holding swab against sound.
    c. Measure distance between end of swab and end of sound.
    d. If the distance is less than 6 cm, expulsion, bleeding, pain, and perforation are more likely.
    e. If the distance is greater than 10 cm, decreased contraceptive effectiveness (increased cavity surface) may occur.
    f. No resistance may indicate perforation.
    g. Leave sound in place for a few seconds to dilate the cervix.
7. Load the IUC device into the inserter barrel under sterile conditions. IUC loading instructions differ in how the T-shaped plastic frame is loaded into the inserter. ParaGard IUC folds the ends of the wings down into the inserter, whereas the Mirena and Skyla IUCs fold the wings up into the inserter as they are pulled through with a gentle tug on the threads. Check the loading instructions on the product packaging before loading the device.
8. Inserter may be slightly bent to conform to the shape of the cervical canal.
9. Apply steady, gentle traction on the tenaculum with nondominant hand.
    a. If it is anteverted, pull downward and outward.
    b. If it is retroverted, pull upward and outward.
10. Introduce the inserter barrel through the cervical canal until the top of the fundus is reached. (The tip of the inserter may be lubricated with sterile, water-soluble jelly.)
11. Release the IUC device from the inserter only after placement at the top of the fundus is confirmed by feeling the fundal walls. (This correct position is essential to maximize protection against pregnancy and minimize the risk of expulsion.)
12. Withdraw the inserter tip ½ inch, enough to allow for release of the IUC's transverse arms from the tube.
13. Transfer the inserter to the nondominant hand, which is also holding the tenaculum.
14. Extract the plunger while gentle pressure is placed on the inserted tube to ensure that the IUC device remains at the top of the fundal cavity. Be careful to prevent impingement of the tail as the tube is removed.
15. Withdraw the inserter tube and the tail of the device, allowing for proper placement.
16. Remove the tenaculum, and observe for any bleeding.
17. If suspected perforation occurs at any point, stop the procedure immediately.
18. Withdraw the plunger, then the barrel of the inserter.

19. Trim string. *Leave 3 to 5 cm. Can trim shorter if needed at later date.*
20. Remove the speculum.
21. Possible causes of disappearance of strings
    a. Drawing up of strings into the cervical canal or uterus
    b. Cut too short during insertion
    c. Rotation of the device within the uterus
    d. If the problem occurs, try to grasp strings with uterine forceps (no further than 1 inch) and pull them down into the vagina.
    e. Performation. Recommend transvaginal ultrasound (3-D is best) and possibly pelvic/abdominal x-ray
22. Assist the woman to a sitting position.
23. Observe for a syncopal episode.
24. Allow her to rest if necessary.

G. Postinsertion instructions
    1. Teach the patient to feel for the string of the IUC before leaving the examining room.
       a. She should be instructed to feel for the IUC string similarly after each menses.
       b. May use a mirror to show the placement in the os.
       c. Instruct the woman how to feel for the string.
          (1) Wash hands
          (2) Assume a comfortable position, either lying down with knees on her chest; standing with one leg on a chair, toilet, or stool; or sitting on the toilet.
          (3) Insert fingers into the vagina, and feel backward toward the cervix.
          (4) Call the clinician if no string is felt. It may simply be curled up in the cervix.
          (5) Avoid tugging on the string.
    2. Call the clinician if moderate to severe uterine cramping occurs.
       a. Mild cramping over 1 to 3 days is normal. Treat the patient with NSAIDs.
       b. May normally occur 1 to 3 months after insertion
    3. Avoid use of tampons for the first 48 hours.
    4. Avoid sexual intercourse for the first 24 hours.
    5. Call the clinician if you miss a period. This can occur normally with the levonorgestrel IUC (Mirena or Skyla).
    6. Always use condoms with a new sexual partner.
    7. Chances of accidental pregnancy, although low, are highest during the first month. The patient may use additional contraception but it is usually not necessary.
    8. A follow-up visit after the first menses may be recommended.
    9. Keep a careful menstruation calendar.
    10. Warn the patient that initially bleeding may normally be heavy for the first few periods.

11. Reinforce that the patient is at greatest risk of infection during the first month.
    a. Patient should observe for early signs of PID, and return immediately if present.
    b. Report increased and abnormal vaginal discharge, fever, or lower abdominal pain.
12. Review need for condoms if at risk for STIs.

H. Post-insertion documentation. Clearly document the following:
1. Teaching and counseling provided
2. Uterine contour
3. Depth of uterine sounding
4. Type of IUC device used
5. Ease of insertion
6. How patient tolerated the procedure
7. Length of string
8. Any pregnancy test results
9. File signed consent form.

III. Management of side effects

A. Increased cramping. If this should occur
1. Avoid strenuous exercise, and rest when possible.
2. Hot water bottle or heating pad placed on lower abdomen may be helpful.
3. Use analgesics (ibuprofen or naproxyn as needed).
4. Call provider if concerned.

B. Partner feels string. Return for evaluation.
1. String too long: Trim shorter.
2. String too short: Remove IUC device and replace.

C. Missed menses. Return for a pregnancy test. May occur with Mirena or Skyla *and is considered normal.*

D. Increased vaginal discharge. Evaluate for vaginitis, cervicitis, PID, and STIs.

E. Heavy menses, anemia. Monitor and work up as indicated.
1. Treat anemia as indicated.

IV. Follow-up visit

A. Schedule after next menses
1. Assess satisfaction with IUC.
2. Review menstruation calendar.
3. Check for the strings and trim if needed.
    a. If no strings are visualized, they can be extracted from the cervical canal by rotating two cotton-tipped applicators or a Pap smear cytobrush in the endocervical canal.
    b. If further maneuvers are required, the clinician should refer the patient to a gynecologist.

      4. Return in 1 year for annual exam (with or without a Pap per the ACS [2012], the ASCCP, and the ASCP Consensus Guidelines as needed, or with concerns.

  B. Elicit information regarding the presence of
     1. Foul-smelling vaginal discharge
     2. Low backache
     3. Menorrhagia
     4. Dysmenorrhea
     5. New sexual partner(s)
     6. Fever

  C. Perform infection evaluation with STI testing, pH, amine testing, and wet mount/vaginal microscopy if infection is suspected.

  D. Patient instructions
     1. Reinforce previous teaching.
     2. Return for annual examination.

V. Removal

  A. Reasons for removal
     1. Patient wishes
       a. Desire to switch to alternative method of contraception
       b. Desires pregnancy
       c. Contraception is no longer required.
       d. Uncomfortable with side effects
     2. Possible medical indications
       a. Accidental pregnancy
       b. Severe anemia resulting from persistent bleeding
       c. PID—controversial
       d. Excessive cramping and bleeding
       e. Development of a malignancy
       f. Pain with intercourse
       g. Partial expulsion of the device
       h. Cervical or fundal perforation
       i. Approximately 7% of women with IUCs will have actinomyces identified on their Pap smears and this may represent colonization, not infection. Symptomatic women with IUCs should have the IUC removed and should receive antibiotics. However, the management of the asymptomatic carrier is controversial because actinomyces can be found normally in the genital tract cultures in healthy women without IUDs. False-positive findings of actinomycosis on Pap smears can be a problem. When possible, confirm the Pap smear diagnosis with cultures.

  B. Technique
     1. Insert speculum and visualize os.
     2. Grasp tail with ring forceps.
     3. If the IUD is embedded, the patient may require hysteroscopy.

4. Apply gentle, steady traction, being careful not to break the strings, and remove.
5. If gentle traction does not lead to IUC removal, refer to gynecologist.
6. Remove the speculum.
7. Examine the device for unusual discharge. *If present, consider sending for culture.*
8. Instruct woman to remain sitting on the table for a few minutes. Observe for any dizziness.

VI. **Management of side effects and complications**
A. Pelvic inflammatory disease
   1. Positive cultures and IUC in place with no symptoms— treat without removal.
   2. If PID, treat per 2010 CDC STI Treatment Guidelines, but if *not* improved within 72 hours, the device may be removed. Prudent clinical judgment must be used.
B. BV: Consider treating the patient with oral antibiotics (metronidazole) to prevent BV-associated endometritis; the IUC may remain in place.
C. Endometritis. Treat per CDC STI Treatment Guidelines for PID.
D. Pregnancy
   1. Risk of pregnancy is very low.
   2. Irregular menses commonly occur. Lack of menses is no longer an indicator of pregnancy.
   3. Routine pregnancy testing is not necessary.
   4. Testing is indicated in a patient who has an abrupt change in bleeding patterns or who develops symptoms of pregnancy.
   5. Women who conceive need to have ultrasonographic localization of the gestational sac to rule out ectopic pregnancy.
   6. In pregnancy the IUC should be removed because the risk of miscarriage, sepsis, premature labor, and delivery increase. Consider referral to gynecologist for IUC removal in this context.
E. Actinomyces
   1. Actinomyces may be found on the Pap smear in up to 7% of IUC users. May be normal colonization (not infection).
   2. If the patient is asymptomatic and the clinical exam indicates no infection, then no treatment is needed and the clinician may leave the device in place.
   3. If the patient is symptomatic, the device should be removed and oral antibiotics should be given. Penicillin 500 mg orally four times a day for 1 month is recommended.
   4. May replace device after repeat culture performed 3 months later shows absence of actinomyces.

VII. Expulsion
   A. Removal of partially expelled IUC
      1. Grasp the string or tip with ring forceps.
      2. Evaluate the patient for infection or pregnancy.
      3. Reinsert another IUC if the woman desires.

Acknowledgment

Thank you to Dr. Joellen Hawkins for her assistance in editing this chapter.

Bibliography

American Heart Association. (n.d.). *New guidelines*. Retrieved from http://circaha journals.org./cgi/reprint/CIRCULATIONAHA.106.183095

Bayer Healthcare. (2013). *Mirena* (product insert). Whippany, NJ: Bayer Healthcare. Retrieved from http://labeling.bayerhealthcare.com/html/products/pi/Mirena_ PI.pdf 2013

Bayer Healthcare. (2013). *Skyla* (product insert). Whippany, NJ: Bayer Healthcare. Retrieved from http://labeling.bayerhealthcare.com/html/products/pi/Skyla_ PI.pdf 2013

Hatcher, R. A., Trussell, J., Nelson, A. Cates, W., Kowal, D., & Policar, M. S. (2011). *Contraceptive technology* (20th ed., pp. 148–149). Cooper Station, NY: Ardent Media.

Inki, P. (2007). Long-term use of the levonorgestrel-releasing intrauterine device. *Contraception, 75*(6 Suppl.), S161–S166.

Peterson, H. B. (2005). Clinical practice. Long-acting methods of contraception. *New England Journal of Medicine, 353*(20), 2169–2175.

Sudhakar, S. S., & Ross, J. J. (2004). Short-term treatment of actinomycosis: Two cases and a review. *Clinical Infectious Diseases, 38*, 444.

Teva. (2013). *Paragard* (package insert). Sellersville, PA: Teva Pharmaceuticals. Retrieved from http://www.paragard.com/images/ParaGard_info.pdf

Westhoff, C. (2007). IUDs and colonization or infection with actinomyces. *Contraception, 75*, S48.

Contraceptive Implants

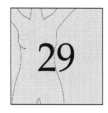

29

R. Mimi Secor, Kahlil A. Demonbreun, and Nancy Gardiner Dirubbo

I. **Etonogestrel Implant (Nexplanon) explained**
   A. Nexplanon (formerly Implanon) is a progestin-only, single-rod, subdermal contraceptive implant that utilizes the third-generation progestin 3-keto-desogestrel (etonogestrel) and has a reported efficacy of up to 3 years.
      1. Over 11 million implants have been inserted worldwide in over 60 countries since 1998.
      2. Etonogestrel Implant was initially approved by the Food and Drug Administration (FDA) in the United States in 2006 and marketed under the product name Implanon. Nexplanon (approved in 2011) differs from Implanon only in that the device is impregnated with barium sulfate, rendering it radiopaque, and utilizes an improved specialized insertion system.
      3. Consists of a 4-cm long by 2-mm diameter (1.57 x 0.078 inch) rod with a rate-controlling membrane of 37% ethylene vinyl acetate (EVA) copolymer, 3% barium sulfate (15 mg), and 60% etonogestrel (68 micrograms)
      4. The progestin is released at a rate of 60 to 70 micrograms initially and then decreases to 25 to 30 micrograms by the third year.
      5. Is a long-acting, low-dose, quickly reversible, progestin-only method of contraception.
      6. Average retail cost ranges from $600 to $850 for the device, and insertion charges range from $125 to $200.
      7. Many private insurers cover all or some of the cost of the device as well as insertion and removal. Merck offers clinicians a program that will investigate individual patient's insurance policies to determine coverage and copays.

8. Many state Medicaid programs cover the device as well as insertion and removal in full.
9. Careful and correct subdermal placement technique is crucial to successful insertion and facilitates removal.
10. All providers must complete a free educational program on Nexplanon provided by the manufacturer per FDA requirements before inserting or removing these implants. For information about training programs go to www.nexplanonusa.com

B. Effectiveness
   1. Six pregnancies were reported in 20,648 cycles. Each conception was likely to have occurred before removal or within 2 weeks after removal.
   2. Cumulative Pearl Index is 0.38 pregnancies per 100 woman-years of use.
   3. No clinical data are available concerning efficacy and overweight or obese women. However, because serum concentrations of etonogestrel are inversely related to body weight, it is possible that the implant is less effective in women who are overweight.

C. Mechanism of action
   1. Primarily inhibits ovulation
   2. Secondarily increases viscosity of cervical mucus
   3. Is not an abortifacient.

D. Indications: Nexplanon can be used by any woman who
   1. Seeks a safe, highly effective, long-term, reversible form of contraception
   2. Cannot take estrogen because of contraindications or intolerance of side effects
   3. Has a history of poor compliance with other methods of contraception
   4. Does not desire future pregnancies but is unsure of permanent sterilization
   5. Because of health problems or medication use should not become pregnant

E. Advantages
   1. Does not contain estrogen so can be used for effective hormonal contraception in women who cannot use estrogen
   2. Can be used postpartum in breastfeeding women. Less than 0.2% estimated absolute maternal dose is excreted in breast milk. Does not affect production or quality of breast milk.
   3. Effective immediately when inserted at the proper time (see manufacturer's insert)
   4. Stable hemoglobin levels with use because menstrual blood loss is less than in women who are not using this method
   5. Highly effective, safe, and rapidly reversible method that requires little adherence from user

6. Free 2- to 3-hour training program to teach product insertion and removal
7. Method is paid for up front. If patient's financial or insurance status changes in those 3 years, contraception is already paid for.
8. Discreet and does not affect spontaneity

F. Disadvantages
1. Predictably unpredictable bleeding patterns throughout the duration of the 3 years of use
2. Weight changes may occur in women who use Nexplanon. Some women gain weight and some women lose weight. The number of women who gain is about equal to the number of those who lose weight. Total weight gain is minimal, that is, less than 2 to 3 pounds per year.
3. Cost can be a disadvantage for some women as all the costs for this method are paid up front.
4. Some women do not like that they cannot start or stop this method without the assistance of a clinician and so feel less in control.
5. Some women do not like the idea of a foreign object being inserted into their bodies.
6. Some women may be able to see the implant slightly under the skin.
7. Implant offers no protection from sexually transmitted infections

G. Irregular bleeding
1. Bleeding is the most common reason for removal. Patient needs to be educated that this is to be expected and that it is normal. If patient is intolerant of irregular bleeding, she may not want to choose implants.
2. Counsel patient that bleeding can be light or heavy, last for a few days or many days in a row, or absent for several months.
3. Bleeding patterns are not necessarily similar to other progestin-only methods of contraception. Patient's experiences with other methods of progestin-only contraception do not predict what her experience with Nexplanon will be.
4. Typically, the mean bleeding days per 90-day reference time show that women using Nexplanon had fewer total bleeding and/or spotting days than women not using any hormones.
5. Prostaglandin inhibitors (nonsteroidal anti-inflammatory drugs [NSAIDs]) or a trial of supplemental estrogen (if applicable) have been shown to be effective in the management of abnormal bleeding.

H. Contraindications/warnings and precautions are summarized in Box 29.1 and Box 29.2.

> **BOX 29.1** *Contraindications of Nexplanon Use*
>
> - Known or suspected pregnancy
> - Hypersensitivity to any components of etonogestrel implant
> - Known, suspected, or past history of breast cancer
> - Current or past history of thrombolytic disease
> - Hepatic tumor or active liver disease
> - Undiagnosed genital bleeding

> **BOX 29.2** *Warning and Precautions for Nexplanon Use*
>
> - Arterial cardiovascular disease
> - History of cerebrovascular accident
> - Systemic lupus erythematosus (antibody positive or unknown)
> - Smoking
> - Diabetes mellitus
> - Severe cirrhosis
> - Current and history of ischemic heart disease

   I. Drug interactions
       1. Women who take drugs that are potent inducers of hepatic enzymes should not use etonogestrel, as these drugs potentially can decrease the efficacy of etonogestrel and therefore may result in an unintended pregnancy.
       2. Examples of these drugs include griseofulvin, barbiturates, rifampin, phenytoin, carbamazepine, felbamate, oxcarbazepine, topiramate, and modafinil.
   J. Special considerations
       1. To assist clinicians in the decision process for providing the etonogestrel implant to women, the Centers for Disease Control and Prevention (CDC) U. S. Medical Eligibility Criteria for Contraception Use (US MEC) defined the following conditions affecting eligibility for the use of progestin-only contraceptive implants.
          a. 1 = A condition for which there is no restriction for the use of the contraceptive method
          b. 2 = A condition for which the advantages of using the method generally outweigh the theoretical or proven risks

      c. 3 = A condition for which the theoretical or proven risks usually outweigh the advantages of using the method

      d. 4 = A condition that represents an unacceptable health risk if the contraceptive method is used

      e. The full summary chart can be obtained from www.cdc.gov/reproductivehealth/UnintendedPregnancy/Docs/USMEC-Color-62012.docx

  2. Recommendations for use in postpartum women (nonbreastfeeding/breastfeeding)

a.	< 21 days	USMEC Category 1/USMEC Category 2
b.	21 days to < 30 days	USMEC Category 1/USMEC Category 2
c.	30 to 42 days	USMEC Category 1/USMEC Category 2
d.	> 42 days	USMEC Category 1/USMEC Category 1

  3. Recommendations for use postabortion

a.	First trimester	USMEC Category 1
b.	Second trimester	USMEC Category 1
c.	Immediate postseptic abortion	USMEC Category 1

II. **Nexplanon insertion: Providers must complete a training program provided free by the manufacturer per FDA regulations before clinicians can insert or remove Nexplanon. To inquire about training, visit www.Nexplanon-usa.com**

  A. Counseling

    1. Appropriate counseling is essential for proper selection of implants for contraception.

    2. It is best to do this during a visit separate from product insertion.

    3. Explain what it is, how it works, its advantages and disadvantages, bleeding patterns, what to expect at insertion and removal, contraindications, and costs.

    4. Informed consent may be obtained at this visit or at time of insertion.

  B. When to insert. Pregnancy must be excluded before insertion.

    1. If patient is not using any hormonal contraception, it can be inserted on days 1 to 7 of her menstrual cycle.

    2. If patient is switching from combined oral contraceptive, Nexplanon can be inserted any time within 7 days from the last dose of active hormone pill.

    3. If patient is switching from a progesterone-only pill and has not skipped any pills that month, Nexplanon can be inserted at any time.

4. If the patient has a Nexplanon that is due for removal and wishes to continue with Nexplanon, a new one can be inserted right after removal through the same incision.
5. If the patient is switching from medroxyprogesterone acetate injections, Nexplanon can be inserted during the 2-week window when the next injection would have been due.
6. Can be inserted within the first 7 days after a spontaneous or induced abortion (USMEC 1)
7. Can be inserted any time postpartum and breastfeeding exclusively (USMEC 2 if less than 1 month postpartum and USMEC 1 if greater than 1 month postpartum).
8. If Nexplanon is inserted according to the preceding guidelines, it is effective immediately.
9. If patient has an intrauterine contraceptive (IUC), Nexplanon can be inserted the same day as the device's removal.
10. If switching from an IUC and the women has had sexual intercourse since the start of her current menstrual cycle and it has been more than 5 days, the following options should be considered
    a. Advise her to retain the IUC for at least 7 days after insertion of the implant.
    b. Advise her to abstain from sexual intercourse or use a barrier contraception for 7 days before removing the IUC.
    c. Advise her to use emergency contraception at the time of IUC removal.
11. If Nexplanon is being inserted outside these guidelines, patient should be advised to use a non-hormonal form of back-up contraception for 7 days.

C. Equipment required
1. Comes in a sterile, disposable, preloaded applicator
2. A comfortable table with support for the patient's arm (a pillow works well) is needed.
3. Sterile gloves, antiseptic solution, local anesthetic, sterile gauze, skin closures, paper tape, and elastic gauze dressing are needed.

D. Insertion procedure
1. Non-dominate arm is used
2. Insertion site is between the biceps and triceps muscle, in midline 8 to 10 cm (3–4 inches) from the medial condyle of the humerus.
3. Insertion is always subdermal.
4. No incision is necessary as insertion is via the trocar.
5. Experienced clinicians can insert Nexplanon in 2 to 3 minutes.
6. Correct placement must be confirmed right after insertion.
7. Careful and correct subdermal insertion is necessary for successful placement and will facilitate removal.

BOX 29.3 *Circumstances for the Removal of Implant*

Nexplanon should be removed
1. If the patient wants to conceive
2. If patient wants to change to another form of contraception
3. If there are side effects, such as unscheduled vaginal bleeding, allergic reaction, or other unexpected adverse reactions

Three years after insertion, if patient wants to continue with etonogestrel implant, a new rod can be inserted at the time of removal of initial rod, at the same site.

   E. Post-insertion complications
     1. Pain at insertion site occurred in fewer than 3% of women.
     2. Redness, swelling, and hematoma were reported in less than 1% of women.

III. **Implant removal procedure**
   A. When to remove: The etonogestrel implant should be removed at the patient's request or when the time period has expired (Box 29.3).
   B. Patient education points
     1. Most removals take about 5 to 10 minutes.
     2. Minor to no discomfort is experienced at the time of removal.
     3. Postremoval the patient may have some bruising and tenderness at the site.
   C. Changing to another method of contraception
     1. Another method of contraception can be initiated immediately post-removal without loss of contraceptive efficacy, that is, oral contraceptives, contraceptive ring, patches, or IUC.

IV. **Patient and provider resources**
   A. The manufacturer has a comprehensive program for provider and patient education and support that can be accessed by calling 1-877-467-5266 or by visiting www.Nexplanon-USA.com.
   B. For full prescribing information, see the package insert available on the manufacturer's website.

Bibliography

American College of Obstetricians and Gynecologists. (2011). ACOG Practice Bulletin No. 121: Long-acting reversible contraception: Implants and intrauterine devices. Retrieved December 23, 2013, from http://www.acog.org/~/media/Practice%20 Bulletins/Committee%20on%20Practice%20Bulletins%20--%20Gynecology/Public/pb121.pdf?dmc=1&ts=20120908T1124504893

Centers for Disease Control and Prevention. (2010, May). U.S. medical eligibility criteria for contraception use, 2010: Adapted from the *World Health Organization medical eligibility criteria for contraceptive use* (4th ed.). *Morbidity and Mortality Weekly Report, 59,* 1–88. Retrieved December 23, 2013, from http://www.cdc.gov/mmwr/pdf/rr/rr59e0528.pdf

Centers for Disease Control and Prevention. (2011). Update to CDC's U.S medical eligibility criteria for contraceptive use, 2010: Revised Recommendations for the use of contraceptive methods during the postpartum period. *Morbidity and Mortality Weekly Report, 60*(26), 878–883. Retrieved December 23, 2013, from http://www.cdc.gov/mmwr/pdf/wk/mm6026.pdf

Centers for Disease Control and Prevention. (2013). U.S. selected practice recommendations for contraception use. Adapted from the *World Health Organization selected practice recommendations for contraceptive use* (2nd ed.). *Morbidity and Mortality Weekly Report, 62*(5), 1–64. Retrieved December 23, 2013, from http://www.cdc.gov/mmwr/pdf/rr/rr6205.pdf

Kapp, N., Curtis, K., & Nanda, K. (2010). Progestin-only contraceptive use among breastfeeding women: A systematic review. *Contraception, 82,* 17–37. doi: 10.1016/j.contraception.2010.02.002

Kittur, N. D., Secura, G. M., Peipert, J. F., Madden, T., Finer, L. B., & Allsworth, J. E. (2011). Comparison of contraception use between the contraceptive CHOICE project and state and national data. *Contraception, 83*(5), 479–485. Retrieved December 23, 2013, from http://www.ncbi.nlm.nih.gov/pmc/articles/PMC3074095/pdf/nihms246992.pdf or doi:10.1016/j.contraception.2010.10.001

Lewis, L. N., Doherty, D. A., Hickey, M., & Skinner, S. R. (2011). Implanon as a contraceptive choice for teenage mothers: A comparison of contraceptive choices, acceptability and repeat pregnancy. *Contraception, 81*(5), 421–426.

Mansour, D. (2010). Nexplanon®: What Implanon did next. *Journal of Family Planning Reproductive Health Care, 36*(4), 297–299. Retrieved December 28, 2013, from http://jfprhc.bmj.com/content/36/4/297.long or doi: 10.1783/147129910793048629

Merck Sharp & Dohme Corp. (2011). *Merck launches Nexplanon® (etonogestrel implant) 68 mg in the United States—A long acting reversible hormonal contraceptive effective for up to three years.* Retrieved December 23, 2013, from http://www.mercknewsroom.com/press-release/prescription-medicine-news/merck-launches-nexplanon-etonogestrel-implant-68-mg-united-

Merck Sharp & Dohme Corp. (2013). *Nexplanon prescribing information.* Retrieved December 23, 2013, from http://www.merck.com/product/usa/pi_circulars/n/nexplanon/nexplanon_pi.pdf

Raymond, E. G. (2011). Contraceptive implants. In R. A. Hatcher, J. Trussell, A. L. Nelson, W. Cates, D. Kowal, & M. S. Policar (Eds.). *Contraceptive technology* (20th ed.). New York, NY: Ardent Media.

Walch, K., Unfried, G., Huber, J., Kurz, C., van Trotsenburg, M., Pernicka, E., & Wenzl, R. (2009). Implanon versus medroxyprogesterone acetate: Effects on pain scores in patients with symptomatic endometriosis—a pilot study. *Contraception, 79*(1), 29–34. doi: 10.1016/j.contraception.2008.07.017

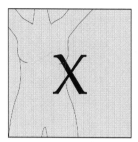

Investigative Procedures

Cervical Cancer Screening

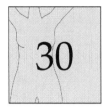

30

Nancy R. Berman,
Rebecca Koeniger-Donohue,
and Alison O. Marshall

I. **Screening for cervical cancer**
   A. According to the American Cancer Society (ACS), globally, cervical cancer is second to breast cancer as the leading type of cancer in women (ACS, 2013a). In the United States, cervical cancer is the second leading cause of death in women 20 to 39 years of age (ACS, 2013b). However, testing now exists that has helped dramatically lower the numbers of women affected by this disease, particularly in the United States.
      1. The Pap smear
         a. The Pap smear cytologic sampling technique, or Pap test, named for Dr. George Papanicolaou, was invented in 1941. It is a screening tool only. It *must* correlate with abnormal tissue in order for the clinician to make a diagnosis of cervical pathology.
            (1) During the Pap test, the clinician collects desquamated cells of the female cervix.
            (2) The sample is sent to a pathologist where the cells are evaluated for size, shape, and regularity. Should an abnormality be reported, the clinician will determine whether a diagnostic procedure is needed.
         b. The most common diagnostic procedure used to confirm the results of the Pap smear is a colposcopy.
            (1) The provider looks through the colposcope at the cervical or vaginal tissue after acetic acid (vinegar) has been applied.
            (2) Directed biopsies can be taken during the colposcopy and the tissue analyzed.
            (3) Treatment decisions are based on the histological results of the tissue biopsy.

    c. The Pap test results are reported using the Bethesda system of cytologic classification (2001, 2002). The gold standard used to interpret the Pap test findings are the algorithms developed by American Society for Colposcopy and Cervical Pathology (ASCCP, 2013).

    d. There are two acceptable ways to prepare the collected cells for examination. The first is the conventional dry slide method and the second is to use a liquid-based medium.

    e. The test is intended to detect changes in cervical cells caused by infection with human papillomavirus (HPV) and are graded according to the degree of abnormality and the cell type that is involved. This may range from an equivocal change to either a low- or high-grade change (precancerous) to cancer.

    f. The Pap smear is a valuable screening test because it is relatively inexpensive and can detect precancerous conditions long before they become cancerous.

    g. Limitations of the Pap smear

        (1) Errors in Pap smear testing can be broadly categorized as errors in sampling and preparation, screening, or interpretation.

        (2) Sampling and preparation represent the greatest limitation because the sample must contain a representative cellular smear.

2. HPV testing

    a. The U.S. Food and Drug Administration (FDA) approved HPV testing along with Pap for screening women 30 and older in 2003.

    b. Testing women for HPV starting at age 30 along with the Pap is called "co-testing."

    c. The peak age for HPV prevalence is in the mid-20s and the majority of infections are cleared by 24 months.

    d. Long-term persistent infection is necessary for the development of significant neoplasia and progression to cancer.

    e. Testing young women under age 30 in screening would find many positive tests due to HPV infections that are transient and will be cleared in a short time. See Section 3, that follows, for an update on primary screening with HPV recently FDA approved.

    f. If a woman 30 and older is positive for HPV, it is more likely a persistent infection.

    g. Co-testing will identify women with persistent infection who may have neoplastic change that was missed by the Pap.

    h. Co-testing will identify women who may develop neoplasia and they should be followed diligently as long as they remain positive.

3. Primary HPV screening for cervical cancer
   a. On April 25, 2014, the FDA approved the Roche cobas HPV test for the primary screening of women 25 and older. This means testing with a stand-alone HPV test first instead of a Pap test.
   b. The Roche cobas test provides a positive or negative result for a panel of 12 HPV types and a separate result for HPV 16 and 18. It also has an internal control for specimen adequacy.
   c. At this time, no other HPV test has received approval for stand-alone primary screening, but three other tests are approved for co-testing along with a Pap test.
   d. The Roche test was approved for primary screening after data from Addressing the Need for Advanced HPV Diagnostics (Athena) Trial was presented to a panel at the FDA. The Athena trial enrolled more than 47,000 women and demonstrated that one in four women who are HPV 16 positive will have cervical disease within 3 years and that nearly one in seven women with normal cytology, who were HPV positive, actually had high-grade cervical disease that was missed by cytology.
   e. Primary screening by HPV testing identifies not only women at risk for disease, but also identifies women who have future risk.
   f. The interim guidelines for management of the results of this testing are awaiting publication as this book goes to press. The guidelines will include strategies for reflexing to a Pap test and referral to colposcopy. (Note: For a full listing of Roche Molecular Diagnostics products, see http://molecular.roche.com.)
4. Statistics
   a. Since 1941 cervical cancer incidence rates have decreased approximately 75% and mortality rates 70%.
   b. The Pap test has reduced the disease burden from cervical cancer by 75% since its introduction. However, cervical cancer continues to be a significant health issue (Box 30.1).
   c. More Black and Hispanic women are diagnosed with cervical cancer and are diagnosed at later stages of the disease than women of other races (incidence rates 10.7 cases/100,000 women and 12.1 cases/100,000 women, respectively), possibly due to decreased access to Pap testing or follow-up treatment (ACA, 2013).
   d. Cancers missed by laboratories represent only a tiny fraction of cervical cancers. Of women who develop cervical cancer, 22% reported no regular Pap smear testing (ACA, 2013).

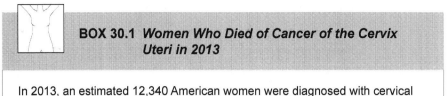

BOX 30.1 *Women Who Died of Cancer of the Cervix Uteri in 2013*

In 2013, an estimated 12,340 American women were diagnosed with cervical cancer, and 4,030 women died of cancer of the cervix uteri (ACA, 2013).

5. HPV epidemiology
   a. HPV is widespread. In the United States, approximately 1,700 new HPV infections occur daily, 6.2 million new infections every year (incidence), and there are 20 million active infections every year (prevalence).
   b. Approximately 75% to 80% of both males and females will be infected in their lifetime.
   c. The Centers for Disease Control and Prevention (CDC) estimates $8 billion per year is spent in direct medical costs for preventing and treating HPV-associated disease.
   d. Up to 40% of women are infected with HPV within 24 months of first sexual intercourse.
   e. Infection rates peak in the mid-20s, with highest prevalence in 20- to 24-year-olds, then decrease as the woman ages. In women ages 14 to 19, the prevalence of HPV infection is 35%. Conversely, the prevalence in women 50 to 65 years is just 6%.
   f. Long-term persistence of HPV infection, that is, greater than 24 months, is necessary for the development of high-grade neoplasia and progression to cancer.
   g. Most lesions caused by HPV will regress spontaneously. Research indicates that 91% of HPV infections in women over the age of 18 resolve within 2 years[*]; 61% of low-grade squamous intraepithelial lesions (LSILs) in young women regress at 12 months, and 91% regress at 36 months; 3% of LSILs progress to high-grade SILs (HSILs).
6. Development of cervical abnormalities: Understanding the transformation zone

---

[*]Author note: Visit the ASCCP website for information on the first HPV genotyping assay, which was approved in March 2009. Based on this approval, ASCCP released the *Management Algorithm for Using HPV Genotyping to Manage HPV High-Risk Positive/Cytology Negative Women 30 Years and Older*. This also includes the descriptions of the new FDA-approved P HPV DNA designed to identify 14 high-risk types of HPV. This test will be marketed under the name Cervista HPV HR for use with ThinPrep samples. Available at www.asccp.org/pdfs/consensus/hpv_genotyping_20090320.pdf. Click on 2009 Algorithm: Use of HPV Genotyping to Manage HPV HR Positive/Cytology Negative Women 30 Years and Older.

a. There are two types of cervical cells
   (1) Columnar epithelial cells: The interior of the cervical canal is lined with columnar tissue that contains mucus-secreting glands.
   (2) Squamous epithelial cells: The knob of the cervix is covered with a different type of flat tissue, called squamous epithelial tissue. This tissue is pink and shiny.
b. These two types of tissue meet at the squamocolumnar junction, or the transformation zone (TZ). The endocervical cells are located in the transformation zone (Figure 30.1).
c. Significance of the transformation zone
   (1) The majority of malignant and premalignant diseases arise in the transformation zone. This is an area of rapidly changing metaplastic cells that varies with hormonal status (Table 30.1).
d. These cells are absent in 10% of Pap smears in premenopausal women and in 50% of postmenopausal women.
e. The transformation zone shifts in response to age and hormone levels.
f. Infection of the cervix with high-risk HPV is a requirement for the development of virtually all cervical carcinomas (squamous cell and adenocarcinoma).
g. HPV has a unique mechanism of infection in that it can only bind to the outermost layer of the cervical epithelium. It then requires capsid proteins to infect deeper layers of the epithelium and complete its life cycle.

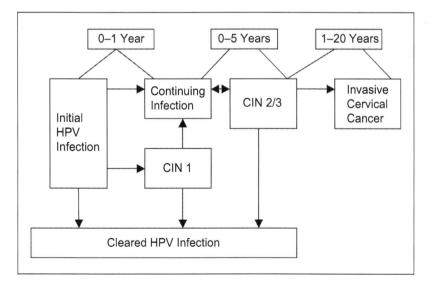

FIGURE 30.1 Progression of invasive carcinoma.

TABLE 30.1 Transformation Zone (Squamocolumnar Junction) Shifts in Response to Age and Hormonal Alterations

DEVELOPMENTAL PERIOD	PATHOPHYSIOLOGIC PROCESS	LOCATION OF TRANSFORMATION ZONE
Puberty	Squamous tissue slowly replaces the glandular tissue on the ectocervix under the influence of estrogen	Junction on the surface of the cervix
Early to middle years	Remains relatively stable	Junction at the cervical os
Menopause	Lack of estrogen causes the squamous cells to migrate up the endocervical canal	Junction recedes inside the os

      (1) LSILs are characterized by abnormalities in the cells of the lower third of the epithelium.

      (2) HSILs occur when *abnormal cells proliferate into the basal layer of the cervical epithelium.*

  h. The addition of cofactors may trigger malignant transformation (Box 30.2)

  i. Of the more than 100 known HPV types that may infect humans, approximately 40 infect the female genital tract. Fourteen of these are considered oncogenic or high-risk carcinogenic types for cervical carcinoma.

  j. Two high-risk types, HPV 16 and HPV 18, account for nearly 70% of cervical carcinomas. Two low-risk types, HPV 6 and HPV 11, cause 90% of anogenital warts.

BOX 30.2 *Co-Factors That Trigger Malignant Transformation*

- Co-infection with or exposure to other sexually transmitted infections
- HIV
- Smoking
- Nutritional deficiencies

    k. HPV testing should target only high-risk carcinogenic cancer–associated types.

    l. Types of cancer detected

        (1) Squamous cell carcinomas: 70%

        (2) Adenocarcinomas: 18%

        (3) Adenosquamous carcinomas: 4%

        (4) Other carcinomas or malignancies: 6.5%

    m. Cervical cancer may progress from HSILs and become invasive (Figure 30.1).

    n. The peak incidence of HSILs occurs between the ages of 35 and 45 years.

    o. It generally takes 10 to 15 years from precancer to the development of invasive cancer. Rapid development of invasive carcinoma is rare (Figure 30.1).

7. Symptoms

    a. Most cervical cancer is asymptomatic.

    b. Abnormal uterine/cervical bleeding is the most significant finding. It is usually associated with friability of the diseased cervix, occurring as postcoital or mid-cycle spotting.

8. Risk factors and prevention

    a. The clinician should assess each patient for cervical cancer risk factors (Box 30.3).

    b. Women should be taught measures to reduce the risk for cervical cancer (Box 30.4).

    c. Clinicians should use strategies for increasing the use of Pap smears.

BOX 30.3 *Risk Factors for Cervical Cancer*

- Unprotected sex, particularly if with multiple partners
- Early coitarche (age of first intercourse < 16 years)
- A sexual partner with more than one sexual partner or a history of multiple sexual partners
- Exposure to or infection with other sexually transmitted diseases
- HPV, particularly if concomitant smoking
- DES exposure
- Previous abnormal Pap smear
- HIV
- Malnutrition

DES, diethylstilbestrol.

BOX 30.4 *Measures to Reduce the Risk of Cervical Cancer*

- Get an HPV vaccine
- Avoid early coitarche (age of first intercourse)
- Limit the number of sexual partners
- Use condoms consistently and correctly with every episode of oral, vaginal, or anal intercourse
- Pap test screening per ASCCP guidelines
- Avoid smoking cigarettes
- Consume a diet rich in vitamins A and C and folate

(1) Speak regularly to all female patients about the risk of cervical cancer and the need for regular screening.
(2) Reduce the costs associated with the procedure.
(3) Provide easy access to screening.
9. Screening
   a. Screening recommendations are age dependent (CDC, U.S. Preventive Services Task Force [USPSTF], ACS, American College of Obstetricians and Gynecologists [ACOG]).
   b. Women under 21 should *not* be tested.
   c. Start screening at age 21, regardless of coitarche.
   d. Age 21 to 29 years
      (1) Screening is recommended with cytology alone every 3 years. Co-testing with Pap and HPV or stand-alone HPV testing is not recommended in this age group.
   e. Age 30 to 65 years
      (1) Preferred screening—Co-testing: Pap test (cytology) with HPV testing every 5 years. There are two options
          • Women who are Pap/negative and HPV/positive
            ▪ Pap and HPV in 12 months
            ▪ If the HPV test is still positive, and the Pap is negative, referral for colposcopy
          • Genotyping may be performed for HPV 16 and 18
            ▪ If positive for 16 or 18, immediate referral for colposcopy
      (2) HPV testing should be performed with an FDA-approved test. There are currently four tests on the market.
          • Hybrid Capture 2 (Qiagen)
            ▪ Tests for a panel of 13 high-risk types
            ▪ Reported as positive or negative for the panel

- Cobas (Roche)
  - Tests for a panel of 12 high-risk types and uses a separate test for 16/18
  - Reported as positive or negative for the panel and individually for 16 and 18
- Cervista (Hologic)
  - Tests for a panel of 14 high-risk types
  - Reported as positive or negative for the panel
  - If the panel is positive, a test for 16/18 may be ordered.
- Aptima RNA
  (3) Acceptable screening—Cytology alone every 3 years
f. Age greater than 65 years
  (1) It is *not* recommended to screen this age group when there has been adequate negative screening in the previous 10 years.
  - Adequate negative screening occurs when there have been three negative Pap tests or two negative co-tests (Pap and HPV) in the past 10 years with no history of an abnormal result during this time.
  (2) Once testing has stopped, it should not be started again.
  (3) Women with a history of treatment for precancer should continue to be tested for at least 20 years after that diagnosis, even if testing continues past age 65 (per ASCCP guidelines).
g. Women exposed to diethylstilbestrol (DES)
  (1) There are differing guidelines regarding the frequency of Pap smears in this group of women. At a minimum, these women should have an annual pelvic, bimanual, and rectal exam. The most frequently these women should have a Pap test is every year, but they may be able to be spaced out as above depending on provider discretion (ACS, 2013).
h. DES offspring
  (1) Use of DES was discontinued by the FDA in 1971; therefore, treatment of DES offspring includes those women who are 43 years of age and older.
  (2) Women whose mothers took DES while pregnant may have a very large area of columnar tissue on the outside of the cervix. The cervix often appears to have a collar. This tissue is more fragile and subject to infection.
  (3) Recommended testing: Yearly cervical and four quadrant vaginal Pap smears. During a four-quadrant smear, the provider is instructed to sample from four different quadrants of the vagina, maximizing the surface area tested.

     i. HIV-infected women
- (1) These women should have biannual Pap smears in the first year of diagnosis and then may reduce to annual Pap smears based on the results.

     j. Women who have undergone hysterectomy
- (1) Elicit reason(s) why the hysterectomy was performed.
  - Benign: ACS, USPSTF, and ASCCP guidelines recommend stopping routine Pap screening for women who have undergone total hysterectomy for benign disease (such as fibroids, uterine prolapse, or endometriosis).
  - Malignancy: Women with hysterectomy resulting from cervical intraepithelial neoplasia (CIN 2) or higher, cervical or vaginal cuff screening can be discontinued once three normal Pap tests have been documented.
  - In women whose cervix remains intact after a hysterectomy, regularly scheduled Pap tests should be performed as indicated, per ASCCP.

    k. A woman who has been vaccinated against HPV should still follow the screening recommendations for her age group.

10. Obtaining the Pap smear
- a. Patient instructions: When the patient schedules her appointment for a Pap test, she should be instructed in the following.
  - (1) Do not schedule a Pap test during menses because the presence of blood may obscure the results.
  - (2) Avoid intercourse for 48 hours before the test.
  - (3) Abstain from vaginal douches, creams, or medications for 48 hours before the test. Douching and medications may remove or contaminate the cells necessary for collection. Pap tests can be obtained under these conditions if absolutely necessary, but the woman must understand that the results may be altered.
  - (4) Postpartum: Schedule the Pap test for 6 to 8 weeks after delivery, by which time the cervix will have undergone reparative changes.
- b. Equipment: The following equipment should be assembled in advance.
  - (1) Nonsterile gloves
  - (2) Speculum (metal or plastic)
  - (3) A good light source (a speculum with a light is ideal)
  - (4) Liquid-based container or one frosted glass slide (some facilities use a two–glass slide system)
  - (5) A pencil for labeling the frosted portion with the woman's name or a label for the liquid-based container

(6) A single or double cardboard slide cover

(7) Ideally a "notched" plastic spatula (Figure 30.2) or an Ayres wooden spatula paired with a cytobrush or a broom. (Cotton swabs are no longer recommended.) A broom may be used alone as it combines endo- and ectocervical sampling.

(8) Aerosol fixative for the conventional smear

c. Liquid-based Pap

(1) The FDA approved a test in May 1996 as a replacement for the conventional Pap test (ThinPrep Pap Test, Hologic Corporation; Surepath, Becton Dickinson Company).

(2) It was the first such advance in 50 years.

(3) Liquid-based testing reduces the chance that the Pap test will need to be repeated, but it does not seem to find more precancers than a conventional Pap test.

(4) The liquid helps remove some of the mucus, bacteria, yeast, and pus cells in a sample. It also allows the cervical cells to be spread more evenly on the slide (monolayer) and keeps them from drying and distorting.

(5) A key point is that the cells kept in the liquid can also be tested for HPV.

d. The technique: Careful sampling techniques are vital to ensure an adequate sample for accurate interpretation by the pathologist. This is true for both liquid-based and conventional Pap testing.

(1) Endocervical brush and spatula protocol
- Insert a speculum (water-soluble gel lubricant can be applied sparingly on the posterior blade of the speculum if needed) .
- Gently open the speculum to visualize the entire cervix and cervical os.

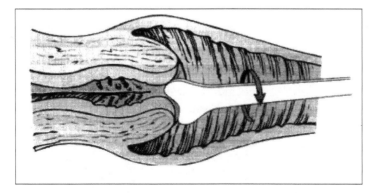

FIGURE 30.2 Collecting an ectocervical sample with a plastic spatula.

- Insert the plastic spatula and, using the contoured end, make contact with the outer surface of the cervix. Keeping firm pressure on the cervix, rotate the spatula 360 degrees around the entire exocervix while maintaining light contact with the cervix.
- Remove the spatula and immediately place it in the vial of solution. Agitate the spatula to remove sample by swirling it vigorously in the liquid 10 times. Discard the spatula.
- Insert the endocervical brush into the vagina. Gently insert the tip of the brush into the cervical os until only the bottom-most fibers are exposed. Slowly rotate one quarter or half turn in one direction. Take care to sample the squamocolumnar junction (Figure 30.3; transformation zone).
- Remove the brush and place it immediately into the same vial of solution. Remove sample from brush by rotating the brush in the solution 10 times while pushing against the vial wall. Swirl the brush vigorously several more times to further release material. Discard the brush.
- Another option: The spatula and brush may be placed into the liquid-based vial and rubbed together 10 times as an alternative mixing option. All mucus may *not* be removed from the brush and this is acceptable.
- Tighten the cap so that the torque line (marker) on the cap passes the torque line on the vial.
- Record the patient's name and ID number on the vial. Record the patient information and medical history on the cytology request form. Place the vial and requisition in a specimen bag for transport to the lab.

(2) Endocervical broom-like device protocol
- Insert a speculum (water-soluble gel lubricant can be applied sparingly on the posterior blade of the speculum if needed) into the vaginal canal.
- Gently open the speculum and visualize the entire cervix and cervical os.
- Insert the central bristles of the broom into vagina and make contact with the cervix. Push the tip of the broom into the endocervical canal deep enough to allow the shorter bristles to fully contact the ectocervix. Push gently, and rotate the broom five times.

- Remove the broom from the vagina and place it immediately in the vial of solution. Agitate the sample off the broom by pushing it into the bottom of the vial 10 times, forcing the bristles apart. As a final step, swirl the broom vigorously in the liquid to remove additional cellular material. Discard the broom. Some labs request the broom tip be included in the vial, so check with your lab.
- Tighten the cap so the torque line marker on the cap passes the torque line on the vial.
- Record the patient's name and ID number on the vial, and the patient information and medical history on the cytology requisition form. Place the vial and requisition in a specimen bag for transport to the laboratory.
- The cells on the slide must be clearly visible to be accurately interpreted. Characteristics of an adequate conventional smear include
  - An adequate number of squamous epithelial cells
  - Lack of excessive amounts of blood, inflammatory exudate, or ovulatory discharge
  - Good fixation of smear, with minimal air-drying artifact
  - Spreading the cells sufficiently thin in a monolayer
- Insert a speculum (water-soluble gel lubricant can be applied sparingly on the posterior blade of the speculum if needed) into the vaginal canal.
- Gently open the speculum; visualize the entire cervix and cervical os.
- Insert the plastic spatula and, using the contoured end, make contact with the outer surface of the cervix. Keeping firm pressure on the cervix, rotate the spatula 360 degrees around the entire exocervix while maintaining light contact with the exocervical surface.
- Hold the horizontal surface of the spatula with the sample on it in the upright position and carefully withdraw from the vagina.
- Place the flat side of the spatula against the labeled glass slide and smear uniformly to create a monolayer across two thirds of the side, using one firm motion. A counterclockwise, circular,

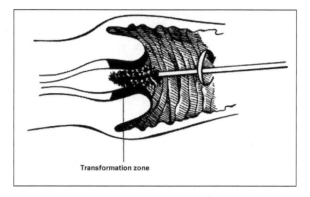

FIGURE 30.3 Ectocervical sampling using a brush to obtain cells from the transformation zone/endocervix.

or zigzag pattern may be used. Avoid excessive pressure because it may alter or destroy the cell structure.

- Insert the endocervical brush into the vagina. Gently insert the tip of the brush into the cervical os until only the bottom-most fibers are exposed. Slowly rotate one-half turn in one direction. Take care to sample the squamocolumnar junction (transformation zone; Figure 30.3).
- Unroll the specimen on the slide in the opposite direction of that taken when collecting the specimen. Add to the remaining third of the slide, being careful not to overlap with the ectocervical sample.
- Apply fixative to the entire slide. Hold the aerosol bottle approximately 6 to 12 inches away from the slide and spray enough times to saturate the sample.

(3) Conventional slide using the broom
  - Insert a speculum (water-soluble gel lubricant can be applied sparingly on the posterior blade of the speculum if needed).
  - Gently open the speculum; visualize the entire cervix and cervical os.
  - With a large swab, carefully clear any excessive cervical mucus from the cervix.
  - Insert the central bristles of the broom into vagina and make contact with the cervix. Insert the tip of the broom into the endocervical canal deep enough to allow the shorter bristles to fully contact the ectocervix. Push gently, and rotate the broom in a clockwise direction five times.

- Transfer the sample to the slide with two single paint strokes, applying first the one side of the bristles, then the other side, painting the slide again in exactly the same area.
- Apply fixative to the entire slide. Hold the aerosol bottle approximately 6 to 12 inches away from the slide and spray enough times to saturate the sample.

e. Follow-up: The system of communicating Pap smear results to women varies by clinic and facility.

  (1) The patient is informed the results may not be known for up to 4 weeks, and in some cases even longer.

  (2) A good practice is to send a negative test result via a letter or secure messaging, with a standardized template. This should be documented in the patient's medical record.

  (3) Abnormal results need to be verbally and clearly communicated by the clinician to the patient as the woman may misinterpret written information or have immediate questions. This should be documented in the patient's medical record.

f. Special considerations

  (1) Because the os tends to bleed with use of the cytobrush, it is best to obtain the ectocervical sample first with the spatula before it becomes obscured with blood.

  (2) If the patient is symptomatic or the vaginal discharge is abnormal, the clinician may consider obtaining a pH test of the secretions and/or performing a (potassium chloride) KOH/amine test and/or a wet mount in addition to the Pap smear. Sexually transmitted infection (STI) testing may also be indicated.

  (3) If an infection is present, the condition should be treated and the woman asked to return for a Pap smear in a month.

  (4) If the examiner is obtaining additional samples from the cervix, obtain the Pap smear first. STI testing may utilize cervical, vaginal, or urine samples.

  (5) Box 30.5 compares the different collection devices.

11. Liquid-based cytology (LBC) versus conventional Pap smears

  a. Pros and cons

    (1) Liquid-based pros

      - Less risk of air-drying artifact
      - More sensitive
      - May have lower risk of "partially obscuring inflammation"
      - HPV testing can be performed from the same specimen.

BOX 30.5 *Comparison of Brush and Broom for Cervical Sampling*

Brush: Advantages and Disadvantages

Advantages

- Highly efficacious for collection of endocervical cells
- Can insert into a narrow os more easily than broom
- Cochrane review found brush is safe in pregnancy

Disadvantages

- May cause more bleeding and discomfort
  Controversy regarding safety in pregnancy
- Manufacturer warns *not* to use brush after 10 weeks of pregnancy

Broom: Advantages and Disadvantages

Advantages

- Causes less bleeding
- Usually effective for endocervical cell collection
- Simultaneously collects both the endocervical and ectocervical sample
- May be used in pregnancy

Disadvantages

- More expensive if must purchase
- May not be as effective in obtaining endocervical cells if narrow cervical os and/or if the transformation zone is high in the canal (common in older women)
- Sampling errors if clinician doesn't complete five rotations

---

    (2) Liquid-based cons
       • May be more false positives
       • Uses more cytopathology resources so more expensive
   b. LBC is *not* more sensitive than conventional Pap smears for the detection of HSIL+ and CIN2+ regardless of age. But, LBC decreases the rate of inadequate smears, has increased rates of low-grade cytology detection for women younger than 40 years of age, and has a decreased total rate of abnormal smears in women older than 40 years of age (Sigurdsson, 2013).
  12. Management of abnormal Pap results using the Bethesda classification system. (Please refer to the end of the chapter for the management of Pap smear results using the 2013 ASCCP algorithms.)
   a. The Bethesda Classification System (2001, 2002) is the most widely used protocol for classifying Pap smears. This is an abbreviated summary.

(1) Adequacy of specimen: Satisfactory for evaluation (endocervical cells [ECs] and TZ present or not) or unsatisfactory for evaluation (reason).

(2) Interpretation/Result: Negative for intraepthithelial lesion or malignancy (NILM). Can include the following findings: *Trichomonas*, bacterial, viral, and fungal infection; nonneoplastic findings including reactive cellular changes associated with inflammation, radiation, and intrauterine devices (IUDs); glandular cells (post-hysterectomy); and atrophy.

(3) Squamous cell abnormalities: Atypical squamous cells (ASC)

- ASC-US: Atypical squamous cells of undetermined significance
- ASC-H: Cannot exclude high-grade squamous intraepithelial lesion
- LSIL: Refers to cervical cancer precursors including HPV, CIN 1, lesion involves the initial one third of the epithelial layer.
- HSIL: Refers to cervical cancer precursors, including CIN 2 (lesion involves one third to two thirds of the epithelial) CIN 3 (lesion involves two thirds to full thickness)
- Squamous cell carcinoma: Malignant cells penetrate basement membrane of cervical epithelium and infiltrate stromal tissues. If advanced can invade other parts of the body proximal and distant.

(4) Glandular cells

- Atypical glandular cell (AGC) specify: Endocervical, endometrial, or not otherwise specified (NOS).
- Atypical glandular cell favor neoplastic: Specify endocervical or NOS.

(5) Endocervical adenocarcinoma in situ (AIS)

(6) Adenocarcinoma

(7) Other

- Endometrial cells: These are cells shed from the lining of the uterus.
  - If the Pap smear was taken during the time of menstruation, this finding is normal.
  - This finding is abnormal in postmenopausal women. Endometrial biopsy and possibly transvaginal ultrasound are necessary to rule out endometrial cancer.

13. Management of cytologic abnormalities: Referral for colposcopy. See ASCCP guidelines.

    a. Management of Pap smear results in algorithmic form by the ASCCP, available at www.asccp.org/Portals/9/docs/Algorithms%207.30.13.pdf

14. Adequate colposcopy

    a. Visualizes the entire transformation zone and the entirety of all lesions

    b. Establishes agreement (accordance) between cytology and histology

    c. Answers whether the severity of screening test matches the diagnosis based on biopsied samples of tissue

      (1) If there is discordance in the results, the cytology sample and/or the histology sample(s) are sent for a second opinion.

15. Beyond the Pap smear

    a. HPV vaccine Gardasil (Merck): Licensed June 2006 for use in females. Approved for use in males in 2011.

      (1) Quadrivalent HPV 6/11/16/18 L1 virus like particle (VLP) vaccine.

        • Each 0.5-mL dose contains HPV types 6, 11, 16, and 18 (20, 40, 40, and 20 Ig L1 protein, respectively).

      (2) Can be administered at same visit as other age-appropriate vaccines (e.g., tetanus, diphtheria, and pertussis [Tdap]; adult diphtheria and tetanus [TD]; meningococcal conjugate [MCV4], and hepatitis B)

      (3) Costs approximately $140.00 per dose (~$420 for full series)

      (4) Not recommended for use in pregnancy

      (5) Can be given to lactating women

      (6) Available in single-dose vial or a refillable syringe

      (7) Store at 2°C to 8°C (36°F to 46°F) and do not freeze.

      (8) Vaccination schedule

        • Routine schedule is 0, 2, and 6 months

        • Minimum intervals

          ■ 4 weeks between doses 1 and 2

          ■ 12 weeks between doses 2 and 3

      (9) Do not restart the series if the schedule is interrupted.

    b. HPV vaccine and cervical cancer screening

      (1) Cervical cancer screening: No change in screening recommendations.

        • The quadrivalent vaccine does not prevent 30% of cervical cancers caused by HPV.

        • Nonvaccine HPV types could subsequently infect vaccinated women.

        • Sexually active women may have been infected before vaccination.

      (2) Educate women who received the HPV vaccine regarding the importance of cervical cancer screening.

(3) Educate women that HPV is the most common sexually transmitted virus. Condoms can reduce the incidence by 70%.
c. Contraindications to vaccination
(1) Moderate or severe acute illnesses: Defer until after illness improves.
(2) Acceptable to administer during minor acute illnesses (e.g., diarrhea or mild upper respiratory infection with or without fever)
(3) History of immediate hypersensitivity or severe allergic reaction to yeast or to any vaccine component.
16. Summary of treatment algorithms and patient education
a. Table 30.2 summarizes the follow-up for a Pap smear.
b. Patient education handouts: Free to download from the CDC
(1) www.cdc.gov/cancer/cervical/basic_info/screening.html
c. Management of Pap smear results in algorithmic form by the ASCCP available at www.asccp.org/Portals/9/docs/Algorithms%207.30.13.pdf

TABLE 30.2 Pap Smear/HPV Follow-Up Guidelines

PAP TEST RESULT	PREFERRED APPROACH	ACCEPTABLE APPROACH
Unsatisfactory cytology		
HPV unknown (any age)	Repeat cytology after 2–4 months	Repeat cytology in 2–4 months
HPV negative (age ≥ 30)	Repeat cytology after 2–4 months	
HPV positive (age ≥ 30)	Colposcopy	
	Management of results per ASCCP guidelines	
Normal but (EC)/(TZ) absent Age 21–29 Age ≥ 30 years	Routine screening	
	If HPV negative, return to routine screening	
	If HPV unknown, order HPV testing	
	Management of results per ASCCP guidelines	

(continued)

TABLE 30.2 Pap Smear/HPV Follow-Up Guidelines (*continued*)

PAP TEST RESULT	PREFERRED APPROACH	ACCEPTABLE APPROACH
Age ≥ 30, normal Cytology/ HPV positive	Repeat co-testing at 1 year	HPV DNA testing?
	Management of results per ASCCP guidelines	Management of results per ASCCP guidelines
Atypical squamous cells of undetermined significance (ASC-US)	HPV testing	Repeat cytology at 1 year
(Management options may vary if pregnant or ages 21–24)	Management of results per ASCCP guidelines	Management of results per ASCCP guidelines
ASC-US or LSIL: Age 21–24	Repeat cytology 12 months	Reflex HPV testing (for ASC-US only)
	Management of results per ASCCP guidelines	Management of results per ASCCP guidelines
LSIL	If negative HPV test (≥ 30 with co-testing), then repeat co-testing at 1 year	If positive HPV test (> 30 w/co-testing) or no HPV test, proceed to colposcopy
	If > ASC or HPV (+) proceed to colposcopy	(manage women 25–29 same)
	Management of results per ASCCP guidelines	Management of results per ASCCP guidelines
LSIL pregnant woman	Colposcopy	Defer colposcopy until at least 6 weeks postpartum
	Management of results per ASCCP guidelines	Management of results per ASCCP guidelines
ASC-H (women > 24 years)	Colposcopy (regardless of HPV status)	
	Management of results per ASCCP guidelines	
ASC-H and HSIL: Age 21–24	Colposcopy (immediate loop electrosurgical excision is unacceptable)	
	Management of results per ASCCP guidelines	

(continued)

TABLE 30.2 Pap Smear/HPV Follow-Up Guidelines *(continued)*

PAP TEST RESULT	PREFERRED APPROACH	ACCEPTABLE APPROACH
HSIL	Immediate loop or electrosurgical excision (*Not if pregnant or age 21–24) or colposcopy with endocervical sampling	
	Management of results per ASCCP guidelines	
Initial workup atypical glandular cells (AGC)	*All subcategories* (except endometrial cells)	
	Colposcopy with endocervical and endometrial sampling	
	If atypical endometrial cells, endometrial and endocervical sampling	
	Management of results by ASCCP guidelines	
AGC subsequent management	If initial cytology AGC-NOS with no CIN2+, AIS or Ca; then co-testing at 12 and 24 months. Any abnormality requires colposcopy.	
	If CIN2+ but no glandular neoplasia, management per ASCCP guidelines	
	Initial cytology AGC (favor neoplasia or AIS), then diagnostic excision is recommended	
	Management of results per ASCCP guidelines	

(continued)

TABLE 30.2 Pap Smear/HPV Follow-up Guidelines (*continued*)

PAP TEST RESULT	PREFERRED APPROACH	ACCEPTABLE APPROACH
Biopsy-confirmed cervical intraepithelial neoplasia—Grade 1 CIN1 preceded by "lesser abnormalities" (*Management options may vary if pregnant or ages 21–24)	Co-testing at 12 months Management of results per ASCCP guidelines	
CIN1 preceded by ACC-H or HSIL	Co-testing at 12 and 24 months Management of results per ASCCP guidelines	
CIN1: Age 21–24	If after ASC-US or LSIL, repeat cytology at 12 months If < ASC-H or HSIL, repeat cytology at 12 months If ≥ ASC, proceed to colposcopy After ASC-H or HSIL, management per ASCCP guidelines	
Biopsy confirmed CIN 2 and 3	If adequate colposcopy, proceed to excision or ablation of the transformation zone If no adequate colposcopy or CIN2,3 is recurrent, proceed to a diagnostic excisional procedure Management of results per ASCCP guidelines	

Note: HPV testing unacceptable for screening women ages 21 to 29 years.

Bibliography

American Cancer Society (ACS). (2013a). *Cancer facts and figures 2013*. Retrieved from http://www.cancer.org/research/cancerfactsfigures/cancerfactsfigures/cancer-facts-figures-2013

American Cancer Society (ACS). (2013b). *Cervical cancer*. Retrieved from http://www.cancer.org/cancer/cervicalcancer/detailedguide/index

American Society for Colposcopy and Cervical Pathology. (2012). *Journal of Lower Genital Tract Disease 16*(3), 00Y00. Retrieved from http://www.cdc.gov/cancer/cervical/pdf/guidelines.pdf

American Society for Colposcopy and Cervical Pathology. (2013). *Journal of Lower Genital Tract Disease 17*(5), S1YS27. Retrieved from http://www.cdc.gov/cancer/cervical/pdf/guidelines.pdf

ASSCP (2013). *Algorithms: Updated consensus guidelines for managing abnormal cervical cancer screening tests and cancer precursors*. Retrieved from http://www.asccp.org/Portals/9/docs/Algorithms%207.30.13.pdf

Bethesda System: Terminology for reporting results of cervical cytology. (2002). *Journal of the American Medical Association, 287*(16), 2114–2119.

Centers for Disease Control (CDC). (2012a). In W. Atkinson, S. Wolfe, & J. Hamborsky (Eds.). *Epidemiology and prevention of vaccine-preventable siseases*. Washington, DC: Public Health Foundation.

Centers for Disease Control (CDC). (2012b). *Cervical cancer screening guidelines for the average-risk woman*. Retrieved from http://www.cdc.gov/cancer/cervical/pdf/guidelines.pdf

Louie, K. S., de Sanjose, S., Diaz, M., Castellsagué, X., Herrero, R., Meijer, C. J., … Bosch, F. X. (2009). Early age at first sexual intercourse and early pregnancy are risk factors for cervical cancer in developing countries. *British Journal of Cancer, 100*(7), 1191–1197.

Massad, S. L., Einstein, M. H., Huh, W. K., Katki, H. A., Kinney, W. K., Schiffman. M., … Lawson, H. L. (2013). 2012 updated consensus guidelines for the management of abnormal cervical cancer screening tests and cancer precursors. *Journal of Lower Genital Tract Disease, 17*(5), S1–S27.

National Institutes of Health. (1996). *NIH Consensus Statement I, 14*(1), 1–38.

Plummer M., Peto, J., & Franceschi, S. (2012). Time since first sexual intercourse and the risk of cervical cancer. *International Journal of Cancer, 130*(11), 2638–2644.

Saslow, D., Solomon, D., Lawson, H., Killackey, M., et al. (2012). American Cancer Society, American Society for Colposocpy and Cervical Pathology, and American Society for Clinical Pathology, Screening guidelines for the prevention and early detection of cervical cancer. *Journal of Lower Genital Tract Disease, 16*, 1–29.

Saslow, D., Solomon, D., Lawson, H. W., Killackey, M., Shalini, K. L., Cain, J., & Myers, E. R. (2012). American cancer society, American Society for Colposcopy and Cervical Pathology, and American Society for Clinical Pathology Screening Guidelines for the prevention and early detection of cervical cancer. *American Journal of Clinical Pathology, 137*, 516–542. doi: 10.1309/AJCPTGD

Schiller, J. T., Day, P. M., & Kines, R. C. (2010). Current understanding of the mechanism of HPV infection. *Gynecologic Oncology, 118*(1 Suppl), S12–S17. doi: 10.1016/j.ygyno.2010.04.004

Schiffman, M., & Castle, P. E. (2003). Human papilloma virus: Epidemiology and public health. *Archives of Pathology & Laboratory Medicine, 127*, 930–934.

Schiller, J. T., Day, P. M., & Kines, R. C. (2010, June). Current understanding of the mechanism of HPV infection. *Gynecological Oncology, 118*(1 Suppl), S12–S17.

Sigurdsson, K. (2013). Is a liquid-based cytology more sensitive than a conventional Pap smear? *Cytopathology, 24*(4), 254–263. doi: 10.111/cyt.12307. Epub Jan 20 .

Solomon, D., Davey, D., Kurman, R., Moriarty, A., O'Connor, D., Prey, M., & Young, N. (2002). The 2001 Bethesda System: Terminology for reporting results of cervical cytology. *Journal of the American Medical Association, 287*(16), 2114–2119.

U. S. Cancer Statistics Working Group Cancer Statistics: 1999–2010 Incidence and Mortality Web-based Report, Atlanta (GA), Department of Health and Human Services, Centers for Disease Control and Prevention and The National Cancer Institute.

Weaver, B. A. (2006). Epidemiology and natural history of genital human papillomavirus infection. *Journal of the American Osteopathic Association, 106*(3 Suppl 1), S2–S8.

Wright, T. C,. Jr., Stoler, M. H., Behrens, C. M., Apple, R., Derion, T., & Wright, T. L. (2012). The ATHENA human papillomavirus study: Design, methods, and baseline results. *American Journal of Obstetrics & Gynecology, 206*(1), 46.e1-e11.

Vaginal Microscopy

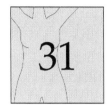
31

Helen A. Carcio and R. Mimi Secor

I. Vaginal microscopy explained

A. The value

1. Vaginal microscopy is an important laboratory tool for the differential diagnosis of vaginitis. It is also used to assess normal vaginal flora. Six common conditions cause the majority of discharge or infection (see Box 31.1).

2. Vaginal microscopy allows observation of living vaginal organisms to study the ecology of the lower genital tract in women.

3. It is a direct, rapid, inexpensive test with low to moderate sensitivity and specificity for diagnosis of vaginal infections.

4. It acts as an accessory tool to patient history, inspection of the vulvar and vaginal mucosa, and pH determination to arrive at a presumptive etiologic diagnosis.

5. The two components involved are saline wet mount and 10% potassium hydroxide (KOH) wet mount.

B. The wet mount

1. Nomenclature: Microscopy involves use of the wet mount.
   a. Other similar terms include *wet smear, wet prep, vaginal smear, vaginalysis,* or *hanging drop.*

2. Basic principles
   a. A 3- to 5-minute microscopic search is necessary before concluding that a slide is negative for a certain condition.
   b. Examination under oil immersion is rarely needed.
   c. The sample should be collected from the lateral vaginal side walls.
   d. The sensitivity depends on the expertise of the clinician and the adequacy of sample and ranges from 60% to 80%.
   e. Remember to consider cervical factors when evaluating patients with vaginal discharge; also consider a cervical wet mount, especially if discharge is yellow, the patient has persistent unexplained white blood cells (WBCs) on microscopy, or cervicitis is noted.

> **BOX 31.1** *The Six Conditions Causing the Majority of Vaginal Discharge or Infection (in Order)*
>
> 1. Bacterial vaginosis (BV)
> 2. *Candida* vulvovaginitis
> 3. Cervicitis (usually caused by chlamydia)
> 4. Excessive but normal secretions
> 5. *Trichomonas* vaginitis
> 6. Vulvovaginal atrophy (VVA), genital atrophy (GA) (atrophic vaginitis)

C. Indications: Vaginal microscopy should be performed
   1. On every patient presenting with vaginal symptoms or with clinical features suggestive of a cervical or vaginal condition
   2. Even if the diagnosis is clinically obvious (such as with a curd-like discharge associated with candidiasis) because many conditions can mimic other conditions and mixed infections are also common
   3. In a patient with urine sediment that contains white cells and many squamous epithelial cells to determine the exact source of infection (vagina or urinary tract)
   4. To determine the reason a routine Pap smear shows an inflammatory response
   5. As a follow-up test in a woman after treatment for a vaginal or cervical infection
   6. During the routine health maintenance visit to assess for normal flora or asymptomatic vaginal infection
   7. As a complement: A thorough and comprehensive health history is necessary to establish a differential diagnosis (Box 31.2). Table 31.1 presents the differential diagnoses.

II. Comments on the vaginal ecology
   A. The vagina has minimal nerve endings; therefore, the symptoms of vaginal disorders may become evident only when the vaginal discharge irritates the sensitive vulvar skin.
   B. Normally, the vagina cleanses itself by the discharge of acidotic secretions.
   C. The pH is acidotic, approximately 3.8 to 4.6.
      1. Organisms live symbiotically in an acid environment.
         a. Factors that increase the glycogen content (high levels of estrogen in pregnancy or medication) increase the acidity of the vaginal secretions.

BOX 31.2 *Key History-Taking Questions and Considerations*

History and chronology
- Onset of symptoms
- Duration of current episode
- Date, diagnosis, treatment, and response of previous infection
- Self-diagnosis and treatment
- Monthly or seasonal variation
- Affect on lifestyle
- Evolution of chronicity
- Sentinel events
- History of IV drug use
- Blood transfusion

Sexual history
- Age of first sexual experience
- Lifelong number of partners, gender, ages
- STI exposure
- Current sexual partner(s), duration of relationship, other partners
- Partner history of STIs, GU symptoms, circumcision
- Sexual practices (i.e., anal intercourse, oral sex, order of activities, hygiene)
- Condom use (percentage of time)
- Sexual devices or toys
- Lubricants (specify brand)
- Date of last coitus or genital contact
- Dyspareunia (superficial, deep; before, during, or after penetration)

Symptoms
- Description (use patient's own words)
- Location (use patient-guided drawing)
- Radiation
- Severity (use a rating scale of 0 to 3+)
- Full review of systems

Obstetric and gynecologic factors
- Last menstrual period
- Duration of menses
- Tampons versus pads
- Dysmenorrhea or dysfunctional uterine bleeding
- Pregnancy, birth, episiotomy, lacerations
- Pain in pregnancy
- Infertility
- Pelvic or genital surgeries
- Pap smear history
- Vulvar care

Aggravating factors
- Allergies
- Activities
- Positions
- Dietary
- Self-treatments
- Prescription and OTC medications
- Clothing
- Sexual activities
  Sex toys
  Hygiene issues

Relieving factors
- Vulvar care measures
- Prescription and OTC medications
- Alternative or home remedies
- Stress reduction measures
- Vitamins, supplements, and diet

GU, genitourinary; IV, intravenous; OTC, over the counter; STI, sexually transmitted infection.

      b. Glycogen present in the epithelial cells is used by the peroxide-producing lactobacilli to produce lactic acid, which maintains an acid environment.

      c. Acidity allows for the overgrowth of the yeast organisms.

   2. This level of acidotic secretions is antagonistic to harmful bacteria.

D. Factors affecting normal vaginal flora

   1. Role of hormones

      a. Estrogen

        (1) Affects vaginal epithelium

        (2) Causes glycogen to be deposited in the vagina, mainly in the intermediate cells

        (3) Glycogen is metabolized to become lactic acid.

      b. Progesterone causes shedding of these glycogen-rich cells into the vaginal pool. (This may be the reason symptoms of candidiasis increase premenstrually and are somewhat relieved after the menstrual flow.)

   2. Effect of medications on the vaginal ecology

      a. Antibiotics may increase the incidence of *Candida* infection. There are many theories

        (1) *Candida* reproduce rapidly because they no longer have the competition from other bacteria, which were destroyed by the antibiotic.

        (2) Secretion of an antifungal substance by bacteria stops when the bacteria are killed (more recent theory).

        (3) Possible direct stimulation of growth of *Candida* by the antibiotic.

        (4) Other theories describe reduction of host defenses, as in human immunodeficiency virus (HIV).

      b. Certain medications can affect the growth of lactobacilli and thus affect the vaginal milieu.

        (1) Anbiotics may have a variable effect on the vaginal milieu such as causing a temporary reduction in lactobacilli, and then a possible increase in lactobacilli.

        (2) Antibiotics may also cause a secondary overgrowth of candidiasis.

        (3) Antifungal agents can temporarily reduce the number of lactobacilli, possibly contributing to the problem of recurrence.

      c. Corticosteroids

        (1) Reduce inflammatory response of host

        (2) Topical steroids do not usually aggravate candidiasis, as previously thought.

TABLE 31.1 Differential Diagnosis of Vaginal Conditions

CONDITION	VULVOVAGINAL SYMPTOMS	VAGINAL DISCHARGE	LACTOBACILLI	pH	MICROSCOPY
Candida albicans	Mild to severe itching Cyclic Marked vulvovaginal erythema	Increased amount White, curdy, cottage cheese-like	Moderate	< 4.7	KOH Hyphae, pseudohyphae, and spores "Spaghetti and meatballs"
C. glabrata and other non-*C. albicans* infections	Mild to moderate burning/itching Chronic, cyclic Mild vulvovaginal erythema	Increased Unchanged to white	Moderate	< 4.7	KOH Spores only Vary in size and shape Need culture to confirm
Bacterial vaginosis (BV)	Mild to moderate itching Absent to mild inflammation Mild vulvovaginal erythema	Adherent, homogenous discharge Appearance of milk poured into vagina Fish odor, particularly after intercourse	Rare	> 4.5	Saline Clue cells, few to many WBCs KOH + Whiff test

(continued)

TABLE 31.1 Differential Diagnosis of Vaginal Conditions *(continued)*

CONDITION	VULVOVAGINAL SYMPTOMS	VAGINAL DISCHARGE	LACTOBACILLI	pH	MICROSCOPY
Cytolytic vaginosis (scant research)	Mild to moderate burning/itching Premenstrual, relieved with menses	Unchanged to increased white	Excessive	$< 3.5–< .7$	Saline Overabundance of lactobacilli Fragments of epithelial cells, Rare WBCs
Lactobacillosis vaginal (scant research)	Itching/burning Chronic, cyclic	Thick White to creamy	Elongated Rare, short rods	4–5	Saline Very long rods Few short rods Rare WBCs
Trichomonas	Severe vulvar itching Petechiae of cervix and vagina Vulvar Erythema	Copious Yellow-green May be frothy Malodorous	Plus or minus	> 4.7	Saline Unicellar trichomonads Many WBCs

(continued)

TABLE 31.1 Differential Diagnosis of Vaginal Conditions *(continued)*

CONDITION	VULVOVAGINAL SYMPTOMS	VAGINAL DISCHARGE	LACTOBACILLI	pH	MICROSCOPY
Vulvovaginal atrophy (VVA)	Pruritus, irritation Vaginal dryness and dyspareunia Smooth vaginal walls	Red, tender vestibule and vagina Scant discharge Lack of rugae	Rare	> 5-6 > 4.7	Saline Parabasal cells Few to many WBCs Few lactobacili
Desquamative inflammatory vaginitis (DIV)	Erythema of vulva, vagina, and cervix Dyspareunia Pruritus or irritation	Thick, profuse No odor	Rare	> 4.7	Saline Basal/ parabasal cells Many WBCs

KOH, potassium hydroxide; WBC, white blood cell.

3. Douching: Decreases normal flora and increases the risk for bacterial vaginosis (BV)
4. Tampon use may also alter normal flora and increase the risk for vulvovaginal infection.

III. **The microscope: The clinician must be familiar with all parts of the microscope and know how to care for it properly.**
   A. Selection of magnification
      1. Low-power objective (10x magnification, eye piece 10x = 100x magnification)
      2. High-power objective (40x magnification, eye piece 10x = 400x magnification)
   B. Light source: Helps increase the examiner's ability to visualize details by controlling the illumination. The examiner must increase or decrease the light transmitted through the preparation. The light source is controlled by the following features:
      1. Intensity setting of the light source
      2. The light shutter
      3. The position of the condenser
         a. For the low-power objective, drop the condenser for a lower intensity setting.
         b. For the high-power objective, increase the condenser for a higher intensity setting.
   C. Mechanics of observing the saline smear. (Always wear gloves.)
      1. Position the slide on the stage of the microscope with saline preparation under the objective and secure with stage clips.
      2. Turn light on under stage.
      3. Click low objective into place over the specimen (obtains a larger view of the slide area, although the images are small).
      4. Turn the condenser to the lowest position; subdued light is best to accentuate fine details. (Try increasing the light by raising the condenser while viewing the specimen to see how the cells and bacteria disappear from view.)
      5. Move objective and slide as close together as possible, until just barely touching.
      6. Adjust the eyepiece until a single round field is seen (interpupillary diameter).
      7. While looking through the eyepiece, turn the coarse adjustment knob in the opposite direction until the microscopic field comes into focus. Use both eyes.
      8. Turn fine-adjust knob back and forth to adjust to the different planes and bring image into sharper focus.
      9. Adjust each eyepiece separately by closing one eye at a time.

10. Turn knob slowly to focus (some microscopes are very sensitive; turning too rapidly may result in missing the proper plane of visualization).
11. Move the saline specimen under the objective and scan the slide at low magnification to locate representative sections.
    a. Scan all fields because characteristic findings may be clumped in one section of the slide.
    b. When the side of the coverslip is reached, move the slide over one field's width, and then start scanning in the opposite direction. It is important to avoid the objective coming in contact with the KOH that might be leaking along the edges of the coverslip. This can cause scratching of the glass surface and require replacement of the objective.
12. Switch to high-power objective (40x $\times$ 10x = 400x) magnification.
    a. Facilitates identification of microbes by further magnifying the specimen
    b. It may be necessary to increase the light source slightly.
    c. Watch stage when switching to make sure that the objective does not break the slide. This should not happen if low power is properly adjusted.
13. Turn fine adjustment back and forth; coarse adjustment should not require readjustment.
14. Using the stage adjustment knobs, move the slide laterally up and down and back and forth to view all fields because pathogens may not be distributed evenly throughout the slide and may be found in a limited number of fields.
15. Scan the slide systematically to evaluate the specimen fully.
16. Move the slide until you have a general impression of the number of squamous cells and any other findings.
17. Evaluate at least 10 to 12 fields.
18. Hint: If you immediately see organisms that might be causing vaginitis, you still should continue to examine the specimen thoroughly to prevent missing a concomitant/mixed infection.
D. Mechanics of observing the KOH preparation. Observe same principles of microscopy described previously.
   1. Move the KOH slide into position on stage.
   2. Switch back to low-power objective to scan fields for yeast forms. Pseudohyphae are easiest to identify on low-power, appearing as "spaghetti and meatballs."
   3. If yeast forms are noted, switch to high power to confirm their presence and type. Observing only buds suggests a possible *C. glabrata* infection, but this should be confirmed by culture, preferably with polymerase chain reaction (PCR) testing.

E. Concluding comments
  1. Thorough observation of both preparations should be undertaken for a minimum of 3 to 5 minutes.
  2. When the procedure is completed, remember to turn off the microscope light source and dispose of the slide(s) in a solid biohazard container as is used for syringe disposal.
  3. Clean the microscope stage if it is soiled, and clean the lenses with special paper or a cotton swab with lens cleaner.
    a. KOH can damage the objective so an effort should be made to avoid liquid leaking onto the microscope objective. Clean microscope promptly and thoroughly if there is leakage.
  4. Record findings, and review the findings with the patient.

IV. Preparation for the wet mount procedure
  A. Patient preparation: Any substance in the vagina can alter the accuracy of the microscopic findings. Instruct the woman in the following preparations.
    1. Explain that the examination is similar to a Pap smear and should not cause discomfort.
    2. Menses cannot be avoided if a woman has symptoms during that time. However, it does make evaluation more difficult because of the presence of red blood cells in the smear.
    3. Avoid coitus or douching for 24 hours before the examination.
    4. Do not use over-the-counter preparations before the examination (avoid for as long as possible).
  B. Perform clinical evaluation. Box 31.3 shows the sequence of the examination.
  C. Observe characteristics of vaginal discharge (Table 31.2).
  D. Equipment
    1. Gloves
    2. Speculum (metal or plastic)
    3. Cotton or Dacron-tipped applicators or a plastic spatula, or both
    4. Frosted-glass slide (1 or 2)
    5. Coverslips (1 or 2 inch)
    6. Bottle of normal saline (slightly warmed if possible)
    7. Bottle of 10% to 20% KOH
    8. Vaginal pH test paper (Nitrazine; Squibb & Sons, or other brand)
    9. Microscope with 10x and 40x objectives
    10. Small test tubes (3 to 4 inches long) with 1–3 mL (or half inch) of saline if saline immersion method is used
  E. Perform pelvic examination (see Chapter 4, "The Physical Examination").

V. Saline wet mount
  A. Obtaining and preparing the sample

> **BOX 31.3** *Sequence of Examination During an Infection Check*

- Obtain a thorough, focused history
- Review procedure and expected outcomes with patient
- Insert speculum
- Inspect genitalia, noting signs of infection
- Determine vaginal pH
- pH should be collected first because cervical specimens may cause cervical bleeding, which might increase the pH level
- Collect sample of discharge from the lateral vaginal walls
- Collect STI cultures from urine, cervical, or cervicovaginal samples, if indicated
- Remove speculum
- Label any specimens
- Perform wet mount evaluation
- Document results
- Review results with patient
- Treat any infection

TABLE 31.2 Analysis of Vaginal Discharge

CHARACTERISTIC	POSSIBLE FINDINGS
Magnitude (quantitate amount)	Stains on undergarment dime size, quarter size
Color	Off-white Creamy Whitish-gray Yellow Greenish Pink-red
Character	Watery thick, curd-like, homogenous
Odor	Fishy foul
Relation to menses	Premenstrual midcycle after menses

Note: A yellow color indicates sloughing of leukocytes; primarily seen with cervicitis and pelvic inflammatory disease (PID).

1. Obtain copious sample from the posterior and lateral vaginal walls using a plastic spatula or a cotton or Dacron swab.
   a. The collection technique may vary with the suspected diagnosis.
2. Place two separate samples of vaginal discharge on the same frosted-glass slide. It takes practice to use only one slide, but

it is time and is cost-effective; therefore, it is probably worth developing the skill. (Saline sample should be thin.)

a. Alternate procedure: Double slide method
  (1) May use two separate slides
  (2) Place smear of sample on one slide and a sample on the second slide. Gently apply the coverslip. Do not press down.
  (3) Blot sides of slide if necessary with paper towel (if leaking out from under the coverslips).
  (4) This method has the advantage of eliminating the possibility of the two solutions contaminating each other.

3. Add one drop of normal saline to thinner sample.
  a. Be careful not to mix the solutions.
    (1) If the solutions are mixed, the sample must be collected again because the KOH will dissolve the cellular material on the saline portion of the slide.
  b. Mix each specimen, thoroughly stirring until smooth, to create a turbid suspension. May use same device if saline is mixed first.
    (1) May use a plastic spatula or the opposite end of a Dacron swab.
    (2) The saline specimen should be fairly diluted to separate the epithelial cells from each other. Sample should appear only very slightly cloudy.
    (3) If the cells are clumped on top of each other, the characteristic of the individual form is difficult to determine and sensitivity is reduced.
  c. Alternate method: Saline immersion
    (1) Some believe that an undiluted smear is often too thick to interpret accurately and dries too quickly.
    (2) Place 7 to 10 drops (0.5 ml) of physiologic saline in a small test tube. (Saline must be room temperature or warmer.)
    (3) Roll a Dacron swab along the posterolateral vaginal walls.
    (4) Immediately immerse applicator into the saline-filled tube (approx. 1–3 mL).
    (5) Place a drop of the suspension on the slide using either method described previously. A plastic dropper works well for this.
  d. Some comments
    (1) Whether the diluted effect of this method affects the sensitivity of this test is controversial.
    (2) It may prevent drying of the specimen; therefore, the examiner may have more time—15 minutes—to read slide.
    (3) This procedure may best be reserved for those examinations when trichomoniasis is suspected to

ensure the motility of the organism or when the examination does not allow the clinician to leave the room immediately.

    (4) KOH is tested by directly mixing vaginal sample with KOH and testing for a positive amine result immediately. KOH added to the test tube sample of saline may produce a false negative result due to the dilution effect.

  4. Immediately place separate coverslips over each specimen just before viewing to prevent drying.

    a. Hold one edge of the coverslip against the slide, and slowly drop (like a hinged door) over the liquid specimen to reduce the number of air bubbles.

  5. If necessary, take a paper towel and gently dab the side of the slide to absorb any excess fluid leaking from the slide.

    a. This helps keep the microscope clean.

  6. Interpret findings immediately, viewing saline slide first (allowing KOH time to lyse).

  7. At least 12 fields should be analyzed for a total of 3 to 5 minutes. If unable to allocate this time, view slide for at least 1 to 2 minutes.

B. Findings on saline wet mount (see Table 31.3)

  1. Vaginal epithelial cells

    a. Slightly grainy cytoplasm-containing vacuoles

    b. Distinct cell walls

    c. Evaluate cells for the following features

      (1) Quantity of mature cells present

      (2) Presence of immature cells and their relative frequency. May indicate

        • Decreased estrogen

        • Significant inflammatory reaction of chronic inflammation

        • Presence of many immature cells indicates a severe inflammatory process of significant duration.

    d. Epithelial cells change as they mature in the presence of estrogen (Table 31.4) (see Chapter 12, "Atrophic Vaginitis, Vulvovaginal Atrophy" and Chapter 32, "Maturation Index").

  2. Presence of significant bacterial adherence to cell surfaces

    a. Often indicative of a virulent organism

    b. Dynamic process involving bacterial fimbriae and epithelial surface characteristic

    c. Attachment depends on pH, hydrophobic properties, and surface secretion.

  3. Lactobacilli

    a. Easily visualized in saline preparation (Figure 31.1)

    b. Pleomorphic, gram-positive, aerobic or facultative anaerobic, nonspore-forming organism

TABLE 31.3 Microscopic Structures That May Be Identified in a Wet Mount Preparation (in Order)

SALINE	KOH
Lactobacilli	Yeast forms
Cocci	Hyphae
White blood cells (polymorphonuclear cells)	Pseudohyphae Mycelia Spores
Squamous epithelial cells (varying degrees of maturity)	Chlamydiaspores Blastospores
Clue cells	
False clue cells	
Trichomoniasis	
Red blood cells	

TABLE 31.4 Characteristics of Epithelial Cells in Relation to Menstrual Cycle

Early proliferative phase (Few cells found in smear because desquamation is slight)	Precornified Polygonal shape Little tendency toward folding of the edges Transparent cytoplasm Nucleus with granular chromatin Normal saline (NS) cells present
Late proliferative phase	Under estrogenic stimulation Small deeply pigmented, homogeneous nuclei Polygonal shape May appear flat or folded Rare PMN cells
Midsecretory phase	Progestational phase Increase in number of desquamated superficial cells Predominately precornified More angular with folded edges Nuclei are vesicular and elongated or oval Cytoplasm contains occasional granules Marked tendency toward folding and clumping Background clear Few PMN cells
Late secretory (premenstrual) phase	Clusters of desquamated, precornified cells Fragments of cytoplasm, mucus, and PMN cells Peak shedding

PMN, polymorphonuclear.

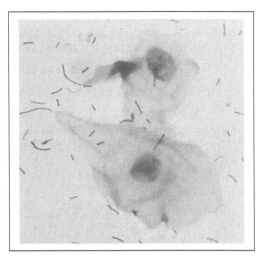

FIGURE 31.1 Lactobacilli.

c. Elongated rod-shaped bacilli that appear as straight rods, which will be motile if smear is made properly and not dried out
  (1) Super-long bacilli may be a normal finding (previously termed *Leptothrix*); they may be longer than the diameter of an epithelial cell.
  (2) May indicate lactobacillosis
d. Lactobacilli usually dominate the flora of the normal estrogenized vagina (96%).
e. Predominance in vagina of acidophilic *Lactobacillus* species
  (1) Eighty species have been identified.
f.. Maintains a low pH of vaginal discharge by making lactic acid, which inhibits adherence of bacteria to epithelial cells.
g. Known to inhibit growth of organisms that may normally be found in the vagina, such as
  (1) *Gardnerella vaginalis*
  (2) *Mycoplasma hominis*
  (3) Certain anaerobes
h. Little effect on candidiasis (may even increase) or trichomoniasis
i. Numbers increase after menarche and markedly decrease after menopause.
4. WBCs (or leukocytes)
  a. Present as dark and granular cells with clearly segmented nuclei
    (1) Termed polymorphonuclear (PMN)
    (2) This lobulated nucleus is often fairly easy to distinguish.
  b. May also appear as cytoplasmic granules with an indistinct nucleus (often with chronic infection)

TABLE 31.5 Significance of White Blood Cells

	NUMBER IN HPF	RATIO OF WBC TO EPITHELIAL CELL
Normal mild	0–4	$< 5{:}1$
Moderate severe	5–10	$> 5{:}1$
	10 or more	$> 10{:}1$

Note: May be influenced by the concentration of the smear. If inflammation is present, observe for the presence or absence of parabasal cells.
hpf, high-power field. WBC, white blood cells.

BOX 31.4 *Causes of the Presence of Leukocytes (White Blood Cells) on Wet Mount*

Moderate increase of leukocytes found with

- IUD use
- Postpartum reparative process
- Atrophicvaginitis, vulvovaginal atrophy (VVA)
- Allergie reaction to spermicides and douches
- Medroxyprogesterone acetate (MPA) (Depo-Provera) users with low estrogen levels

Marked increase of leukocytes found with

- Trichomoniasis
- Candidiasis
- Chlamydia or gonorrhea
- Atrophic vaginitis with bacterial superinfection (common)

Note: If many leukocytes are seen but neither *Candida* nor *Trichomonas* are present, consider an STI culture for infections, such as chlamydia or gonorrhea. Also consider dysplasia or metaplasia as a possible cause. IUD, intrauterine device.

---

    c. Slightly larger than the nucleus of a mature epithelial cell
    d. Immobile trichomonal organisms are more similar to a teardrop in shape and slightly larger than mobile organisms; however, they may be difficult to distinguish from PMN cells.
    e. The number of WBCs helps determine extent of inflammation (Table 31.5).
    f. Increased in many conditions (Box 31.4)
  5. Motile trichomonads
  6. Clue cells
  7. False clue cells
  8. Immature squamous epithelial cells (see Chapter 12, "Atrophic Vaginitis, Vulvovaginal Atrophy").

9. The presence of eosinophils may indicate an allergic response.
10. Mobiluncus
   a. Easily visualized; be careful not to confuse with the rod-shaped lactobacilli.
   b. Comma-shaped, highly motile bacteria
   c. Seen at one point as black dots that bounce off the coverslip and elongate in an eyelash shape
   d. Gram stain is negative.
11. Red blood cells: Visible as small concave spheres
C. Normal findings include
   1. Absence of or less than five WBCs/high-power field (hpf)
   2. pH less than 4.7
   3. Presence of moderate amounts of lactobacilli
   4. Absence of demonstrable pathogens, such as *Trichomonad* or clue cells
   5. Figure 31.2 shows the characteristics of a normal smear.
D. Hints for interpreting a saline smear
   1. Evaluate systematically (as with an electrocardiogram—each part is looked at; for example, the QRS complex rather than the whole rhythm strip).
   2. Picture the smear as an ocean (fluid medium) dotted with islands (vaginal epithelial cells) and boats or rafts that may be in the ocean or dotting the shores of the island.
      a. The boats can come in many sizes and shapes, and they may represent WBCs or trichomoniasis; smaller rafts represent cocci and rods.
   3. Ask yourself the following questions:
      a. Are there any islands? How many in each field? What do they look like? Are the edges clear or obscured? If they are obscured, are they obscured by dots or rods?

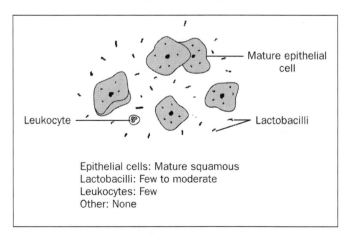

Epithelial cells: Mature squamous
Lactobacilli: Few to moderate
Leukocytes: Few
Other: None

FIGURE 31.2 Normal flora.

    b. What is in the ocean surrounding the islands? Are there rods or cocci, or a mixture of both? Adequate numbers? Too few? Too many?

    c. Is there anything swimming in the ocean (extracellular spaces)? Are there any motile trichomonads or mobiluncus?

    d. Are there any WBCs? How many?

VI. KOH

A. Some comments

    1. Dissolves leukocytes, *Trichomonas,* and background debris, making identification of fungal structures easier

    2. Effects on epithelial cells

        a. KOH breaks down the cell wall, changing the wall from cuboid and translucent to ovoid and transparent.

        b. Epithelial cells become enlarged and faint; called "ghost" cells, a mere shadow of their former selves.

    3. Branching and budding hyphae are alkali resistant and stand out in sharp contrast.

    4. Higher sensitivity for *Candida* using KOH than with saline preparations

        a. Some sources believe that KOH is rarely necessary if the observer is skilled in the evaluation of saline preparations.

B. Obtaining and preparing the sample

    1. Use Dacron swab or plastic spatula to collect specimen from lateral vaginal walls.

        a. Cotton may contaminate the sample with fiber artifact.

        b. If vulvar sample, use plastic spatula or cytobrush to scrape erythematous border.

    2. Dot onto slide or mix sample into KOH placed on slide before mixing.

        a. Material should be fairly thick with epithelial cells clustered to concentrate the yeast forms.

        b. This is in contrast to saline, in which the sample should be relatively thin.

    3. Add a drop of KOH (10%).

        a. Be careful not to mix with saline solution if a single slide is used for both preparations.

        b. Use the solution mixed by the laboratory's own pharmacy or order a premixed bottle.

    4. Mix with the wooden end of a cotton swab or spatula to create a turbid mixture.

    5. Perform the whiff test.

        a. Volatile amines are released into the air when anaerobic bacterial overgrowth comes in contact with an alkaline solution such as KOH.

BOX 31.5 *Artifacts That May Interfere With the Interpretation of* Candida *Species on Wet Mount*

In identification of spores

- White blood cells
- Nuclei of epithelial cells (particularly if clumped together)
- Powder granules from gloves (resemble umbilicated marshmallows)
- Tiny bubbles of emulsified vaginal creams (must elicit possibility of presence by history)
- Dust on microscope lenses
- Red blood cells (round, all similar size shape, convex)

In identification of filaments

- Cotton fiber from cotton-tipped swab, undergarments, or tampons

---

    b. Amines are produced by converting lysine to cadaverine, arginine to putrescine, and trimethylamin oxide to trimethylamine.

    c. Immediately after mixing sample with KOH, smell the collection device (no need to bring entire slide to nose).

    d. Note the presence of a foul or fishy odor.

    e. If odor is present, it is recorded as a positive result. A positive result indicates an imbalance of the vaginal flora in which anaerobes dominate.

    f. Usually indicates the presence of BV but may also indicate the presence of trichomoniasis. Negative if atrophic vaginitis or yeast vaginitis.

  6. Blot the side of the slide with a paper towel, if any excess fluid.

    a. KOH can damage the objective.

  7. If a vulvar sample is obtained, consider heating the slide slightly by passing it under a lighted match to dissolve the keratin.

C. Findings on KOH wet mount

  1. Wait 2 to 3 minutes, allowing time for the KOH to dissolve the cellular structures.

    a. Examine the saline mixture during this time.

  2. Scan slide.

    a. Low power (10x): Locate sections of yeast forms, which may appear as thin sticks, or elongated circus balloons, or sausage links.

    b. High power (40x): Focus on buds and pseudohyphae for further confirmation of morphologic characteristics. Note the presence of any yeast forms.

  3. Artifact may interfere with interpretation of the wet mount (Box 31.5)

D. For summary flow sheet instructions, see Tables 31.6A and 31.6B.

TABLE 31.6A Vaginal Microscopy: Secor Flow Sheet Instructions

Date	
History	Brief history of symptoms, including self-care, medications
LMP, last coitus	LMP, last coitus, dyspareunia
Vulva, vagina, cervix	Erythema, lesions, tenderness
Vaginal mucus	Amount and characteristics pH (4.0–7.5)
Cervical mucus	Color, quality, and amount
(4 = normal)	Use 1 in. strip of pH paper (Nitrazine or ColorpHast paper; dip pH paper into vaginal mucus collected on swab, spatula, or from speculum
Amine test (KOH)	Using spatula containing sample, stir x 5–10 times into 20% KOH on glass slide
Wet mount saline (dilute w/ scattered ECs)	Using spatula containing sample, stir x 1–3 times into saline solution on glass slide
Low-power (quality) magnification	Note general appearance and quality of sample, for example, proper concentration, too dilute, too concentrated
High-power (detail) magnification Lactobacilli (0–5+) appear as rods	Identify organisms and morphology 1+ = few, 2+ = dominant, 3+ = false clue cells
Bacteria: Anaerobes (0–5+) appear as tiny dots	1–+[RR7] = few 2+ = dominant background 3+ = clue cells
WBCs (0–3+): Lobulated nucleus	1+ = 1:1 ratio to ECs; 2+ = 5:1 ratio to ECs; 3+ = 10:1 or greater ratio to ECs
Other	ECs (true clue cells, false clue cells, grainy, furry) yeast, *Trichomonas*, *mobiluncus*, sperm, red blood cells, medications, artifact
Wet mount (KOH) (very concentrated)	ECs look like round, faint balloons, called ghost cells
Low power	Hyphae forms (cobwebs) visible but not buds
High power	Hyphae look like elongated circus balloons Buds look like spherical glass beads
Assessment	Specify, including rule outs, list in order of most likely to least likely
Plan	Diagnostic tests, including yeast cultures, medications, education, and follow-up

EC, epithelial cell; KOH, potassium hydroxide; LMP, last menstrual period; WBC, white blood cell. Adapted from the Secor Scale. Used with permission.

TABLE 31.6B Vaginal Microscopy: Secor Flow Sheet

Date
HPI
LMP, last coitus
Vulva, vagina, cervix
Vaginal mucus
Cervical mucus
pH (4.0–7.5) 4 = normal
Amine test (KOH)
Wet mount (saline)
Low power (quality)
High power (detail)
LB (0–3+)
Bacteria (0–3+)
WBCs (0–3+)
Other
Wet mount (KOH)
Low power
High power
Assessment
Plan

KOH, potassium hydroxide; HPI, history of present illness; LB, lactobacilli; LMP, last menstrual period; WBC, white blood cell.

VII. pH

A. Some comments about pH

1. pH is representative of the acidity or alkalinity of the vagina, as determined by the presence of lactobacilli and other organisms.

2. Exacerbation or amelioration of clinical disease in relation to the menstrual cycle is a function of pH.

3. Correlate pH findings with microscopic examination and clinical assessment.

4. Evaluation of pH of the vaginal secretions is a valuable diagnostic tool.

5. It is easy to perform and is inexpensive, with a high predictive value.

TABLE 31.7 pH in Relation to Life Cycle Changes Affected by the Presence or Absence of Lactobacilli

PHASE OF REPRODUCTIVE LIFE CYCLE	pH
Preadolescence	7.0
Reproductive years	3.8–4.6
Postmenopausal years	4.7–7.0

   6. Women should avoid intravaginal medication and sexual activity 2 to 3 days before the visit.
   7. pH of the vagina varies with the amount of vaginal estrogen during the various reproductive cycles of women (Table 31.7).
   B. Vaginal pH paper (many brands)
      1. Scale must begin at 4.0 at minimum
      2. Record range of pH, as determined by the color of the tape, compared with the manufacturer's chart.
   C. Collection: Cut off strip before inserting speculum.
      1. Use ½- to 1-inch strip of pH paper.
      2. Collect the sample from the upper lateral wall because it is less likely to be mixed with cervical mucus.
      3. Obtain sample directly from pH paper strip applied to vaginal wall or to discharge from the collecting spatula, or dip pH strip into discharge pooled on the upper blade of the vaginal speculum. Sample from a swab or spatula may also be applied to the pH paper.
         a. Keep the speculum in the sink in the event that additional samples are needed.
            (1) Avoids woman having to undergo subsequent pelvic examination.
   D. Interpretation of results
      1. Acidic finding (< 4.7) indicates the presence of vaginal lactobacilli in the vaginal flora.
      2. A pH less than 4.7 effectively excludes
         a. *Neisseria gonorrhoeae*
         b. *Gardnerella vaginalis*
         c. *Haemophilus influenzae*
         d. *Trichomonas vaginalis* (not always)
         e. Vulvovaginal atrophy (VVA), genital atrophy (GA), and atrophic vaginitis
      3. *T. vaginalis* thrives on an alkaline milieu; *Candida* is inhibited.
      4. Factors that interfere with the determination of pH, which, if present, eliminate use of pH as a diagnostic tool
         a. Menses: > 7.2
         b. Semen: > 7
         c. Cervical mucus: alkaline: > 7

TABLE 31.8 Measurement of Vaginal Ph

pH	CONDITION	COLOR CHANGE
4.0–4.6	Normal flora Cytolytic vaginosis Small number of immotile trichomonads may be present (not clinically significant)	Light yellow
4.0–4.6	Vulvovaginal candidiasis (not as diagnostic) Group A or B beta-hemolytic streptococcus	Medium to dark yellow
4.7–6.0	Bacterial vaginosis	Light to dark olive green
4.7–6.0	Trichomoniaisis Significant inflammation (i.e., chlamydia)	Bluish

    d. Lubricant from speculum
    e. Intravaginal medications
    f. Lubricating jelly
    g. Tap water
  E. Summary of findings (Table 31.8)

VIII. Candidiasis explained
  A. The *Candida* species
    1. More than 200 different strains of *Candida* species
    2. Fungi share characteristics of both plants and animals but are classified into their own kingdom.
    3. They reproduce sexually by producing spores and asexually by budding.
    4. Their growth is best supported in an environment that is warm, moist, and dark.
    5. They rely on sugar as their major source of energy (glycogen in the female vagina).
    6. Differentiation of terms: Yeast, fungus, mycoses, monilia, *Candida* are used interchangeably.
    7. Candidiasis is not considered a sexually transmitted disease.
  B. Six genera most typically inhabit the vagina (in order of occurrence)
    1. *Candida albicans* (in 65% of cases, this is the cause of vulvovaginal candidiasis)
      a. They are dimorphic. They form both blastospores and mycelia (filaments, hyphae, and pseudohyphae; Figure 31.3).
      b. Sometimes referred to as "spaghetti and meatballs"
    2. *Candida tropicalis* (23%): Dimorphic
    3. *Candida glabrata* (previously called *Candida torulopsis)* (5–10%): Monomorphic. Forms only spores (buds). Must be confirmed with PCR culture if suspected.

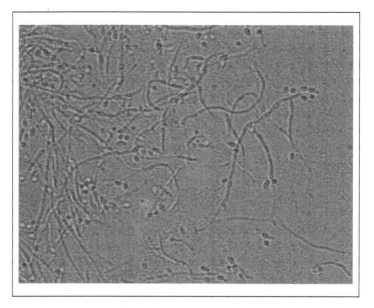

FIGURE 31.3 *Candida albicans.*

    4. *Candida krusei*
    5. *Candida parapsilosis*
    6. *Candida pseudotropicalis*
 C. Relationship to estrogen
    1. There is some evidence that there are estrogen receptors on
    C. albicans and that any condition that increases estrogen may
    increase risk for development of candidiasis, such as
      a. Pregnancy
      b. Estrogen replacement therapy, either systemic or vaginal
      c. Birth control pills (New, lower dose pills do not seem to be
      as much of a problem.)
 D. Relationship to pH
    1. Presence does not usually change the acidity of the vaginal
    secretions
 E. Predisposing factors for the development of candidiasis
    1. Resistance altered by immune status of the body
      a. HIV
      b. Pregnancy, corticosteroids, and stress may lead to depressed
      immunity.
    2. Vaginal allergens cause a chemical vaginitis (Box 31.6).
    3. Increased vaginal glycogen from sugar sources, such as artificial
    sweeteners, wine, fruit juices, and processed sugar
 F. Clinical features of *C. albicans*
    1. Subjective findings
      a. Inflammatory response on the walls of the vagina

> **BOX 31.6** *Substances That May Cause Chemical Vulvovaginitis*
>
> **Substances associated with laundering**
> - Chlorine bleach
> - Laundry detergent
> - Fabric softeners
>
> **Intravaginal preparations**
> - Propylene glycol found in spermicides, lubricants, and vaginal medications
>
> **Feminine hygiene products**
> - Deodorant tampons, liners, and sanitary napkins
> - Douches and vaginal sprays
>
> **Body secretions**
> - Semen
> - Saliva
>
> **Vulvar or vaginal medications**
> - Antifungals
> - Lidocaine
> - Crotamiton
> - Estrogen creams and suppositories
> - Antibiotic preparations
>
> **Clothing**
> - Fabric dyes, especially in colored underwear
> - Nylon (can give off formaldehyde vapors)
> - Fiberglass particles on underwear (residual in washing machine after washing fiberglass)

     b. Produce erythema, edema, intense pruritus, pain, anodyspareunia
       (1) Reactive increase in the production of PMN leukocytes
     c. Clump-like cottage cheese on undergarments
     d. Adherence to cells is necessary for symptomatic disease.
       (1) *C. albicans* adheres more than other species.
       (2) This characteristic may explain why this species is more frequently found.
  2. Objective findings
     a. Invasion of *C. albicans* causes increased shedding, which leads ultimately to the thick curd-like discharge (sample for wet mount is best if taken from that discharge).
       (1) Variable: Present 20% to 50% of the time
       (2) Loosely adherent to the vagina or vestibule

          (3) White or yellow

          (4) May coat entire vagina or stick like patches of a rolled-up piece of tissue paper

          (5) Will scrape off with a spatula

    b. External dysuria (burning when the urine touches the vulva)

    c. Excoriation from scratching of affected tissues

    d. Minimal odor

G. Diagnosis

    1. Use of vaginal microscopy in the diagnosis of candidiasis is about 60% sensitive.

    2. Yeast forms seen more easily with KOH preparation than with saline.

    3. Plastic spatula best to obtain sample because use of a cotton swab may create a fiber artifact, leading to an incorrect diagnosis.

    4. Observations using saline

        a. Presence of varying numbers of leukocytes (PMN)

          (1) Helps determine the extent of inflammation

          (2) Number increases with inflammation

        b. Lactobacilli are present in moderate numbers.

        c. Negative whiff test

        d. Possible concomitant infection

          (1) Rare

          (2) Determine whether pH is increased.

        e. Presence of yeast forms

          (1) *Tinea cruris* may have only hyphae.

        f. Abundance of epithelial cells (increase in exfoliation)

          (1) Many clumps are only sheets of sloughed squamous epithelium.

          (2) Carefully examine edges of these sheets for protruding *Candida* pseudohyphae.

    5. Observations using KOH

        a. Blanches cell wall transparent, making yeast forms more apparent

        b. Note the presence of yeast forms (other yeast forms are described in Table 31.9).

H. pH less than 4.7 unless concomitant BV, trichomoniasis, or VVA is present

I. Fungal cultures. PCR culture is more accurate and quick, within 3 to 5 days.

    1. Usually unnecessary because wet mount is moderately diagnostic

    2. Yeast cultures with speciation are expensive and may cause a delay in treatment.

    3. Indicated if the diagnosis is suspected but no yeast forms are seen on wet mount or if symptoms are recurrent especially over time

TABLE 31.9 Candidal Forms in Relation to Species

YEAST FORM	DESCRIPTION	SPECIES NAME
Pseodohyphae	Long segmented sausages	*Candida albicans*
Hyphae	Long continuous fllaments	*C. tropicalis*
Chlamydiaspores	Clusters of glass beads at terminal ends of the hyphae Uniform in size, associated with hyphae forms	*C. albicans*
Blastospores	Budding ovoid spores of variable size 2–10 microns Round to ovoid; no filaments	*C. glabrata*
	May be budding or grouped in clusters interspersed with filaments Smaller than red blood cells Located at the proximal branches, appearing much like a fern Tiny glass beads	*C. tropicalis*

4. More sensitive than wet mount but may confuse diagnosis
   a. *Candida* may be part of normal vaginal flora, known as commensal colonization.
   b. A positive culture does not indicate the presence of infection, especially if noted on a Pap smear. If patient is asymptomatic, there may be no need for treatment.
   c. The culture may be positive in up to 20% of women not infected with *Candida.*
5. Nickerson or Sabaroud's culture
   a. Standard medium for *Candida* growth
   b. Most sensitive
   c. PCR yeast cultures are available now through various commercial labs and allow quick and accurate diagnosis with speciation of yeast.
J. Gram stain may be positive when wet mount is negative because of excessive cellular debris.
K. Pap smear
   1. Sensitivity is 50%.
   2. Not routinely used as a diagnostic tool
   3. Asymptomatic *Candida* infection may be picked up on a routine smear. No need to treat if symptoms are absent.
   4. A Pap smear should not be performed when *Candida* infection is suspected because presence of an inflammatory process will alter results.

IX. BV explained

A. Description of terms

1. "*–osis*" means in excess of; "*–itis*" means inflammation of.
2. Previously referred to over the years as haemophilus vaginitis, cornybacterium vaginitis, *Gardnerella,* nonspecific vaginitis, anaerobic vaginosis, BV—now, vaginal bacteriosis is being used more frequently.
3. The term is defined as an excess of vaginal bacteria, with little or no inflammation.

B. Some comments

1. It is the most common cause of vaginal complaints, occurring twice as frequently as candidiasis.
2. It is a surface bacteria and does not usually invade vaginal tissues or cause an inflammatory reaction.
3. It is the most symptomatically benign of the common infections.
   a. It may have serious implications, such as premature labor, increased risk of sexually transmitted infections (STIs) including HIV, postsurgical gynecologic infections, cystitis, and pelvic inflammatory disease (PID).
   b. An estimated 50% of women with BV do not have symptoms.
4. The condition can coexist with trichomoniasis.

C. Risk factors

1. Sexual activity, particularly multiple partners (may also be found in women never sexually active), or a new sex partner, including new female partner
2. Often coined as a "sexually associated disease"
   a. Can be cultured from the prepuce of sexual partners
   b. Treating male partners has not increased the cure rate in women, or reduced recurrent infections.
3. Douching, which may alter the vaginal environment and push bacteria into the upper reproductive tract
4. Presence of an intrauterine contraceptive (IUC)
5. Not using condoms

D. Pathogenesis

1. Decrease in lactobacilli, particularly hydrogen-peroxide producing
2. Increase in various anaerobic bacterial pathogens (often by a factor of 100–1,000-fold)
3. Lack of inflammation
   a. *Mobiluncus* and *Bacteroides* produce succinic acid, which may inhibit leukocyte formation, producing infection without inflammation: In mild BV, there is less inhibition of leukocytes; therefore, inflammation may be visible.

E. Clinical features

1. Subjective findings
   a. Increase in vaginal discharge

b. Fishy odor, particularly after intercourse, due to presence of alkaline secretions that release amines
   (1) Semen has a high pH (7–9)
2. Objective findings
  a. Uniform discharge that adheres to the vaginal walls like "spilled milk"
  b. Mild erythema or absence of inflammation of vulvar or vaginal tissues
F. Diagnosis: Requires three of the following four criteria (Amsel's criteria):
  1. pH 4.7 or higher
    a. Highest sensitivity
    b. Lowest specificity because it can be elevated in concomitant infections, semen, medications, douching, and blood
  2. KOH: Positive whiff test—amine volatilized when the pH is increased
  3. Uniform, homogenous vaginal discharge
  4. Presence of "clue cells" in saline preparation (Figure 31.4).
    a. Stippled or granular mature epithelial cells that appear speckled rather than translucent, resembling fried eggs sprinkled with pepper
    b. The nucleus remains distinct, thus aiding identification of the cell.

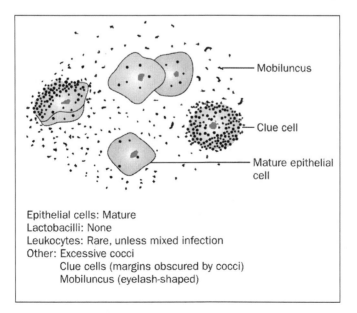

Epithelial cells: Mature
Lactobacilli: None
Leukocytes: Rare, unless mixed infection
Other: Excessive cocci
    Clue cells (margins obscured by cocci)
    Mobiluncus (eyelash-shaped)

FIGURE 31.4 Bacterial vaginosis (BV).

     c. Small, pleomorphic, gram-negative coccobacilli adhering to surface of epithelial cells so that the cell wall becomes indistinct (75% of cell margin obscured)

       (1) May be confused with vacuolated squamous cells, which also contain small, dark spots

       (2) Focus up and down to distinguish between coccobacilli stuck on the surface of the cell with BV, and vacuoles found within the cell itself.

     d. Often comprise between 10% and 50% of epithelial cells. Greater than 20% clue cells suggests BV. Always consider Amsel's criteria.

     e. High sensitivity (91.2%) and specificity (94.3%)

  5. Additional findings

     a. Absence or relative scarcity of lactobacilli

     b. Possible presence of *Mobiluncus* species, such as *Mobiluncus curtisii* or *Mobiluncus mulieris*

       (1) Highly motile, anaerobic, gram negative

       (2) Short-curved, "comma" cells

       (3) Present in 50% to 100% of patients

     c. Few leukocytes (unless a concomitant infection is present, such as trichomoniasis)

       (1) Ratio of PMN cells to epithelial cells is less than or equal to 1.

     d. Floating background bacteria between epithelial cells, which usually outnumber lactobacilli

G. Gram stain

  1. Not usually necessary because wet mount study is often diagnostic

  2. The diagnosis is based on the stippled appearance of epithelial cells due to uniformly spaced coccobacilli, a reduction of *Lactobacillus* morphotypes, and an increase in small gram-negative rods and gram-positive cocci.

H. Cultures

  1. Not helpful

  2. Anaerobes can be recovered from healthy women.

I. Pap smear

  1. Unreliable for diagnosis of BV. Correlate with Amsel's criteria and do not use as sole criteria for diagnosis per the 2010 CDC STI Guidelines.

X. Trichomoniasis explained

  A. Some comments

     1. Causes about 10% of all cases of vaginitis; however, prevalence seems to be decreasing

     2. Almost exclusively sexually transmitted; present in 30% to 40% of sexual partners of infected women

      3. Can cause nongonococcal urethritis

      4. Chronic trichomoniasis can reduce the glycogen content of the cells, causing vaginal lining to become thinner and more prone to ulceration.

      5. Primarily affects the vagina but can affect the cervix, Bartholin's glands, urethra, and bladder, including the Skene's ducts

      6. Many infections are asymptomatic especially in older women; prevalence up to 22% of high-risk teenagers and up to 13% of women older than 45 years of age.

      7. May be asymptomatic for decades

B. Identification of trichomoniasis

      1. Trichomonads are unicellular, anaerobic protozoans.

      2. Actively motile by virtue of four filaments of equal length

         a. One to two times the length of the organism itself

         b. Protrude from the forward end of the trichomonad

      3. Teardrop shape of various sizes

         a. A little larger than PMN leukocytes

         b. Smaller than a mature epithelial cell but larger than its nucleu

C. Replication

      1. Binary division

      2. Transfer from one host to another only in the presence of moisture

D. Effects of pH

      1. If less than 4.7, the organism is rounded. It is difficult to distinguish.

      2. Usually pH is greater than 4.7 (pH less than 4.7 virtually eliminates the possibility of trichomoniasis).

E. Predisposing factors

      1. Hypoacidity of vaginal secretions due to an increase in cervical mucus production (cervical mucorrhea; estrogen effect) or menstruation

      2. Exogenous estrogen, including estrogen replacement therapy, estrogen creams, and oral contraceptives (possibly)

F. Clinical features

      1. Subjective findings

         a. Profuse, often malodorous discharge

            (1) Variable appearance

            (2) Classic appearance: Frothy, yellow to green

         b. Pruritus, vaginal burning

      2. Objective findings

         a. Vulvar edema and erythema

         b. Strawberry cervix (ecchymotic petechiae) occasionally present (30% risk).

G. Diagnosis

      1. Observations using saline

         a. Patience and diligence at the microscope are often necessary.

    b. Trichomonads visible only in saline; lysed in KOH
    c. Time is a critical factor.
        (1) Susceptible to oxygen, cool temperature, and drying. (This may be another reason to examine the saline slide first.)
        (2) If wet mount cannot be performed immediately, place cotton-tipped applicator with vaginal secretions in a test tube with 0.5 inch normal saline.
        (3) The organisms will remain motile for at least a half hour unless they dry out or the saline is old (must change saline every 3 months or else it becomes hypertonic).
    d. May warm slide slightly by passing a match under it to increase motility. Microscope light may warm.
    e. Squamous epithelial cells present
        (1) Immature parabasal and intermediate cells may be present with marked or chronic infection.
    f. Polymorphonuclear leukocytes are increased due to the inflammation (may be dramatic).
    g. Lactobacilli may be present.
    h. *Candida* may be noted concomitantly (uncommon).
  2. Characteristics of trichomonads in saline
    a. Flagella never visible under low power and sometimes visible under high power
    b. Healthy trichomonads undulate, jerk, or twitch or actively move in the direction of the flagellae.
    c. Unhealthy trichomonads assume a rounded shape, are more difficult to identify, are sluggish, and usually are visible only under high power.
    d. Mobility is reduced when cold or if the sample dries.
        (1) Keep the saline warm, and view immediately.
        (2) Motility may be hampered by large numbers of PMN leukocytes.
    e. Trichomonads assume a rounder shape when they are dry or drying.
    f. Trichomonads can provoke a strong WBC response. Carefully examine clumps of WBCs that may surround and attach to a trichomonad.
    g. Figure 31.5 demonstrates characteristics of trichomoniasis.
  3. Observations using KOH preparation (Figure 31.6)
    a. Trichomonads are lysed.
    b. Possible presence of amine odor (50%)
  4. Pap smear
    a. Usually does not reveal trichomonads because they are immotile by the time they are evaluated
    b. Positive predictive value only 40%

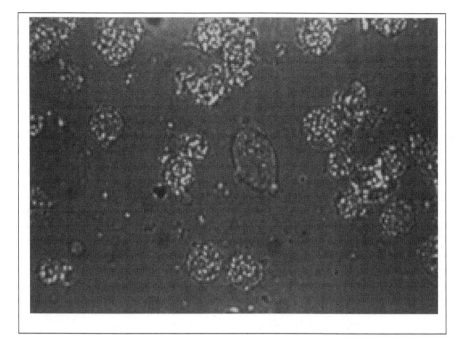

FIGURE 31.5 Characteristics of trichomoniasis.

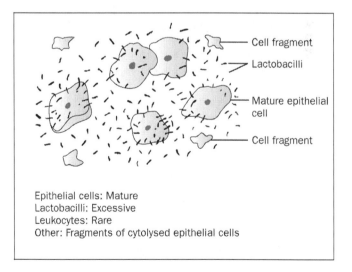

FIGURE 31.6 Cytolysis.

5. Gram stain
   a. Trichomonads can be identified by Gram stain but offers no real advantage over a careful wet mount.
   b. More difficult to distinguish from PMNs by this method

6. Culture: *Trichomonas*
   a. Most sensitive (95%)
   b. Easy to perform
   c. Not readily available
   d. Limit use to those in whom diagnosis is suspected but not seen on wet mount
7. Gonorrhea culture
   a. Perform on all women with trichomoniasis because up to 60% of women with trichomoniasis may also have gonorrhea.
8. Urinalysis: Organism may be clearly visualized due to lack of other cellular debris.

XI. **Cytolytic vaginitis explained; controversial and unproven with scant research**
   A. Some comments
      1. Caused by destruction of vaginal epithelial cells by the acid environment caused by the overgrowth of lactobacilli
      2. Previously termed *Döderlein's cytolysis* after the Döderlein species of lactobacilli
         a. Over 100 different species of lactobacilli have been discovered.
      3. This infection is often confused with candidiasis because symptoms are similar, especially if premenstrual and chronic. However, microscopic findings are much different.
      4. Controversial and unproven; very little research to support this condition
   B. Clinical features
      1. Subjective findings
         a. Pasty discharge
         b. Pruritus, vulvar dysuria
         c. Symptoms worsen during the luteal phase.
         d. Low-grade burning or discomfort; increased with sexual activity
         e. Lack of odor
      2. Objective findings
         a. Vulvar tissues may be erythematous and edematous.
         b. Discharge may be thick or flocculent (clumpy).
   C. Diagnosis
      1. Observations of saline preparation (see Figure 31.6)
         a. Large number of epithelial cells
         b. False clue cells
            (1) Long rods (lactobacilli of varying lengths)
            (2) May be adherent to epithelial cells (intermediate)
            (3) May be confused with the clue cell of BV
         c. Contains cytoplasmic debris from fragments of epithelial cells destroyed by acid environment

    d. Stippled nuclei
    e. Negative for *Candida,* trichomonads, and clue cells
    f. Rare leukocytes
  2. Observations of KOH preparation
    a. Bacteria lysed
    b. Negative odor
  3. pH is low (3.5–4.0)
  4. Culture recommended to rule out *Candida* infection
  5. Pap smear
    a. Shows cytolysis on routine smears
    b. Should not be used as a diagnostic tool because wet mount is reliable and readily available
 D. Treatment consists of increasing the pH of the vagina by means of sodium bicarbonate douches or baths; self-correcting with menses.
  1. Recommend 30 to 60 g per 1 L of warm water two to three times per week, then once weekly as needed.

XII. **Lactobacillosis explained; controversial and unproven with scant research.**
 A. Some comments
  1. Condition characterized by an increase in vaginal discharge and discomfort
  2. May occur after antimycotic treatment after treatment of a *Candida* infection
  3. The incidence is unknown because of scant research; condition is poorly understood.
  4. Bacteria elongates, particularly anaerobic lactobacilli
 B. Clinical features
  1. Features resemble those of candidiasis
    a. Thick, white, creamy, or curdy discharge
    b. Associated with vaginal itching, burning, and irritation
  2. Symptoms tend to occur 7 to 10 days before menses (second half of menstrual cycle), reaching a peak shortly before menstruation, after which it disappears after menses, only to recur before the next menses.
 C. Diagnosis
  1. Saline
    a. Many long (40–75 μm) serpiginous rod-like lactobacilli, previously termed *Leptothrix*. Normal rods are between 5 and 15 μm.
    b. May be confused with filaments of candidiasis (thinner strands)
    c. Mature epithelial cells are present with few PMN cells.
  2. Differs from cytolytic vaginitis in that rods are longer and less abundant
 D. Treatment with amoxicillin and clavulanate is clinically successful in 100% of patients. Baking soda douche is not as effective as it is with cytolysis.

XIII. Desquamative inflammatory vaginitis (DIV) explained
A. Some comments
1. Associated with overstimulation of vaginal mucosa from unknown causes
a. May be associated with lichen planus of the mouth and genitals
b. Overabundance of squamous cells, which act as a substitute for bacteria
c. Commonly misdiagnosed as *Trichomonas* infection; must rule out cervical cancer
2. Incidence may be underestimated
B. Clinical features: May resemble trichomoniasis or atrophic vaginitis with bacterial infection
1. Subjective findings
a. Thick, profuse discharge accompanied by dyspareunia and pruritus
b. No odor
2. Objective findings include ecchymotic and petechial lesions on the vulva, vagina, and cervix.
C. Diagnosis
1. Wet mount
a. Many PMN cells
b. Many basal and parabasal cells (hallmark of the disease)
c. Few mature epithelial cells
d. Naked nuclei
e. Negative clue cells, yeast forms, or trichomoniasis
f. Absent lactobacilli with few microorganisms
g. Red blood cells may be present.
2. KOH
a. Negative whiff test
3. pH: More than 4.5
4. Culture and Gram stain
a. Gram-positive cocci (mainly Group B streptococci)
D. Treatment options include intravaginal clindamycin or intravaginal steroid creams. Relapses are more common with clindamycin. Local estrogen may also be effective. Use of intravaginal steroid cream is typically preferred starting with hydrocortisone 25-mg suppositories at bedtime for 2 to 4 weeks. Dose may be increased. Consultation with an expert is recommended.

XIV. Atrophic vaginitis explained (see Chapter 12, "Atrophic Vaginitis, Vulvovaginal Atrophy")
A. Some comments
1. Inflammation of the vaginal epithelium occurs due wholly and in part to a lack of estrogen.

2. Found in breastfeeding women and those who underwent natural or surgical menopause, or in patients taking antiestrogen medications
3. Epithelium is thin and lacks glycogen because of a decrease in endogenous estrogen.

B. Clinical features
1. Subjective findings
   a. Vaginal dryness
   b. Dyspareunia
   c. Vulvar and vaginal irritation and burning
   d. Possible spotting
   e. Vulvodynia (see Chapter 14, "Assessment of Vulvar Pain and Vulvodynia")
2. Objective findings
   a. Thin and smooth vaginal walls; lack of rugae
   b. Inflammation or exudate may be present.
   c. Smooth, shiny vulva with adherence of labia
   d. Urethral caruncle or prolapse
   e. Microscopy finding (Figure 31.7)

C. Assessment of the maturation index in the diagnosis of atrophic vaginitis (see Chapter 32, "Maturation Index")

XV. Vaginal cultures
A. Procedure: An adjunct to the wet mount; is needed only if the wet mount is inconclusive. Often performed too frequently.
1. Wipe cervix free of discharge (particularly if copious, slippery estrogenic mucus may make collection of columnar cells difficult).
2. Observe any special instructions or precautions from the laboratory.

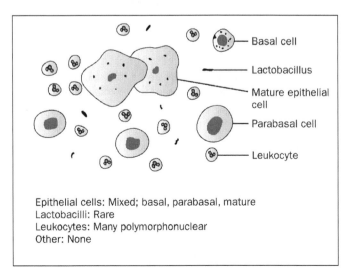

Epithelial cells: Mixed; basal, parabasal, mature
Lactobacilli: Rare
Leukocytes: Many polymorphonuclear
Other: None

FIGURE 31.7 Atrophic vaginitis, vulvovaginal atrophy (VVA), and genital atrophy (GA).

3. STI cultures may be taken from cervical, vaginal, cervicovaginal, or urine samples. Vaginal samples are preferred and provide the highest accuracy.
   a. Withdraw sample and place in specified tube or container.
   b. Label with name and presumptive diagnosis.
4. Vaginal culture: Take sample from vaginal pool; label

XVI. Gram stain of vaginal secretions
  A. The procedure
   1. Briefly heat-fix the slide that contains the smear of vaginal secretions.
   2. Flood the slide with gentian violet stain solutions for 10 seconds.
   3. Wash the slide in water.
   4. Flood it with Gram's iodine solution for 10 seconds.
   5. Rinse it again with water.
   6. Decolorize it with acetone and alcohol solutions for 10 seconds.
   7. Flood it with safranin stain for 10 seconds.
   8. Wash it in water a third time.
   9. Cover with a glass coverslip, and view it under a microscope.
   10. Add a drop of saline on top of the coverslip to use the oil immersion lens (without having to add oil).
  B. Stain of various organisms
   1. Gonorrhea: Intracellular gram-negative diplococci
   2. BV: Small pleomorphic gram-negative coccobacilli
   3. Trichomoniasis
      a. Pale staining
      b. Pear-shaped parasites

Bibliography

Agnew, K. J., & Hillier, S. L. (1995). The effect of treatment regimens for vaginitis and cervicitis on vaginal colonization by lactobacilli. *Sexually Transmitted Diseases, 22*(5), 269–273.

Allsworth, J. E., & Peipert, J. F. (2007). Prevalence of bacterial vaginosis: 2001–2004 National Health and Nutrition Examination Survey data. *Obstetrics and Gynecology, 109*(1),114–120.

Forna, F., & Gülmezoglu, A. M. (2003). Interventions for treating trichomoniasis in women. *Cochrane Database of Systematic Reviews, 2,* CD000218.

Hainer, B. L., & Gibson, M. V. (2011). Vaginitis: Diagnosis and treatment. *American Family Physician, 83*(7), 807–815.

Hensel, K. J., Randis, T. M., Gelber, S. E., & Ratner, A. J. (2011). Pregnancy-specific association of vitamin D deficiency and bacterial vaginosis. *American Journal of Obstetrics and Gynecology, 204*(1), 41.

Horowitz, B. J. (2001). *Vaginitis and vaginosis: Recurrent and relapsing vaginitis.* New York, NY: Wiley-Liss.

Horowitz, B. J., Mardh, P. E., & Nagy, E. (1994). Vaginal lactobacillosis. *American Journal of Obstetrics and Gynecology, 170,* 857–861.

Lamont, R. F., et al. (2012). Rescreening for abnormal vaginal flora in pregnancy and re-treating with clindamycin vaginal cream significantly increases cure and improvement rates. *International Journal of STD & AIDS, 23*(8), 565–569.

Lowe, N. K., Neal, J. L., & Ryan-Wenger, N. A. (2009). Accuracy of the clinical diagnosis of vaginitis compared with a DNA probe laboratory standard. *Obstetrics & Gynecology, 113,* 89.

Mylonas, I., & Bergauer, F. (2011). Diagnosis of vaginal discharge by wet mount microscopy: A simple and underrated method. *Obstetrics and Gynecologic Survey, 66*(6), 359–368. doi: 10.1097/OGX.0b013e31822bdf31

Oduyebo, O. O., Anorlu, R. I., & Ogunsola, F. T. (2009). The effects of antimicrobial therapy on bacterial vaginosis in non-pregnant women. *Cochrane Database of Systematic Reviews, 3,* CD006055.

Pappas, P. G., Kauffman, C. A., Andes, D., Benjamin, D. K. Jr, Calandra, T. F., Edwards, J. E. Jr, … Infectious Diseases Society of America. (2009). Clinical practice guidelines for the management of candidiasis: 2009 update by the Infectious Diseases Society of America. *Clinical Infectious Diseases, 48*(5), 503–535.

Raphaelidis, L., & Secor, R. M. (2006). Bacterial vaginosis update. *Women's Health Care, 5*(3), 21–29.

Secor, R. M. (1994). Bacterial vaginosis: A common infection with serious sequelae. *Advances for Nurse Practitioner, 2*(4), 11–16.

Secor, R. M. (1997). Vaginal microscopy: Refining your technique. *Clinical Excellence for Nurse Practitioners, 1,* 29–34.

Secor, M., & Coughlin, G. (2013). Bacterial vaginosis: Advances in the diagnosis and treatment of acute and recurrent infections. *Advanced Healthcare Network for NPs & PAs, 4(8),* 23-26.

Sibley, L. J., & Sibley, L. J. (1991). Cytolytic vaginosis. *American Journal of Obstetrics and Gynecology, 165,* 1245–1249.

Maturation Index

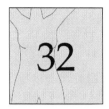

32

Helen A. Carcio

I. **Effects of estrogen on epithelial cells**
   A. The presence of estrogen promotes the maturation of the epithelial cells lining the vaginal mucosa.
   B. Cells begin their journey at the level of the basement membrane.
   C. They evolve to mature forms that build on top of each other increasing the thickness of the vaginal walls.
   D. Types of cells that are in the epithelium
      1. Basal cells
         a. Least mature, less differentiated
         b. Represent a single layer of cells from which all others grow and mature
         c. Rarely visible unless ulceration exists down to the basement membrane
      2. Parabasal cells
         a. Adjacent to the basal cells
         b. Represent the next ring on the ladder
         c. Nucleus fills a large portion of cells
         d. Round
         e. Often become the top layer in the thin, atrophic vagina
      3. Intermediate cells
         a. Nucleus becomes smaller and the amount of cytoplasm increases
         b. Become flatter and more cuboidal
      4. Superficial cells
         a. Outer layer of cells that line the well-estrogenized vagina
         b. Represent a mature, well-differentiated epithelium
         c. Composed of larger, flat, squared-off cells with even smaller nuclei and increasing amounts of cytoplasm
         d. Normally shed in the latter half of the menstrual cycle and comprise normal vaginal discharge

    e. Represent the outer layer of cells most commonly visible on cytolytic examination

    f. Maturation normally occurs in 7 to 10 days.

II. **The maturation index documents the differentiation of the immature squamous cells toward their most evolved forms, from parabasal to intermediate cells, to the mature superficial cells, each representing a cellular layer (Figure 32.1).**

  A. Laboratory examination of vaginal cells was routinely evaluated by a pathologist for many years. Technique can be easily modified to be done in every practice setting by the examiner, providing immediate results.

  B. The microscopic examination

    1. Obtain the vaginal smear from the lateral fornix and upper third of the vaginal wall because it is considered to be most reflective of the hormonal state of the cells. The posterior fornix is not a good site since the cervical cells tend to pool there.

      a. Use a wooden spatula to gently scrape the walls of the vagina or collect the cells as the speculum is withdrawn. Secretions will pool in the tip.

      b. Save these pooled secretions in case more cells are needed to review.

      c. A vaginal pH can also be tested for this sample.

      d. Dip a saline-moistened cotton-tipped applicator into the sample.

      e. Apply a small dot to the slide.

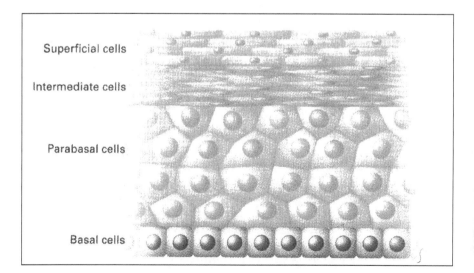

Superficial cells

Intermediate cells

Parabasal cells

Basal cells

FIGURE 32.1 Layers of the vaginal epithelium.

   f. Add enough saline to dilute sample and create a turbid suspension.
   g. It is important to dilute the sample in order to separate the epithelial cells from each other for better viewing.
   h. Place coverslip over sample and blot with paper towel to stabilize mixture and protect the microscope from contamination.
   i. View six to eight fields under 40x magnification.
   j. Count the number of each type of cells viewed.
      (1) Vaginal epithelial cells are easy to identify and characteristically have a slightly grainy cytoplasm.
      (2) The cells walls are distinct.
2.
   a. The index represents the relative number of each kind of cell per hundred cells counted (see Box 32.1 for a comparison of the type of cell in each cell layer). The index measures the estrogen effects of a representative sample of epithelial cells lining the vagina and documents the ratio of the various cells types to each other.
   b. Expressed in a ratio of parabasal to intermediate to superficial cells and read from "left to right"
      (1) 0:0:100—superficial cells—well estrogenized because there are all superficial cells present

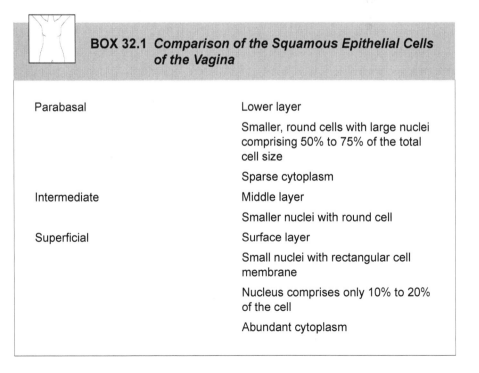

BOX 32.1 *Comparison of the Squamous Epithelial Cells of the Vagina*

Parabasal	Lower layer
	Smaller, round cells with large nuclei comprising 50% to 75% of the total cell size
	Sparse cytoplasm
Intermediate	Middle layer
	Smaller nuclei with round cell
Superficial	Surface layer
	Small nuclei with rectangular cell membrane
	Nucleus comprises only 10% to 20% of the cell
	Abundant cytoplasm

(2) 0:100:0—intermediate cell atrophy—minimal atrophic vaginitis

(3) 100:0:0—parabasal cell atrophy—marked atrophic vaginitis because there are no mature epithelial cells, only parabasal cells (Note: The presence of any parabasal cells on a wet mount may be considered documentation of atrophic vaginitis.)

Bibliography

Bachmann, G. A., & Nevadunsky, N. S. (2000). Diagnosis and treatment of atrophic vaginitis. *American Family Physician, 61,* 3090–3096.

Carcio, H . A. (1999). The maturation index. In *Advanced health assessment of women* (Vol. 12, pp. 226–228). Baltimore, MD: Lippincott.

Carcio, H. A. (2009). Urogenital atrophy: A new approach to vaginitis diagnosis. *Advance for Nurse Practitioners, 10*(10), 40–47.

MacBride, M. B., Rhodes, D. J., & Shuster, L. T. (2010). Vulvovaginal atrophy. *Mayo Clinic Proceedings, 85,* 87–94.

Management of symptomatic vulvovaginal atrophy: 2013 position statement of the North American Menopause Society. *Menopause, 20,* 888–902.

Sonohysteroscopy (Fluid Contrast Ultrasound)

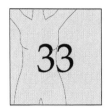

33

Helen A. Carcio

I. **Sonohysteroscopy explained**
   A. Sonohysteroscopy is the infusion of sterile saline though the cervix and into the uterus, after which the area is imaged by transvaginal ultrasound examination.
      1. The saline distends the normally collapsed uterus, allowing for a more accurate view of the inner surfaces.
         a. Reveals the presence of any abnormalities lining the uterus or in the cavity itself
         b. Is an adaptation of standard pelvic ultrasonography
      2. Provides a three-dimensional view of the uterine cavity and ovaries
      3. Has the potential to replace the more invasive diagnostic methods, such as hysteroscopy and endometrial biopsy surgery
      4. Is usually less costly and easier to perform than hysteroscopy, and is well tolerated by the patient
      5. Findings are immediately viewed on a monitor, often making instant diagnosis possible.
      6. Can be done in an office setting without the use of anesthesia
      7. Uses sound waves that are reflected from the tissue back to a receiver that records the different tissue densities
   B. Indications
      1. To evaluate uterine bleeding in postmenopausal women
      2. To investigate dysfunctional uterine bleeding in reproductive-age women if an area is unable to be visualized clearly with sonography
      3. To monitor endometrial thickness in a patient undergoing tamoxifen therapy
      4. To assess endometrial carcinoma

5. To investigate recurrent pregnancy loss in which uterine anomalies contribute to habitual abortion
6. To evaluate tubal infertility
   a. Infusion contains albumin or lactose particles
   b. Can actually view the proximal portion of the tube
7. Preoperative assessment of leiomyomata
   a. Determines the exact size of uterine fibroids
   b. Provides an excellent delineation of fibroid contour
8. Sonographic indications
   a. Thickened or poorly defined endometrium in patients with abnormal uterine bleeding
C. Uterine abnormalities detectable by saline infusion sonography
   1. Endometrial cancer
   2. Endometrial hyperplasia
   3. Endometrial polyps
      a. Sensitivity: 86%
      b. Specificity: 81%
   4. Dyssynchronous endometrium
   5. Uterine fibroids: Intraluminal, submucosal
      a. Sensitivity: 87%
      b. Specificity: 92%
   6. Tamoxifen-induced changes
   7. Intrauterine synechiae
   8. Intrauterine fluid accumulation due to cervical stenosis
D. Potential diagnostic and therapeutic applications
   1. Directing endometrial biopsy
   2. Identifying asymptomatic disease during routine examinations
   3. Determining depth of invasions and sites of attachment of endometrial carcinomas
   4. Retrieving "lost" intrauterine devices (IUDs)
E. Comparison with other diagnostic methods
   1. Hysterosalpingography
      a. Necessitates use of radiation and iodinated contrast material
      b. Provides only indirect information about the uterine cavity
      c. Is more expensive
   2. Hysteroscopy
      a. Provides an accurate topographic map of the cavity itself
      b. Cannot determine the extent of submucosal myomas or the thickness of endometrial layers
      c. Necessitates distention of the uterine cavity with liquid medium or gas
      d. May necessitate anesthesia
   3. Magnetic resonance imaging (MRI)
      a. Provides excellent images of the uterus
      b. Lesions within the uterus can be obscured.
      c. Expensive

BOX 33.1 *Optimal Timing of Sonohysterography*

- Midfollicular phase of a spontaneous menstrual cycle
- At least 4 days after a progestin-induced menstrual flow
- After the progestin phase in women taking cyclic hormone replacement therapy
- Anytime for women using combined continuous regimens

II. **The procedure**
   A. Patient preparation
      1. Antibiotic prophylaxis in women with a history of mitral valve prolapse or regurgitation or joint replacement or other orthopedic hardware. Take 1 hour before saline-infusion sonography.
      2. The woman should take a nonsteroidal anti-inflammatory agent 1 hour before the procedure to alleviate any discomfort.
      3. The woman should void immediately before the procedure.
      4. Determine that the woman is free of active pelvic inflammatory disease or vaginitis.
         a. Perform wet mount before scheduled procedure.
         b. Reschedule procedure if purulent discharge or cervical motion or adnexal tenderness is present.
   B. Timing: It is essential to avoid encountering blood clots that can be interpreted as diseased (Box 33.1).
   C. Equipment
      1. Open-sided speculum: Advantages
         a. User friendly
         b. Does not dislocate the intrauterine catheter when it is removed
   D. Position
      1. Place the patient in the dorsal lithotomy position.
      2. If uterine retroversion is present, place the patient in the left lateral recumbent position.
   E. The technique
      1. Must flush catheter to remove air bubbles because they can produce misleading images
      2. Visualize the cervix through a vaginal speculum.
      3. Cleanse the cervical os with betadine solution.
      4. Insertion may be difficult because of adhesions or stenosis (common in postmenopausal women).
         a. Place tenaculum on cervix.
         b. Instruct woman to cough or perform the Valsalva maneuver while the catheter is placed on the anterior lip.
         c. Distraction technique seems to minimize the patient's pain

        d. For marked stenosis, the clinician can use a dilator through the external and internal catheter that has been placed in freezer (becomes stiffer).

    5. Marked retroversion

        a. Grasp the posterior lip of the cervix to straighten the uterine axis and to facilitate catheter placement.

    6. Withdraw speculum, and replace with the ultrasound probe.

        a. Anteverted uterus: Anterior to the catheter

        b. Retroverted uterus: Posterior to the catheter

F. Instillation

    1. Watch monitor closely during instillation because sonohysterography is a dynamic procedure that momentarily distends the uterus and thereby reveals any endometrial disease.

    2. Slowly inject 10 to 20 mL saline. The slow rate helps minimize discomfort.

        a. The saline causes the normally collapsed uterus to distend.

        b. It allows polyps and fibroids to be seen with greatly enhanced clarity.

        c. Optimal uterine distention is very important.

        d. Infusion rate depends on three factors

            (1) The size of the uterus

            (2) Amount of backflow into the vagina

            (3) Patient discomfort

    3. Place absorbent towels under the patient's buttocks.

G. The scan

    1. Move slowly from cornu to cornu in the long axis to measure the endometrial echo.

    2. Rotate the probe 90 degrees, and scan from the endocervix to the fundus.

    3. Note

        a. Echotexture and echogenicity of the endometrium

        b. Symmetry of the myometrium

    4. Visualize the adnexa in the semicoronal place, using one hand to gently palpate and push the adnexa toward the probe.

    5. If fallopian tubes are to be visualized, use Albunex (CSL Limited), a new ultrasound imaging agent that can enhance image clarity in fallopian tube studies when added to the saline.

    6. View the cervix and cul-de-sac as the probe is removed.

    7. Document the size, location, and characteristics of any masses.

    8. The study usually requires less than 10 minutes.

III. Conclusion

A. The advanced practice clinician is in an advantageous position to learn this new technique and offer it to patients.

B. Although the advanced practice clinician can certainly learn the technique of inserting the catheter and instilling the solution, a physician certified in ultrasound interpretation is required for diagnosis.

Bibliography

Ashley, D. (1997). Sonohysterography in the office: Instruments and techniques. *Contemporary OB/GYN, 4*, 95–99.

Bradley, L. D., & Andrews, B. J. (1998). Saline infusion sonography for endometrial evaluation. *Female Patient, 123*(1), 12–25.

Breitkopf, D., Goldstein, S. R., & Seeds, J .W. (for the ACOG Committee on Gynecologic Practice). (2003). ACOG technology assessment in obstetrics and gynecology. Saline infusion sonohysterography. *Obstetrics & Gynecology, 102*, 659–662.

de Kroon, C. D., de Bock, G. H., Dieben, S. W., & Jansen, F. W. (2003). Saline contrast hysterosonography in abnormal uterine bleeding: A systematic review and meta-analysis. *British Journal of Obstetrics and Gynecology, 110*, 938–947.

Dijkhuizen, F. P., Mol, B. W., Bongers, M. Y., Brolmann, H. A., & Heintz, A, P. (2003). Cost-effectiveness of transvaginal sonography and saline infused sonography in the evaluation of menorrhagia. *International Journal of Gynecolology & Obstetrics, 83*, 45–52.

Mihm, L. M., Quick, V. A., Brumfield, J. A., Connors, A. F., Jr., & Finnerty, J. J. (2002). The accuracy of endometrial biopsy and saline sonohysterography in the determination of the cause of abnormal uterine bleeding. *American Journal of Obstetrics and Gynecology, 186*, 858–860.

Parsons, A. K., & Lense, J. J. (2003). Sonohysterography for endometrial abnormalities: Preliminary results. *Clinical Ultrasound, 21*, 87–95.

Pfenninger, J., & Fowlers G. C. (2011). *Sonohysteroscopy: Procedures for primary care;* Tuggy Garcia *Atlas of Essential Procedures* (3rd ed., pp. 977–985). Philadelphia, PA: Saunders.

Rasmussen, F., Lindequiest, S., Larsen, C., & Justesen, P. (2001). Therapeutic effects of hysterosalpingograph: Oil versus water soluble contrast media—A randomized prospective study. *Radiology, 179*, 75–81.

Genetic Testing for Hereditary Breast and Ovarian Cancer

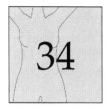

34

Constance A. Roche

I. **Introduction and overview: Cancers of the breast and ovary impose a significant burden on women's health.**
   A. Most cancers are sporadic (noninherited, occurring by chance, and due to cellular changes) and there is limited ability to predict who will be affected.
   B. Family history of cancer is common, but specific features in the family pedigree can suggest a hereditary pattern and increased cancer risk for family members.
   C. Approximately 5% to 10% of breast and ovarian cancers are hereditary, due to a single gene germline mutation.
      1. *BRCA1* and *2* gene mutations are responsible for hereditary breast and ovarian cancer syndrome, accounting for a large percentage of heritable cancers of the breast and ovary. A mutation in one of these genes has a profound impact on cancer risk.
      2. Mutations in other highly penetrant genes are also associated with less common cancer syndromes that predispose carriers to breast and/or ovarian cancers. These include *PTEN* (Cowden Syndrome), *TP53* (Li-Fraumeni Syndrome), *STK11* (Peutz-Jeghers Syndrome), *CDH1* (Hereditary Diffuse Gastric Syndrome), and *MLH1, MSH2, MSH6*, or *PMS2* (Lynch Syndrome).
      3. Lower penetrant genes also contribute to cancer risk
         a. Testing of additional genes is now possible and may be warranted based on personal and family history
   D. Identification and screening of high-risk women are essential skills for health care practitioners.

495

1. Cancer morbidity and mortality in high-risk women can be reduced with implementation of tailored screening, prevention, and treatment.

II. **Facts about breast and ovarian cancer**
   A. Breast cancer is the most frequently diagnosed cancer in women in the United States.
      1. According to the American Cancer Society, approximately 232,340 new cases were diagnosed in 2013.
      2. The average woman has a 12.5% risk of developing breast cancer in her lifetime (1 in 8).
   B. Breast cancer is the second most common cause of cancer death in women.
      1. An estimated 39,620 women died of the disease in 2013.
   C. Ovarian cancer is the nineth most common cancer in American women.
      1. An estimated 22,240 cases were diagnosed in 2013.
      2. The average woman has a 1.5% (1 in 72) lifetime risk of developing the disease.
   D. Ovarian cancer ranks fifth in cancer deaths among women.
      1. An estimated 14,240 women died of the disease in 2013.

III. **Facts about *BRCA1* and 2**
   A. *BRCA1* cloned in 1994; *BRCA2* cloned in 1995
   B. Two copies of these genes in every human cell (one copy inherited from each parent)
   C. Autosomal dominant pattern of inheritance
      1. Child of mutation carrier has 50% chance of inheriting the mutation
   D. Classified as tumor suppressor genes
      1. Gene products involved in DNA repair
   E. Hundreds of mutations have been found in each of these genes
   F. Prevalence of 1/300 to 1/800 in the general population
      1. Some populations at higher risk due to founder effects: Ashkenazi Jewish (1/40), Dutch, Icelandic, and others
   G. Commercial testing became available in 1996.
   H. Lifetime cancer risk estimates high for *BRCA* mutation cancers (Table 34.1)
      1. One 2007 meta-analysis found risk to age 70
         a. *BRCA1*
            Breast: 57%
            Ovary: 40%

TABLE 34.1 Lifetime Cancer Risk for *BRCA* Mutation Carriers

Breast cancer risk: 41%–90%
Ovarian cancer risk: 8%–62%

   b. *BRCA2*
   Breast: 49%
   Ovary: 18%
I. Features associated with *BRCA* mutations
   1. Many family members affected with breast and/or ovarian cancer
   2. Young age at diagnosis (particularly breast cancer)
   3. Bilateral breast cancer
   4. Multiple primary cancers in single individual
   5. Male breast cancer
   6. Multiple generations affected
J. *BRCA1* and 2 grouped and tested together, but some differences in phenotype
   1. *BRCA1* mutation carriers
      a. Younger onset breast cancers
      b. Triple negative (negative for estrogen and progesterone receptors and not overexpressing HER2/neu) breast cancer more common
   2. *BRCA2* mutation carriers
      a. Breast cancer age at onset similar to that of sporadic cancers
      b. Histology similar to sporadic; more likely estrogen and progesterone receptor positive
      c. Higher rate of male breast cancer, melanoma, and pancreatic cancer

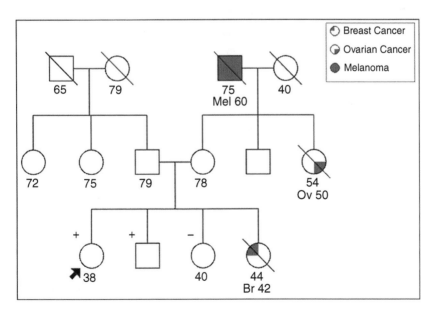

FIGURE 34.1 An example of a pedigree for patients with a familial risk for hereditary breast and ovarian cancer.

IV. Identification of women who may be candidates for testing
   A. Obtain personal and family history (minimum three-generation pedigree is recommended; see Figure 34.1 for an example of pedigree with history of ovarian and breast cancer) to include
      1. Cancers in the family
         a. Both maternal and paternal lineage
      2. Note whether bilateral disease
      3. Age at diagnosis
      4. Relevant surgical history (e.g., oophorectomy and reason for surgery)
   B. Candidates for testing
      1. Individual whose relative has a known *BRCA* mutation
      2. Always preferable to first test family member affected with cancer
         a. Counsel or refer women with
            (1) Breast cancer diagnosed at age 45 or younger
            (2) Bilateral breast cancer
            (3) Breast cancer in Ashkenazi Jewish woman
            (4) Triple negative breast cancer diagnosed before age 60
            (5) Breast cancer and relatives with breast or ovarian cancer
            (6) Any woman with ovarian cancer
            (7) Male with breast cancer
            (8) See National Comprehensive Cancer Network guidelines, updated annually.
      3. When no affected relative able to have testing
         a. Counsel or refer unaffected woman
            (1) With close relatives meeting above criteria
            (2) With elevated risk as calculated by risk models such as BRCAPRO, Tyrer-Cuzick, Claus
            (3) The National Cancer Institute Breast Cancer Risk Assessment Tool (based on the Gail model) is not useful for assessing hereditary risk.
      4. Consider factors impacting the pedigree.
         a. Limited family structure
            (1) Young age at death due to noncancerous causes
            (2) Few females in the family
            (3) Paternal lineage with few females
         b. Unknown or inaccurate history
      5. Testing is not recommended for individuals younger than age 18.
      6. Provide or refer for counseling any woman whose quality of life is affected by her anxiety about cancer risk, regardless of objective assessment.

V. Pretest education and counseling
   A. Should be provided by health care professional with expertise and experience in cancer genetics
      1. Educate and counsel about hereditary cancer and the rationale, logistics, risks, and benefits of testing.

2. Identify most informative family member to have testing.
   a. Once a familial mutation is identified, other family members can be tested for that family-specific mutation and obtain a definitive result.
3. Discuss insurance implications.
   a. GINA (Genetic Nondiscrimination Act) and state laws prohibit health insurance discrimination.
   b. Life, long-term, and disability insurers may use genetic information to change or deny coverage.
4. Determine which genetic test(s) appropriate to consider.
5. Counsel about medical management.
   a. Discuss screening and prevention measures.
6. Assist in formulating plans for management if positive.
7. Discuss importance of sharing with family members and assist as needed.
8. Obtain informed consent.
9. Disclose and interpret results.
10. Provide emotional support and guidance.

VI. **Interpretation of *BRCA* test results**
   A. Deleterious mutation
      1. Breast cancer risk: 41%–90%
      2. Ovarian cancer risk: 8%–62%
      3. No prediction if or when cancer might occur
         a. Penetrance may be mutation specific and/or affected by additional genetic or environmental factors.
      4. Increased risk for melanoma and pancreatic cancer (also prostate)
      5. Family members at risk; first-degree relatives have 50% risk of carrying the mutation.
   B. No mutation
      1. True negative: If known mutation in family
      2. Uninformative negative: If no known mutation in family
   C. Variant of uncertain significance (VUS)
      1. Occurs in 3% to 5% overall
      2. Majority will be reclassified, most as benign polymorphisms/ not disease causing

VII. **Management options for the unaffected woman who tests *BRCA* positive**
   A. Management of cancer risk (Table 34.2)
      1. Breast

TABLE 34.2 Recommended Lifestyle Factors to Reduce Breast Cancer Risk

Achieve and maintain normal weight
Exercise: 150 minutes of moderate intensity exercise per week
Limit alcohol to no more than one drink per day

    a. Breast awareness/breast self-exam beginning at age 18

    b. Clinical breast examination, every 6 to 12 months, beginning at age 25

    c. Mammogram and MRI screening annually, beginning at age 25, or individualized based on earliest age of breast cancer diagnosis in the family

    d. Discuss risk-reducing mastectomy.

      (1) Reduces risk by 90%

      (2) Counsel regarding effectiveness, limitations, reconstruction options and psychological impact.

    e. Consider chemoprevention with tamoxifen or raloxifene.

      (1) Both demonstrated to reduce risk in high-risk women

      (2) Limited data on effect in *BRCA* mutation carriers

  2. Ovary

    a. Recommend risk-reducing salpingo-oophorectomy between age 35 and 40, and after childbearing is complete. May individualize based on earliest age of ovarian cancer onset in family.

      (1) It is believed that many ovarian cancers develop in the fallopian tube.

      (2) No reliable screening for early detection

        (3) Reduces risk of *BRCA*-associated gynecologic cancer by 80% to 85%; there is residual risk of primary peritoneal cancer.

        (4) Reduces risk for breast cancer by 50% when premenopausal at time of surgery

        (5) Counsel regarding health risks of surgically induced early menopause: Vasomotor and vaginal symptoms, osteoporosis, and increased risk for cardiovascular disease.

        (6) Short-term use of hormone replacement therapy (HRT) does not appear to mitigate the reduction in breast cancer risk.

        (7) Due to high rate of occult ovary or fallopian tube cancer, attention to sampling and pathologic review are important

    b. If risk-reducing salpingo-oophorectomy not elected, or pending surgery, consider transvaginal ultrasound and CA-125 every 6 months starting at age 30, or 5 to 10 years younger than earliest age at ovarian cancer diagnosis in the family.

      (1) Counsel that this has not been demonstrated to be an effective screening strategy nor a substitute for surgery.

    c. Oral contraceptives

      (1) Reduce ovarian cancer risk by 50% in *BRCA* mutation carriers as well as in general population

      (2) May increase breast cancer risk after 5 years of use

      (3) Consider pending surgery; weigh pros and cons

3. If childbearing age, consider referral to discuss prenatal diagnosis and/or preimplantation genetic testing
4. Provide or refer for psychological counseling as needed for assistance with coping strategies
5. Provide or refer for community resources such as FORCE (www.facingourrisk.org)

VIII. **Management options for the woman with breast or ovarian cancer who tests *BRCA* positive**
A. Tested at time of breast cancer diagnosis
 1. Higher risk of ipsilateral breast tumor recurrence and contralateral breast cancer
  a. Consider bilateral mastectomy or recommend MRI screening
 2. Tailored treatment options or clinical protocol may be available.
 3. Counsel regarding risk-reducing salpingo-oophorectomy posttreatment.
  a. Postsurgery HRT not recommended
  b. Oral contraceptives not recommended
 4. Address implications for family members.
B. Tested at time of ovarian cancer diagnosis
 1. Tailored treatment options or clinical protocol may be available.
 2. Counsel regarding prophylactic mastectomy or screening with MRI.
 3. Address implications for family members.
C. Tested following treatment for breast and/or ovarian cancer
 1. Consider surveillance and screening options in context of cancer history, prognosis, age, and life expectancy.
 2. Address implications for family members.
D. Provide or refer for counseling as needed.

IX. **Implications of a negative test or VUS**
A. True negative: Negative result when known mutation in family
 1. Negative test indicates the woman is at population risk for cancer.
 2. Counsel regarding continued risk of sporadic cancer.
 3. Psychological adjustment to the change in risk status
 4. Possible "survivor guilt"
 5. Refer for counseling as needed.
B. Uninformative negative: Negative results when no family member is known to have a mutation
 1. Risk assessment and management based on personal and family history
C. VUS
 1. Risk assessment and management based on personal and family history

2. May warrant additional evaluation by an individual trained in cancer genetics

X. **Consider syndromes other than *BRCA*, hereditary breast and ovarian cancer**
   A. Family history should also be assessed for less common syndromes associated with breast and ovarian cancer.
      1. Cowden syndrome
         a. Result of mutation in the *PTEN* gene
         b. Features include follicular thyroid cancer, breast cancer, endometrial cancer, macrocephaly
      2. Li-Fraumeni syndrome
         a. Result of mutation in the *TP53* gene
         b. Young-onset cancers including soft tissue sarcoma, brain tumor, acute leukemia, breast cancer
      3. Peutz-Jeaghers syndrome
         a. Result of mutation in the *STK11* gene
         b. Increased risk for breast, ovary, colon, small bowel, testicular, and other cancers
      4. Hereditary diffuse gastric cancer syndrome
         a. Result of mutation in the *CDH1*
         b. Stomach cancer, breast cancer (lobular)
      5. Lynch syndrome
         a. Result of mutation in the *MLH1, MSH2, MSH6,* or *PMS2* gene
         b. Features include colon cancer, endometrial cancer, ovarian cancer; possibly breast

XI. **Expanded testing options with next generation gene sequencing**
   A. Multigene panels
      1. Evolving technology changing landscape of genetic testing
      2. Panels identify genetic variation in multiple genes (20–40) at the same time
      3. Many moderately penetrant genes included to test for a range of genetic related cancers
      4. May be considered as second-tier test when *BRCA* negative, or when family history suggests greater than one cancer syndrome
      5. No guidelines for eligibility, insurance reimbursement
      6. Limited data about risks associated with mutations with many of these genes
      7. Lack of clear guidelines for medical management for carriers of mutations in low or moderately penetrant genes
      8. Should be interpreted by individuals trained in cancer genetics
      9. Research and increased use will elucidate risks and implications

B. Family pedigree with *BRCA* mutation
  1. No living affected family member, so proband had BRCA testing and deleterious *BRCA2* mutation found. Mother is unaffected and likely demonstrates incomplete penetrance. Inheritance potentially from maternal grandmother's lineage (she died young), or maternal grandfather (melanoma). Brother tested to provide information for future children, but also is at increased risk for breast cancer as well as melanoma and prostate cancer.

Acknowledgment

Special thanks to Dr. Quinetta Edwards for her special expertise in reviewing and editing this chapter.

Bibliography

Aiello-Laws, L. (2011). Genetic cancer risk assessment. *Seminars in Oncology Nursing, 27,* 13–20.

Berliner, J. L., Fay A. M., Cummings, S. A., Burnett, B., & Tillmanns, T. (2013). NSGC practice guideline: Risk assessment and genetic counseling for breast and ovarian cancer. *Journal of Genetic Counseling, 22,* 155–163.

Domchek, S. M., Friebel, T. M., Singer, C. F., Evans, D. G., Lynch, H. T., Isaacs, C., … Rebbeck, T. R. (2010). Association of risk-reducing surgery in *BRCA1* or *BRCA2* mutation carriers with cancer risk and mortality. *Journal of the American Medical Association, 304,* 967–975.

Euhus, D. (2001). Understanding mathematical models for breast cancer risk assessment and counseling. *The Breast Journal, 7,* 224–232.

FORCE/Facing Our Risk Empowered. (2013). Retrieved December 20, from http://www.facingourrisk.org

Ford, D., Easton, D. F., Bishop, D.T., et al. (2007). Meta-analysis of *BRCA1* and *BRCA2* penetrance. *Journal of Clinical Oncology, 25,* 1329–1333.

Grann, V. R., Patel, P. R., & Jacobson, J. S. (2011). Comparative effectiveness of screening and prevention strategies among *BRCA1/2*-affected mutation carriers. *Breast Cancer Research and Treatment, 125,* 837–847.

Hilbers, F. S., Vreeswijk, M. P., van Asperen, C. J., & Devilee, P. (2013). The impact of next generation sequencing on the analysis of breast cancer susceptibility: A role for extremely rare genetic variation? *Clinical Genetics, 84,* 407–414.

Lynch, H. T., Snyder, C., & Casey, J. (2013). Hereditary ovarian and breast cancer: What have we learned? Annals of Oncology, 24 (Suppl. 8), 83–95.

National Comprehensive Cancer Network. NCCN Clinical Practice Guidelines in *Oncology.* (2013). *Genetic/familial high-risk assessment: breast and ovarian* (V4). Retrieved December 20, from http://www.nccn.org/professionals/physician_gls/pdf/genetics_screening.pdf

Oncology Nursing Society. (2012). *Oncology nursing: The application of cancer genetics and genomics throughout the oncology care continuum.* Retrieved December 31, 2013, from https://www.ons.org/about-ons/ons-position-statements/education-certification-and-role-delineation/oncology-nursing

Rebbeck, T. R., Friebel, T., Wagner, T., Lynch, H.T., Garber, J.E., Daly, M.B., ... Weber, B.L. et al. (2005). Effect of short-term hormone replacement therapy on breast cancer risk reduction after bilateral prophylactic oophorectomy in BRCA 1 and BRCA2 mutation carriers: The PROSE study group. *Journal of Clinical Oncology, 23,* 7804–7810.

Robson, M. E., Storm, C. E., Weitzel, J., Wollins, D. S., Offit, K., & American Society of Clinical Oncology. (2010). American Society of Clinical Oncology policy statement update: Genetic and genomic testing for cancer susceptibility. *Journal of Clinical Oncology, 28,* 893–901.

Urinalysis

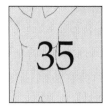

35

Helen A. Carcio

I. **Some comments related to urinary tract infection (UTI)**
   A. UTI is 50 times more common in women than in men.
   B. Ten percent to 20% of women develop a UTI at least once in their lives; 80% of these women develop a second infection.
   C. *Escherichia coli* (*E.coli*) causes 75% to 90% of all acute, uncomplicated infections.
   D. Definitions
      1. Urethritis: Inflammation of the urethra
      2. Cystitis: Inflammation of the bladder.
      3. Pyelonephritis: Inflammation of the kidney
   E. Many factors may predispose a woman to the occurrence of a UTI (Table 35.1).
   F. Symptoms of cystitis include abrupt onset of
      1. Dysuria: Pain or stinging while urinating
      2. Urinary frequency: Voiding small amounts; producing only small amounts
      3. Urinary urgency
      4. Suprapubic pain, ache, pressure
      5. Gross hematuria
      6. Pyuria, odor, milky
      7. Rare systemic symptoms but may occasionally present with low-grade fever (< 101°F)
      8. Confusion and fatigue in women

II. **Urinary evaluation**
   A. Assessment of urine in women in a primary care setting is often performed to identify or rule out UTI in the evaluation of dysuria, frequency, and suprapubic pain. Other conditions that relate specifically to the vulvovaginal area, such as those caused by *Candida, Chlamydia, Neisseria gonorrhoeae,* or *Trichomonas,* may also present with similar symptoms and must be explored.

TABLE 35.1 Factors That Contribute to Infection of the Urinary Tract

FACTOR	RESULT
Sexual activity	Introduction of bacteria into the urethra
Poor hygiene habits	Bacteria multiply in area of the urethra
Wiping from back to front	Introduces bacteria from the rectum into the urethra
Excessive use of caffeine	Causes urinary irritation and diuresis
Excessive stress	Reduces immune response
Contraception: Diaphragm use	Use of diaphragm may press on bladder, causing stasis of urine Spermicides inhibit growth of lactobacilli
Voiding habits	Stasis of urine
Waiting long periods of time between urinating	Decreases flushing of bacteria from bladder

    B. A urine culture does not need to be ordered in young women with a history of previous uncomplicated UTIs who present with the usual symptoms. A dipstick test is sufficient.

    C. Urinary assessment may include a comprehensive health history, physical examination, a urine dipstick test, microscopy, or culture.

    D. A thorough evaluation should be performed.
        1. For an initial episode
        2. If diagnosis is uncertain
        3. As an initial prenatal screen
        4. In elderly women, particularly if a cystocele is present
        5. In immune-compromised women

    E. A physical examination should include the following
        1. Vital signs, especially temperature
        2. Abdominal examination to palpate the suprapubic area for tenderness
        3. Percussion of costal vertebral angle (CVA) tenderness (present in pyelonephritis)
        4. Pelvic examination: Essential to rule out pelvic inflammatory disease, vaginitis, or sexually transmitted infections.
        5. Wet mount, if history or physical exam indicates risk factors for sexually transmitted infection

    F. The female anatomy predisposes a woman to bladder colonization with pathogens. This is related to
        1. Short urethra (2.5 cm)
        2. Proximity to the anal area
        3. Pregnancy: Bladder enlarged with decreased tone; unable to empty completely
        4. Older age: Lack of estrogen may cause urethral atrophy.

BOX 35.1 *Solutes in Random Urine*

- Various solutes normally appear at different times of the day
- Glucosuria: More often after meals
- Proteinuria: After activity or assumption of othostatic position from a recumbent position
- Hemoglobinuria: After severe physical exertion, such as working out at a gym

---

III. **Principles related to the procurement of urine**

   A. Freshly voided concentrated specimen provides more useful information than a diluted specimen

      1. Use the first morning urine. However, a random specimen is more convenient (Box 35.1).

      2. Bacteria must have been in the bladder at least 4 hours for accuracy.

   B. Test within a few minutes of collection. (If this is not possible, cover tightly and refrigerate at 5°C [41°F].)

   C. Do not allow specimen to stand at room temperature. Urine that is allowed to stand at room temperature begins to grow bacteria within 30 minutes; if more than 2 hours elapses, it will be highly contaminated by bacteria.

   D. As urine sits, it becomes alkaline, decomposing important sediment.

   E. Red blood cells and casts lyse quickly in diluted or alkaline urine.

IV. **The clean catch: In women, a clean catch is more difficult to obtain than in men, because external genitalia or vaginal discharge often cause contamination of the sample.**

   A. Equipment

      1. Sterile urine container

      2. Three wipes saturated with soap

   B. The following steps should be explained.

      1. Wash hands thoroughly to remove any potential sources of contamination.

      2. Remove the cover of a sterile specimen container, and put down with the lid side up. (Emphasize not to touch the inside of the lid or specimen container.)

      3. Spread the labia with the nondominant hand, and hold until after the specimen is collected.

      4. Using the dominant hand, wipe one side of the vaginal area with a cleansing towelette.

      5. Always use a single stroke, wiping the cleansing towelette from front to back.

      6. Cleanse the opposite side of the labia with the second towelette.

7. Cleanse the center area directly over the urethra, downward.
8. Release a small amount of urine into the toilet to flush any bacteria from the distal portion of the urethra.
9. Place the specimen container under the urethra (be careful not to touch the vulva), and urinate into the sterile cup while the labia remain separated.
10. If there is heavy vaginal discharge, a tampon should be worn to absorb the vaginal secretions in an attempt to avoid contamination of the urine sample.
11. Perform the urinalysis immediately, or refrigerate the urine sample.

V. **The chemical analysis: The complete analysis of urine is a simple, noninvasive, and inexpensive means of detecting abnormalities of the genitourinary tract. It is the single most important quantitative assessment of adequacy of renal function.**
   A. The dipstick: Analysis of the urine is performed with the dipstick, a chemically impregnated plastic strip. When the dipstick is placed in urine, the color changes in the various reagent strips provide an approximate quantification of the amount of substance present.
      1. Principles
         a. Detects the presence of protein, occult blood, glucose, nitrites, and ketones in the urine
         b. Determines the urinary pH
         c. Color changes may be compared against a chart provided by the manufacturer.
         d. Store in a cool dry place and use before the expiration date.
      2. Technique: There are many rapid agent tests for routine and special urinalyses. Most require dipping the stick into fresh, unspun urine and comparison of each reagent area with the corresponding colored area on the strip at varying suggested intervals (seconds to minutes).
   B. Odor: Fresh urine is aromatic; stale urine smells ammonia-like. It may adopt the odor of certain ingested substances.
   C. Turbidity
      1. Description: Many normal urine samples appear cloudy.
      2. Normally, cloudy urine is often caused by the presence of phosphates and carbonates if the specimen is alkaline. It will clear as the urine cools.
      3. Significance: Abnormal turbidity may be caused by red blood cells (RBCs), white blood cells (WBCs), and bacteria, and may suggest a UTI.
      4. Vaginal discharge may also cause cloudiness.
   D. Color: Urine is often described as "straw colored" or yellow.
      1. Description: The amount of color depends on the density of urochromes (pigments formed by metabolism of bile). The

intensity of the color is due to the concentration of the urine. Many substances may change the color of urine.

2. Normal color ranges from almost colorless to deep yellow, depending on the concentration of urochrome pigment.
3. Significance: May be a sign of disease or may indicate the presence of a pigmented drug, dye, or food (Table 35.2).

E. Specific gravity (SG): Measures urine directly relative to the density of water
1. Description: SG is used as in indirect measure of the kidneys' ability to concentrate the urine. The normal range is 1.010 to 1.025, with urine isotonic to plasma.
    a. Diluted: Under 1.010
    b. Concentrated: Over 1.025
2. Significance: If a first morning specimen is SG 1.025 or greater, it is generally taken as evidence of adequate concentrating ability and, therefore, adequate renal function.

F. pH
1. Description: The dipstick is impregnated with various dyes that respond with different color changes to a pH in the range of 5

TABLE 35.2 Appearance of Urine in Relation to Products

URINE APPEARANCE	ASSOCIATION
Colorless	Dilute urine associated with water diuresis or diabetes mellitus or insipidus
Red	Red blood cells (RBCs) or large amounts of free hemoglobin or myoglobin, bile pigments, food dyes, anthrocyanin (pigment in beets and blackberries)
Red-brown	Porphyria, urobilinogen, bilimbin
Orange	Fever and dehydration
Yellow	Normal due to the presence of a yellow pigment, urochrome
Yellow-red	Pyridium, vegetables, or phenolphthalein
Blue or green	Beets, methylene blue in IV
Brown or black	Porphyrins, melanin, acidification of hemoglobin content, rhubarb
Turbid	Frequently secondary to urates or phosphates (benign), RBC, white blood cells (WBCs)
Foamy	Protein, bile acids
Milky white	Heavy WBC content or precipitation of amorphous phosphate salts in alkaline urine
Cloudy	Pyuria

to 11. Measurement of pH on random urine samples has little clinical value.

2. The normal range of urine pH is 4.5 to 8.5. The urine pH in a freshly voided urine sample from a woman on a healthy diet is about 6.0. Stale urine becomes alkaline.
   a. Diffusion of carbon dioxide into the air
   b. Bacteria converts urea to ammonia

3. Significance: If fresh urine is alkaline, a UTI urea-splitting organism (e.g., *Proteus, Klebsiella, Escherichia coli*) or bicarbonate excretion (e.g., renal tubular acidosis) must be considered.

G. Protein
   1. Description: The dipstick is sensitive to as little as 5 to 20 mg/dL of albumin (the prominent protein in renal disease); normal: Less than 50 mg/day
   2. Significance
      a. Persistent proteinuria usually indicates renal disease.
      b. Transient proteinuria may be associated with orthostasic proteinuria, which results from prolonged standing after being in a recumbent position. Stress, cold, and contamination of the specimen with menstrual blood are other possible causes.

H. Nitrites
   1. Description: Many practitioners use the dipstick as a screening test for occult bacteriuria. It is an insensitive screening test for women who do not have symptoms. It provides an indirect method of detecting bacteriuria because many organisms contain enzymes that reduce nitrate in the urine to nitrite.
   2. Significance: Any degree of pink should be considered positive for the nitrite test, suggesting the presence of 10^5 per mL. Negative nitrate tests do not always mean that no bacteria are present because some strains do not produce the necessary enzymes to convert to nitrites *(Streptococcus faecalis* and gonococci).
   3. Use of a random urine sample is not acceptable because sufficient time would not have passed for conversion of nitrate to nitrite.

I. Ketones: Ketosis is seen in starvation (fad diets) and with alcoholism, as well as in individuals with poorly controlled diabetes mellitus.

J. Blood: Normal—RBCs may normally be seen in extremely small numbers in normal urine, particularly after strenuous exercise.
   1. The normal level is two or fewer RBCs per high-powered field.
   2. Significance: Hematuria is virtually always significant (Table 35.3).

K. Sugar

TABLE 35.3 Hematuria Differential Diagnosis: Red to Brown Discoloration

SYMPTOM	DIAGNOSIS
Without urinary tract pain	Renal or vesicle diseases
	Absence of RBC casts—tumor of bladder or kidney RBC casts—glomerulonephritis Stones, polycystic disease, renal cysts, sickle cell disease, hydronephrosis
Renal colic	Ureteral stone
Dysuria	Bladder infection or lithiasis

1. Description: Can detect 100 mg/dL of glucose because the reaction relies on the enzyme glucose oxidase. However, results are qualitative.
2. Normal: The absence of detectable glucose (negative dipstick) is considered a normal result.
3. Significance: The dipstick method is extremely sensitive and specific for glucose. This test is the main method for the diagnosis of the common disease diabetes mellitus.

VI. **Microscopic examination (see Chapter 31, "Vaginal Microscopy")**
   A. Description: Evaluation of sediment for cellular elements, casts, crystals, and microorganisms
   B. Caution
      1. Microscopic analysis is unreliable if more than 2 hours have elapsed between collection and evaluation.
      2. If specific gravity is below 1.010, sample must be examined immediately after collection.
   C. Principles
      1. Turn condenser down to distance it further from the slide. Use varying light intensities to pick up subtle changes in various elements.
      2. Use low power first, to identify elements in various fields.
      3. Examine near the four edges of the coverslip, where casts accumulate.
      4. Go to high power for cell counts and identification of casts and debris.
      5. If the urine specimen is purulent or bloody, remember to look at an unspun specimen first.
   D. The technique
      1. Pour 10 to 15 mL of freshly voided urine into a conical test tube.
      2. Check SG in remainder.
      3. Using dipstick, check for pH, protein, sugar, ketones, and heme in the remainder.

4. If a UTI is suspected (leukocytes or nitrates present as seen by dipstick), check Gram stain of unspun specimen.
5. Prepare spun specimen.
6. Spin at 1,000 to 2,000 rpm for 3 to 5 minutes.
7. Pour off top supernatant and discard, leaving one to two drops of urine at the bottom. A pellet is usually visible at the bottom.
8. Resuspend pellet immediately in the remaining urine (flick the bottom of the test tube several times with your fingers or tap it against a countertop).
9. Place two drops on a glass slide to dry for Gram stain.
10. While the Gram stain preparation dries, place two to three drops of sediment on another glass slide.
11. Cover the second slide immediately with a coverslip and examine under low power.
12. Use low power and scan entire slide to locate casts that may be present in only a few fields.
13. Examine under high dry power (never oil). Note presence of WBCs and vaginal cells.
14. Scan at least 10 to 15 high-power fields. Squamous epithelial cells are clearly visualized in urine without other vaginal contaminants.
15. Average the number of cells in the fields examined and record.

VII. The sediment
A. Common sediment in women (Table 35.4)
B. Casts
1. Description: Casts usually occur in the distal convoluted tubule of the nephron and are so called because they are casts of the nephron. They are distinguished from other debris by smooth, parallel sides (which may show the trapezoidal narrowing of the nephron collecting system).
2. Rarely normal. Significance: They are often difficult to interpret. They may indicate renal disease.
a. RBC casts indicate proliferative glomerular disease orvasculitis.
b. Hyaline casts that indicate proteinuria can be normal in concentrated urine.
c. WBC casts indicate interstitial nephritis or pyelonephritis.
d. Broad casts indicate tubular atrophy, with waxy casts indicating nephron death. Both are the successive changes in degeneration of cellular casts seen in renal failure.
C. Crystals
1. Description: Crystals occur because of precipitated chemicals and cellular debris. Their interpretation depends on the clinical presentation involved and is beyond the scope of this chapter.

TABLE 35.4 Common Urinary Sediment

SEDIMENT	DESCRIPTION	CLINICAL SIGNIFICANCE
RBCs	Normal: Presence of 0–3/ hpf; pale, biconcave discs; no nuclei; can be crenated; menses can contaminate and give false-positive results	Hematuria Cystitis most common cause of hematuria; can occur secondary to exertion, trauma, stress; may be confused with yeast
WBCs	Normal: Presence of 0–5/hpf Polymorphonuclear leukocyte most common Segmented nuclei 1½ times as large as RBCs Cytoplasmic granules	Pyuria
Renal tubular epithelial cells	Round, single nucleus slightly larger than WBCs	Renal tubular damage
Bladder epithelial cells	Varied shape: Flat to cuboidal; larger than renal cells	Normal
Squamous epithelial cells	Rectangular to round, flat cells; single small nuclei	Normal; usually due to vaginal contamination
Bacteria Gram stain	Normal urine does not contain bacteria	Significant bacteria may indicate a urinary tract infection
	Very small; difficult to identify microscopically Bacilli: Short rods Cocci: Tiny dots more difficult to identify	Presence of WBCs may differentiate between an infection and contamination; almost always found but does not always indicate significant bacteriuria; presence in unspun specimen is significant and provides presumptive evidence of UTI; indicate presence of UTI or contamination; send for culture and sensitivity if suspicious; if count is low and symptoms present, may be UTI
Yeast cells	May be seen in urine (diabetics) Ovoid, budding Variable size Similar in size to RBCs	*Candida* or contamination from vulvovaginal candidiasis If unable to differentiate from the RBC, drop acetic acid; RBCs will lyse, leaving the yeast intact

(continued)

TABLE 35.4 Common Urinary Sediment *(continued)*

SEDIMENT	DESCRIPTION	CLINICAL SIGNIFICANCE
Trichomonas	Most frequently seen parasite in urine Unicellular, ovoid with flagellate Undulates	Can be found in urine or urine contaminated from vaginal *Trichomonas*
Spermatozoa	Ovoid to round, with long tails; forward trajectory, spinning, immobile	May be seen after contamination by vaginal intercourse
Artifact	Starch granules (powder); cotton filbers	

hpf, high-powered field; RBC, red blood cell; UTI, urinary tract infection; WBC, white blood cell.

    2. Crystals are formed in normal (alkaline) urine as the specimen cools.

    3. Significance: Many different types of crystals are found in urine; however, a full discussion is beyond the scope of this chapter. Note: Normal urine contains no more than one or two RBCs, WBCs, and epithelial cells per high-powered field. An occasional hyaline cast may be seen.

VIII. Gram stain

    A. Description: The Gram stain technique can be used in the office setting. The preparation is more time-consuming than microscopy; however, additional information can be obtained to help with diagnosis. The highlighting of cells and organisms during the staining process makes them easier to identify and facilitates making a diagnosis. The following are enhanced by the colors they become

        1. Gram-negative organisms appear pink.

        2. Gram-positive organisms appear purple.

        3. Cells stain purple.

        4. Bacteria may be pink or purple.

        5. WBCs: Unstained at first, nuclei develop a red-blue stain with red cytoplasm.

        6. Hyaline cast: Bright blue

        7. Fine, granular casts: Bright red

        8. *Trichomonas:* Usually do stain but may appear bluish.
          Note: Some clinicians believe that the Gram stain is not necessary for diagnosis of most forms of vaginitis.

    B. Technique

        1. Spread a thin smear of urine sediment on a glass slide.

        2. Allow to air dry.

3. Fix by passing the underside of slide through a flame several times. Allow to cool.
4. Flood the slide with Gram crystal violet.
5. Wait 10 seconds, and rinse with tap water.
6. Repeat step 5, rinsing again.
7. Rinse the slide with decolorizer until all the violet has been rinsed away (fluid is colorless).
8. Immediately rinse again with tap water.
9. Flood the slide again with Gram safranin. Wait 10 seconds and rinse with tap water.
10. Dry or blot dry.
11. Place slide under microscope and put a small drop of oil on the stained specimen.
12. Using high-power objective with bright field illumination (diaphragm open), examine the slide.
13. View several fields.
14. Record findings.

C. Common errors leading to unsatisfactory urine sediment examination
1. Contamination of collecting vessel with foreign material
2. Inadequately resuspended sediment
3. Failure to use both high- and low-power magnification
4. Too much or too little light
5. Dried specimen
6. Artifacts such as cotton fibers from swabs or powder crystals
7. Vaginal contamination

IX. **Urine culture (see Table 35.5 for the interpretation of WBC count in relation to symptoms)**

TABLE 35.5 Significance of WBCs in Urine Culture in Relation to Symptoms

WBCs	WBC COUNT	SYMPTOMS
100,000/mL	10^5	Significant bacteriuria
10,000/mL	10^4	No symptoms Significant asymptomatic bacteriuria symptoms Treat
1,000 to 10,000/mL	10^3–10^4	Contamination of external source Dilute urine Been in the bladder only a short period of time Early days of treatment with antibiotic No infection

WBC, white blood cell.

X. **Management of positive findings (see Table 35.6 for differential diagnoses)**
   A. Uncomplicated UTI
      1. Usually easy to cure because the infection is superficial and a high concentration of the antibiotic is readily achieved in the urine. Long courses of antibiotics are no longer necessary.
         a. Symptoms disappear 1 to 2 days after beginning treatment.
         b. Encourage the patient to continue medication even though symptoms are gone.
         c. Warn the patient that vulvovaginal candidiasis may develop secondary to antibiotic therapy. Tell her to call if she notices any vulvar itching or burning.
      2. Single-dose therapy
         a. Amoxicillin, 3 g
         b. Sulfamethoxazole/trimethoprim (Bactrim), two tablets
         c. Ofloxacin (Floxin), 100 to 250 mg
      3. Three-day regimens (slightly increased efficacy)
         a. Bactrim DS twice a day
         b. Nitrofurantoin macrocrystals (Macrobid) two times a day (somewhat decreased incidence of concurrent candidiasis)
         c. Amoxicillin, 500 mg three times a day

TABLE 35.6 Differential Diagnosis of Conditions That Affect the Urinary Tract

CONDITION/SYMPTOMS	DIAGNOSIS	DESCRIPTION
Cystitis (most common)	10^5 Micro: 8–10 WBCs per hpf	Infection of the superficial mucosa of the lower urinary tract
	Red blood cells	Triad of symptoms
	Bacteria	Urinary urgency Frequency Dysuria
Upper urinary tract (pyelonephritis)	Involves renal parenchyma	Systemic manifestations of chills, fever, flank pain
Asymptomatic bacteriuria	10^3/mL of bacteria in the absence of symptoms	Negative symptoms
Acute urethral syndrome	Negative culture	Dysuria, frequency, urgency
Interstitial cystitis	Negative culture	Urgency and frequency associated with diminished bladder capacity

Note: If large numbers of vaginal epithelial cells are present, it may indicate contamination. A vaginal wet mount must be done to eliminate vaginal discharge as the primary source of the WBCs. hpf, high-power field; WBC, white blood cell.

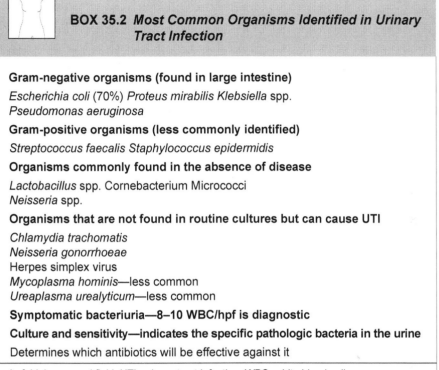

BOX 35.2 *Most Common Organisms Identified in Urinary Tract Infection*

Gram-negative organisms (found in large intestine)
Escherichia coli (70%) *Proteus mirabilis Klebsiella* spp. *Pseudomonas aeruginosa*

Gram-positive organisms (less commonly identified)
Streptococcus faecalis Staphylococcus epidermidis

Organisms commonly found in the absence of disease
Lactobacillus spp. Cornebacterium Micrococci *Neisseria* spp.

Organisms that are not found in routine cultures but can cause UTI
Chlamydia trachomatis
Neisseria gonorrhoeae
Herpes simplex virus
Mycoplasma hominis—less common
Ureaplasma urealyticum—less common

Symptomatic bacteriuria—8–10 WBC/hpf is diagnostic

Culture and sensitivity—indicates the specific pathologic bacteria in the urine
Determines which antibiotics will be effective against it

hpf, high-powered field; UTI, urinary tract infection; WBC, white blood cell.

    d. Ciprofloxacin (Cipro), 250 mg two times a day
    e. Ofloxacin (Floxin), 400 mg two times a day
  4. Box 35.2 summarizes those organisms found in urine cultures.
 B. Complicated cystitis
  1. Use of the medications mentioned in Section X, A; increase use to 7 to 10 days.
  2. Needs further evaluation
 C. If pylonephritis is suspected, continue the aforementioned regimens for 14 days.
 D. May prescribe phenazopyridine (Pyridium) 100 mg three times a day to relieve dysuria by preventing bladder spasm.

Bibliography

Echeverry, G., Hortin, G. L., & Rai, A. J. (2010). Introduction to urinalysis: Historical perspectives and clinical application. *Methods in Molecular Biology, 641,* 1.

National Kidney Foundation. (n.d.). *What you need to know about urinalysis.* Retrieved December 5, 2010, from http://www.kidney.org

Wu, X. (2010). Urinalysis: A review of methods and procedures. *Critical Care Nursing Clinics of North America, 22*(1), 121.

The Simple Cystometrogram

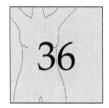

36

Helen A. Carcio

I. **Simple cystometrography (CMG) explained**
   A. Cystometrography is an important first step in the evaluation and management of bladder dysfunction.
   B. It is an appropriate diagnostic test when there is no access to complex cystometrography during urodynamic testing
   C. It is emerging as a reliable indicator to determine a diagnosis of overactive bladder, urinary incontinence, and interstitial cystitis.
   D. The patient must complete a 3-day voiding diary before the test (see Chapter 18, "Urinary Incontinence").
   E. Typical complaints that may lead to simple CMG testing include
      1. Incontinence, stress, and urge
      2. Nocturia
      3. Frequency
      4. Urgency
      5. Pelvic pain
      6. Slow stream

II. **Patient assessment**
   A. Assessment of strength of the pelvic floor muscles
      1. Insert the index finger and middle fingers approximately 2 cm through the vaginal orifice (to the first knuckle).
      2. Palpate the band of muscle located just inside the vagina in the 5 o'clock and 7 o'clock positions.
      3. Ask the woman to squeeze and hold the contraction.
      4. Note the strength of the contraction and the number of seconds she is able to hold the contraction.
      5. Ask the woman to squeeze her pelvic floor muscle tightly several times.
      6. Note strength of the squeeze.
      7. Compare the strength of contralateral sides.

8. The palpable contraction should be strong and sustained with fingers deflected upward and inward.
9. Decreased strength may signify weakened pelvic floor muscles and cause incontinence.

B. Measure postvoid residual (PVR).
1. Have the woman void immediately before the test.
2. The residual is the result of bladder contractility and urethral resistance.
3. Should be obtained within 5 minutes of voiding
4. A high residual may indicate a hypotonic bladder or an inability to contract against an increase in urethral pressure.
5. A PVR of 25% or less of voided volume is acceptable.

III. **The procedure**
A. Patient preparation
1. Patient should be mobile and alert.
   a. The bowel should be as empty as possible.
   b. An enema is not necessary.
2. Explain the various phases of the testing procedure and show the equipment to be used to decrease any anxiety.
3. Patient should not have taken any medications that may alter bladder function, such as an anticholinergic.
4. It is imperative that measures be done to help patients relax because a tense patient is often unconsciously bracing against any leaking.
5. Reassure the patient that every effort will be made to make her comfortable during the procedure.
   a. The procedure only takes 15 minutes.
   b. It is not uncomfortable.
6. Ask client to respond to sensations during filling and to report any urgency or discomfort.

B. Supplies
1. Twelve- to 14-French red rubber catheter
2. A 60-mL catheter-tipped syringe without piston
3. A liter bottle of sterile water at room temperature
   a. Cold water may stimulate the bladder to contract.
4. Absorbent pads

C. The test
1. Catheterize patient and measure and record the PVR.
2. Attach the 60-mL syringe (without the piston) to the red rubber catheter.
3. Hold the syringe 10 to 12 inches above the pubic bone (the syringe acts as a funnel to fill the bladder).
4. Slowly fill the bladder with warm, sterile water, 50 mL at a time (Figure 36.1).
5. Pinch the tube off between each aliquot to prevent putting air into the bladder.

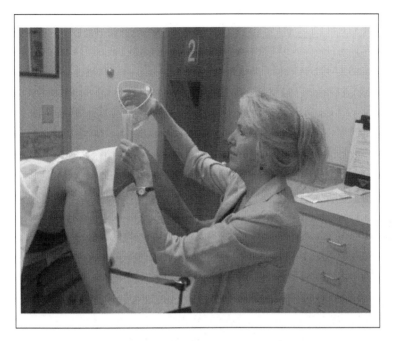

FIGURE 36.1 Performing a simple cystometrogram: After the patient is catheterized, the syringe acts as a funnel to fill the bladder.

6. Note the presence or absence of involuntary bladder contractions.
    a. Noted as an upward movement of the column of fluid in the syringe with each bladder contraction.
7. Record fluid volume at which any contractions occur.
8. Perform provocative maneuvers to elicit potential leaking with each 100 mL of fluid instilled.
    a. Running water
    b. Jingling of keys
    c. Cough
9. Record any leaking or contractions with these maneuvers and the volume at which they occur.
10. The contractions may be accompanied by leaking around the catheter or actual expulsion of catheter if the contractions are strong enough.
11. The examiner must also observe for the presence of any abdominal straining, which would alter the test results.
12. Sensation is the subjective response to bladder filling as communicated by the patient. The patient is asked to respond to three sensations:
    a. First sensation: The first indication of the need to urinate
    b. Second sensation: A point in bladder filling when the patient would actually consider looking for a bathroom

TABLE 36.1 Grading of Responses

SENSATION	OBSERVED RESPONSE	NORMAL RANGE (mL)
First sensation	First inclination to void	90–150
Second sensation	Normal desire to void Can be delayed	200–300
Third sensation	Strong and persistent desire to void Maximum capacity at which the patient feels she can no longer hold her urine or when the bladder spontaneously empties	400–550

    c. Third sensation: A point at which the patient can no longer hold the urine

    d. Table 36.1 summarizes these responses.

13. Note compliance
    a. Observe the stretch ability of the bladder to accommodate the increasing volumes of water.
    b. A normal bladder distends and stretches with filling.
    c. Instilled fluid flows in evenly.

14. Capacity
    a. The optimal amount of fluid the bladder can hold
    b. Normal capacity of 300 to 500 mL

15. Results
    a. Contractions or severe urgency at relatively low bladder volumes (250 mL) suggest urge incontinence
    b. Severe urgency at 150 mL and a volume less than 350 mL suggest interstitial cystitis.
    c. Provocative maneuvers may evoke a bladder contraction or an episode of leaking. Document which maneuver triggers leaking.
    d. Uninhibited detrusor contractions and urge incontinence may be stimulated by triggers.
    e. Instilled fluid that flows slowly through the catheter suggests a noncompliant bladder that will not easily stretch with expanding volumes and suggests interstitial cystitis.
    f. Small bladder capacity suggests detrusor instability, low bladder compliance or insterstitial cystitis.
    g. Leaking with straining or coughing suggests stress incontinence.
    h. Maximum bladder capacity is recorded at the end of the test. It measures the size of the bladder when full.
    i. Drain the bladder when test is complete.

BOX 36.1 *Simple Cystometrography (CMG) Evaluation Form*

Name _____ Date of birth _____ Age _____

Date of service _____

Assessment summary: Urinalysis _____

_____

_____

_____

Filling CMG

Capacity: Amount instilled _____ mL

Compliance

First sensation _____ mL (90–150 mL)

Second sensation _____ mL (200–300 mL)

Third sensation (max) _____ mL (400–550 mL)

Uninhibited contraction _____ mL

Leaking _____ Provocative maneuver _____

Postvoid residual (PVR) _____ (25% or less of voided volume)

❑ Bladder diary completed

Clinical impression _____

Follow-up _____

_____

Provider _____

IV. **After the procedure**
  A. Results are immediate and can be explained to the patient.
  B. Inform the patient that she may note some burning with urination and blood in the urine for the first 24 to 48 hours.
    1. This is normal and expected due to the insertion of the catheter and should spontaneously disappear.
    2. The patient should call the physician if burning and frequency, blood in the urine, or dysuria remains beyond 48 hours because this may indicate a urinary tract infection.
  C. Record findings (see Box 36.1 for a sample form).
  D. Refer for complex CMG if findings are inconclusive.

Bibliography

Bergman, J., & Elia, G. (1999). Effects of the menstrual cycle on urodynamic work-up: Should we change our practice? *International Urogynecology Journal and Pelvic Floor Dysfunction, 10*(6), 375–377.

Burden, H., Warren, K., & Abrams, P. (2013, November). Diagnosis of male incontinence. *Current Opinion in Urology, 23*(6), 509–514.

Carcio, H. A. (2005). Urodynamic testing: A reliable indicator of urinary dysfunction. *Advance for Nurse Practitioners, 13*(10), 45–49.

Carcio, H. A. (2007). Mixed signals: Treating overlapping symptoms of urinary incontinence. *Advance for Nurse Practitioners, 12*(10), 32–36.

Dillon, B. E., & Zimmern, P. E. (2012, October). When are urodynamics indicated in patients with stress urinary incontinence? *Current Urology Reports, 13*(5), 379–384.

Ouslander, J. G., Abelson, S., Staskin, D. R., & Blaustein, J. (1989). Simplified tests of lower urinary tract function in the evaluation of geriatric urinary incontinence. *Journal of the American Geriatrics Society, 37*(8), 706–714.

Patel, B. N., & Kobashi, K. C. (2013, June). Practical use of the new American Urological Association adult urodynamics guidelines. *Current Urology Reports, 14*(3), 240–246.

Pelvic Floor Electrical Stimulation

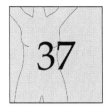

Helen A. Carcio

I. **Urinary incontinence (UI) is a common condition defined as an involuntary leakage of urine.**
   A. Women are twice as likely to be affected as men, and prevalence increases with age.
   B. The severity of incontinence affects quality of life and treatment decisions. The types of urinary incontinence include stress, urge, overflow, functional, and postprostatectomy incontinence (see Chapter 18, "Urinary Incontinence").
   C. Nonsurgical treatment options may include pharmacological treatment, pelvic muscle exercises (PME), bladder training exercises, and electrical stimulation.
   D. Pelvic floor stimulation is proposed as a nonsurgical treatment option for women with pelvic floor dysfunction.

II. **Pelvic floor electrical stimulation (PFES)**
   A. Involves the electrical stimulation of pelvic floor muscles (PFM) through a battery-powered control unit that initiates and regulates the output of electrical stimulation to the electrodes (Figure 37.1)
      1. Affects the smooth muscles of the pelvic floor (levator ani muscle groups), the striated muscles of external urethra and anal sphincters, and the bladder (detrusor)
      2. Sensors: Two types
         a. Vaginal or anal insert device with embedded electrodes
         b. Surface electrodes placed around the anus
         c. Note: Probes are more generally used and will be discussed below.
   B. The principle
      1. A mild electric current passes through an electrode that is in direct contact with the muscles of the pelvic floor.

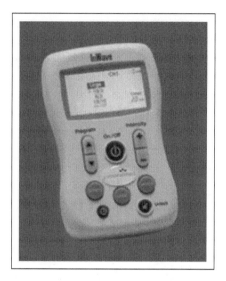

FIGURE 37.1 An electrical stimulation unit that is easy to program.

2. Activation of the motor units produces a passive reflex muscle contraction without any effort by the patient.
3. Stimulates the afferent fibers of pudendal nerve, which tones the levator ani and periurethral musculature group, which may have been dormant for years
4. This neuromuscular stimulation hypertrophies ("bulks up") and strengthens the pelvic floor muscle, which leads to improved urethral closure, improving incontinence.
5. Increased sympathetic tone to the bladder directly inhibits unwanted detrusor muscle contractions, which relax the bladder, reducing the sensation of urinary urgency and frequency.
   a. Reflex inhibitory signals are simultaneously relayed via the afferent pudendal nerve to the bladder, causing the muscle to relax.
6. Additionally PFES is thought to improve partially denervated urethral and pelvic floor musculature by enhancing the process of reinnervation (nerve growth).
7. Passive contractions help to reeducate the user to increase awareness of the location of the pelvic floor muscles to aid in the identification of the correct muscles to contract for Kegel exercises and pelvic floor rehabilitation (PFR) (see Chapter 38, "Pelvic Floor Rehabilitation")
8. Recommend use in conjunction with and as an important adjunct to pelvic floor rehabilitation
9. Research suggests PFES may be effective in up to 87% in treatment of UI.
10. It is a safe procedure with no serious reported side effects.

BOX 37.1 *Contraindications to Electrical Stimulation*

- Dementia
- Absent or diminished sensation (denervation of the pelvic floor)
- Demand cardiac (heart) pacemaker
- Unstable cardiac arrhythmias
- Pregnancy or planning/attempting pregnancy
- Irritated perianal, vulvovaginal skin
- Rectal bleeding/inflamed hemorrhoids
- Short vaginal length
- Prolapse (Grade I)
- Severe atrophic vaginitis
- Vaginal or urinary infection
- Recent pelvic surgery

C. Indications: PFES is indicated for patients with
  1. Stress incontinence
  2. Urge incontinence
  3. Overactive bladder
  4. Mixed incontinence (a combination of both stress and urge incontinence)
  5. Pelvic pain
     a. Interstitial cystitis
     b. Chronic pelvic pain syndrome
     c. Dysparunia (painful intercourse)
     d. Vestibulitis, vulvodynia
D. Components: The PFES equipment comes with settings, which need to be adjusted for the woman's comfort and expected response.
  1. The current is delivered either during a period of stimulation followed by a period of rest, or continuous stimulation.
  2. Amplitude: The intensity of the electrical current
  3. Ramping: A change in the ability of the electrical current to reach the muscle fibers. May ramp up or down. Should be done slowly to avoid patient discomfort.
  4. Frequency rate: The rate or frequency refers to the number of pulses that are generated per unit of time (seconds). This is reported as Hz (hertz). The frequency rate is contingent on the diagnosis.
     a. Low Hz (10–20 Hz): Calms detrusor muscle to decrease unwanted bladder contractions associated with UI
     b. Medium high Hz (50–100 Hz): Strengthens and bulks up muscle, increases urethral closure
     c. Mixed

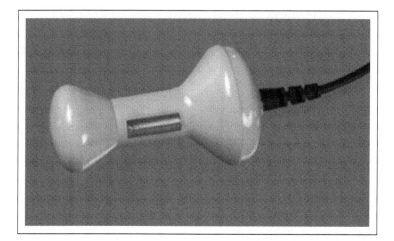

FIGURE 37.2 A vaginal sensor to be used with electrical stimulation. Note the silver sensor, which lies against the pelvic floor muscle just inside the introitus.

E. Preparation: Insert to hub only (Figure 37.2).
  1. Do not use lubricant as it may interfere with impulse.
  2. Electrical current is transmitted to the tissues
  3. Silver sensors should rest on the pelvic floor muscles, which lie 2 to 2.5 cm within the vagina (to first knuckle).
  4. Slowly increase the electrical current (ramping) in accordance with the user's tolerance, until a contraction (tugging) is felt.
  5. The more gradual the current rises to the preset amplitude or threshold level, the more comfortable the stimulation will feel to the person.
  6. Initially may feel prickling but must actually feel the contraction
  7. May adjust the current upward as the patient becomes more accustomed to the initial current
  8. Alert: The nerve endings in the vulvovaginal area are mainly clustered at the vaginal opening. The patient will experience a severe increase in discomfort should the sensor inadvertently slide out beyond the introitus at Hart's line.
     a. Always keep an eye on the location of the sensor in the vagina.
     b. May have to gently hold or ask the patient to hold the sensor in place in a lax vagina.
F. Removal: The device must be turned off before the sensor is removed. This will prevent the strong electrical current from touching the delicate nerves immediately outside the vagina.
G. Electrical stimulation is used either in a practice or clinic setting or can be used at home.

    1. Some insurance may pay for the rental or purchase of the device and probes.

H. Attainable results

    1. Increases the number and strength of slow-twitch fibers of the pelvic floor muscle, thus improving resting urethral closure and coordination and strength of the pelvic floor muscles

    2. Able to isolate the pelvic floor muscles from accessory muscles (diaphragm, buttocks, thighs)

    3. Improves recruitment and holding ability (endurance) of pelvic muscle fibers when doing voluntary pelvic muscle contractions.

    4. Can relax and inhibit bladder activity or bladder contractions that cause urinary urgency, frequency, and urge incontinence

    5. Guides patient from dysfunctional to functional well-being

Bibliography

Alves, P. G., Nunes, F. R., & Guirro, E. C. (2011). Comparison between two different neuromuscular electrical stimulation protocols for the treatment of female stress urinary incontinence: A randomized controlled trial. *Revista Brasileira de Fisioterapia, 15*(5), 393–398.

American Urologic Association (AUA). (2012). *Treatment guidelines for overactive bladder.* Retrieved from http://www.aua.org

Bent, A. E., Sand, P. K., Ostergard, D. R., & Brubaker, L. (1993). Transvaginal electrical stimulation in the treatment of genuine stress incontinence and detrusor instability. *International Urogynecology Journal, 4,* 9–13.

Coyne, K. S., Payne, C., Bhattacharyya, S. K., Revicki, D. A., Thompson, C., Corey, R., & Hunt, T. L. (2004). The impact of urinary urgency and frequency on health-related quality of life in overactive bladder: Results from a national community survey. *Value in Health, 7*(4), 455–463.

Fall M., & Lindström, S. (1991). Electrical stimulation: A physiologic approach to the treatment of urinary incontinence. *The Urologic Clinics of North America, 18*(2), 393–407.

Herderschee, R., Hay-Smith, E. J., Herbison, G. P., Roovers, J. P., &Heineman, M. J. (2011). Feedback or biofeedback to augment pelvic floor muscle training for urinary incontinence in women. *Cochrane Database of Systematic Reviews, 7,* CD009252

Monga, A. K., Tracey, M. R., & Subbaroyan, J. (2012). A systematic review of clinical studies of electrical stimulation for treatment of lower urinary tract dysfunction. *International Urogynecology Journal, 23*(8), 993–1005.

Sievert, K. D., Amend, B., Toomey, P. A., Robinson, D., Milsom, I., Koelbl, H., … Newman, D. K. (2012). Can we prevent incontinence? ICI-RS 2011. *Neurourology and Urodynamics, 31*(3), 390–399.

Pelvic Floor Rehabilitation

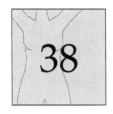

38

Helen A. Carcio

I. **Pelvic floor rehabilitation explained**
   A. Pelvic floor rehabilitation is a nonsurgical training program to strengthen the muscles the pelvic floor.
      1. Combines use of Kegel exercises and biofeedback protocols
      2. Designed to strengthen pelvic floor musculature (PFM) and relax bladder contractions
      3. Treats symptoms of pelvic floor dysfunction
      4. Usually consists of a series of four to eight visits over a period of 4 to 12 weeks
      5. The program is progressive in nature.
      6. Treatment should advance from least invasive (lifestyle changes, behavioral therapies, medications) to more invasive therapies.
      7. It may take a few weeks before a woman notices any improvement. It is important to point out that she has had the condition a long time and it will take a long time to reverse old habits.
      8. Studies indicate a 60% to 90% improvement in the symptoms of urinary and fecal urgency, frequency, and incontinence.
      9. Program is individualized, based on the woman's underlying condition and response to exercise training regimes
   B. Electromyography (EMG) of the pelvic floor muscles
      1. Provides an objective measurement in the evaluation of pelvic floor dysfunction
      2. Evaluation of the PFM is necessary in order to correctly diagnose pelvic floor dysfunction prior to the initiation of pelvic floor rehabilitation.
      3. EMG is interpreted in light of the woman's symptoms, physical findings, and other urological or urodynamic findings.
      4. An exercise protocol is designed based on the results of the EMG.

C. Biofeedback program
   1. Uses computerized technology to assist the woman in isolating her PFM
   2. Increases proprioception and muscle awareness
D. Electrical stimulation of the pelvic floor is often used concurrently (see Chapter 37, "Pelvic Floor Electrical Stimulation").
E. Goals of pelvic floor rehabilitation
   1. Assist women of all ages to strengthen the muscles in their pelvic area, which affect the proper functioning of the bladder and rectum
   2. Improve vaginal muscle tone through a step-by-step exercise program
   3. Prevent or diminish episodes of leaking with activities
   4. Hasten recovery following pregnancy, childbirth, or pelvic surgery
   5. Prevent or reduce pelvic organ prolapse, such as a "dropped" bladder or uterus
   6. Enhance the ability to control urinary and fecal incontinence
   7. Restore normal muscular function of the pelvic floor
   8. Increase sexual satisfaction for those with decreased libido or leaking with sexual activity
   9. Conditions treated (see Table 38.1)
F. Requirements for successful pelvic floor rehabilitation
   1. Intact nervous system
   2. Intact urinary system
   3. Absence of pathology

TABLE 38.1 Conditions Treated With Pelvic Floor Rehabilitation

Stress incontinence	Leaking with coughing, sneezing Leaking with impact
Irritative voiding symptoms	Urinary frequency Overactive bladder
Pelvic pain	Interstitial cystitic Vestibulitis, vulvodynia Pudendal neuralgia Dyspareunia Bladder pain
Voiding and defecation disorders	Urinary retention Constipation Irritable bowel syndrome Fecal incontinence
Postpartum related	Pelvic pain Muscle weakness Urinary problems

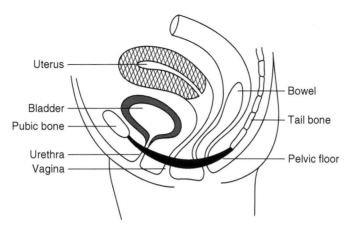

FIGURE 38.1 Note the pelvic floor muscles stretch like a strap from the pubic bone to the tailbone.

II. **Pelvic floor EMG explained**

   A. Anatomy and physiology of the pelvic floor musculature should be thoroughly explained.

   B. Some comments

   1. The pelvic floor muscles are composed of skeletal muscles in the levi ani group and the striated muscle of the urethral sphincter (see Figure 38.1).

   2. Many factors can weaken pelvic floor muscles, including pregnancy, childbirth, age, weight, and lifestyle.

   3. Skeletal muscles atrophy with disuse and denervation.

   a. Inactive muscles can lose 80% of their bulk.

   b. Active muscles only lose 20%.

   4. There are two types of pelvic floor skeletal muscles (Table 38.2). Each has different characteristics and each responds to a specific form of muscle activation.

   a. Type I: Slow-twitch muscle fibers

   (1) Fatigue resistant: Can chronically contract for long periods of time

TABLE 38.2 Types of Skeletal Muscles

NUMBER	DESCRIPTION	LOCATION	
Slow twitch	60%–80% of pelvic floor musculature	Contracts at slow, constant levels Fatigue resistant	Pelvic diaphragm
Fast twitch	20%–40% of pelvic floor musculature	Intense, rapid Fatigue quickly	Urogenital diaphragm sphincter

      (2) Have a slow, but consistent contraction speed
      (3) Similar to a long-distance runner
      (4) Usually recruited to maintain long periods of muscle activity
  b. Type II: Fast-twitch muscle fibers
      (1) Contract rapidly and forcefully
      (2) Fatigue quickly
      (3) Usually recruited for actions that require strength
      (4) Compared to a "sprinter"
  5. Increase in muscle strength improves effectiveness of continence mechanisms
    a. Muscle hypertrophy increases anatomical support of the pelvic structures.
    b. Closing pressure increases as the muscles "bulk up" in the periurethral striated sphincter musculature.
  6. EMG is measured using similar principles as those used for measuring an electrocardiogram (EKG). The heart is a muscle just as the pelvic floor muscles are.
  7. Woman should remain as still as possible as any movement artifact is picked up by the sensors and may interfere with interpretation.
  8. Over time, when the pelvic floor muscles weaken from disuse or injury, other muscles compensate and take over in an attempt to control leaking. (Table 38.3 lists the most common accessory muscles.) Note: The disuse has probably been going on for years, further causing the pelvic muscles to weaken.
C. Measurement: Waveform tracings represent the firing of individual motor units.
  1. There are physiologic phases of muscle contraction (see Figure 38.2).
    a. Baseline (Figure 38.2 [1]): Resting period with minimal activity
      (1) Motor units fire while at rest and often give a "saw-toothed" appearance to a Pelvic Muscle Contraction

TABLE 38.3 Accessory Muscles to a Pelvic Muscle Contraction

Abdominals
Adductor (thighs)
Gluteal (buttocks)
Must stress "no abs, hips, or butts"!

Note: Goal is to isolate use of the pelvic floor muscles from the accessory muscles; should not be recruited.

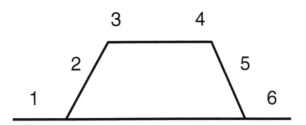

FIGURE 38.2 Characteristics of a contraction (1) baseline (2) recruitment, (3) amplitude, (4) endurance, (5) decruitment, and (6) baseline.

   b. Recruitment (Figure 38.2 [2])
     (1) Ability of the muscle units to fire simultaneously and immediately when asked to contract. Determines how quickly the waveform goes up.
     (2) Often described in terms of quick or slow
   c. Amplitude (Figure 38.2 [3])
     (1) Number of motor units firing in response to a contraction of the pelvic floor
   d. Endurance (Figure 38.2 [4])
     (1) Ability to hold contraction over a 10-second period
     (2) Describe in terms of muscle fatigue at 5-second intervals
     (3) The timing of a muscle until it fatigues
   e. Strength: Height of the waveform of the contraction at its highest point above baseline; maximum contraction that a muscle can generate
   f. Decruitment (Figure 38.2 [5])
     (1) Speed of release of contraction back to baseline
     (2) Described as quick of slow
   g. Baseline (Figure 38.2 [6]): Return to resting baseline after a period of contractions
  D. Sensors: Electromyography uses external or internal surface electrodes to assess the pelvic floor muscle activity from underlying skeletal muscles that initiate muscle contraction.
   1. Surface sensors
    a. Sensors pick up the slight amount of electrical activity (firing of motor units) from the muscle lying below the skin.
    b. Converts to waveforms visible on a computer screen whose tracings provide meaningful information that is then interpreted by the user
    c. Placement of surface electrode: Consists of three electrodes
     (1) Wipe skin with alcohol and allow to dry.
     (2) Place electrodes along the long axis of the muscle.

    d. Sensors are applied to a skin surface as close to the muscle being studied as possible.
        (1) Can be placed on either the abdominal, gluteal, or adductor muscles to pick up erroneous use of that particular accessory muscle group during a PFM contraction
        (2) Abdominal placement is the most common since the majority of women use these muscles as compensation.
        (3) Place midway between the umbilicus and the iliac crest or 2 inches below the umbilicus.
        (4) The three skin sensors are attached to three different colored wires. The black ground wire should be in the middle and the white and red wires on either side (Figure 38.3). Place over the iliac crest bone.
    e. Goal is to isolate the levator muscle and eliminate use of accessory muscles
  2. Internal sensors: Consist of surface electrodes embedded in a probe that is inserted in the vagina up to the hub (refer to Figure 37.2)
    a. Types of single-use sensors
        (1) Vaginal
        (2) Anal
            a. A smaller version of the vaginal sensor
            b. Most often used vaginally in those women having a short vagina
            c. Vaginal placement rather than anal placement is preferred by most women and both correctly assess the strength of the pelvic floor muscle.
    b. Technique
        (1) Wash before insertion.
            a. Dry thoroughly.
            b. Do not use lubricant as it will interfere with accuracy of tracings.

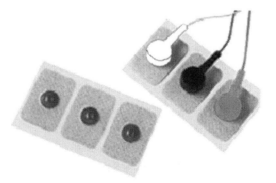

FIGURE 38.3 An example of a skin sensor.
Photo courtesy of PersonalMed.

(2) Insert probe into the vagina only to the "hub."

(3) Arrow on hub to point down to the floor (toward tailbone)

(4) Silver area on the sensor should rest against the levator muscle of pelvic floor.

(5) Wash with warm soap and water on removal.

E. Recording device

1. Once the vaginal and surface electrodes are in place, they are plugged into the recording device. The computer has been preprogrammed and the impulses are transferred to the computer screen for interpretation (Figure 38.4).

III. Kegel exercises

A. Kegel exercises explained

1. In 1951, Arnold Kegel wrote a paper describing the relationship of pelvic floor muscle strength to symptoms related to urinary incontinence.

2. Purpose is to restore tone and function to the weakened pelvic muscle

3. Repeated contractions strengthen the voluntary urinary sphincter and the levator ani muscles, increasing the closing force of the urethra.

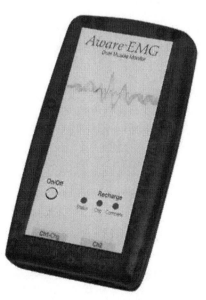

FIGURE 38.4 The Aware device picks up the signals from the muscles and converts them to waveform tracings visible on the computer screen. *Note*: This particular devise is wireless and can be held in the palm of the hand.

Photo courtesy of PersonalMed.

    4. It is important to teach women the proper way to do Kegel exercises.
       a. Studies document that 60% of women do not know how to perform Kegels correctly.
    5. There are many variations and approaches as how best to practice Kegel exercises.
    6. Exercises are first done lying on the back since this puts less gravitational pressure on the pelvic floor.
       a. It is more difficult to contract an overstretched muscle.
       b. Do not practice on the toilet.
    7. Progress to sitting and standing position as the pelvic floor becomes stronger, as muscles contract differently in each position.

B. Technique. Woman is asked to
    1. Relax her abdominal and gluteal muscles and place her hands lightly on the abdominal muscles to monitor for even the slightest movement that would indicate she is engaging them along with her pelvic floor
    2. Tighten her anal sphincter and "draw in" as if attempting to prevent passing gas
    3. Will note a lifting sensation in the vaginal area as the pelvic muscle pulls and tightens against the pubic bone. Breathe regularly throughout the contraction and relaxation cycles.

C. Timing
    1. Long holds: Engage slow-twitch fibers
       a. Begin with 5-second contraction
       b. Goal is to maintain a 10-second hold, alternating with a 10-second relaxation
       c. The time of contraction should equal the time of relaxation.
       d. Must relax completely between contractions
       e. Repeat 10 times in a row, three times a day.
       f. It is a good idea to use triggers to remember to practice (see Appendix to this chapter).
    2. Short holds: Engage fast-twitch fibers
       a. Also called "quick flicks"
       b. Hold squeeze for 2 to 3 seconds, 10 times in a row two to three times a day.
       c. Relax completely between each contraction.

D. Follow-up
    1. Should note a change in 3 to 4 weeks
    2. Once muscles are strengthened, the woman should continue daily exercises to maintain muscles strength and prevent incontinence.
    3. If the woman does not notice much improvement in symptoms after 4 weeks of exercise, she should begin biofeedback, which is the next phase of pelvic floor rehabilitation.

IV. **Biofeedback**
  A. Biofeedback explained
    1. Biofeedback is a training method for urinary incontinence that gives quick and accurate information about the woman's ability to contract and relax her pelvic floor muscles.
    2. Based on the principle that the use of visual information and positive reinforcement can train a woman to correctly identify her pelvic floor muscles and return them to their normal level of function
    3. It is not a treatment per se but a teaching technique, which uses the tracings seen on the computer screen from both the surface and internal sensors to change or modify behavior.
    4. Provides immediate feedback on when to alter a physiologic response
    5. The woman can "see" and control the correct activation of the selected muscles.
      a. When a woman contracts her pelvic floor muscle against the sensor, the computer screen displays a PFM contraction as the tracing rises in response.
      b. Once found, the correct innervation can be linked with the corresponding body feeling, which again effectively trains the body awareness ("muscular reeducation").
  B. Training session
    1. Woman is seated comfortably in front of the computer screen with skin electrodes and vaginal sensors in place (Figure 38.5).
    2. When a woman performs a rectal squeeze, the muscles contract against the silver plate and show a simultaneous rise in the waveform tracing as displayed on the computer screen (see Figure 38.6).

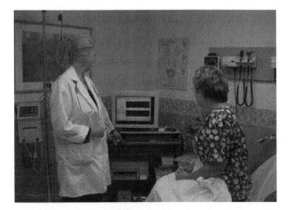

FIGURE 38.5 Training session.
Photo by author.

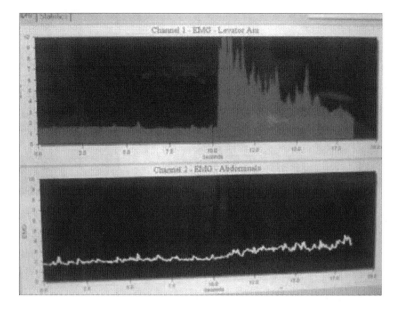

FIGURE 38.6 Sample tracing. The top screen shows muscle activity from the internal vaginal sensor. The woman relaxes for 10 seconds and then tightens and holds for 10 seconds. The contraction diminishes as the woman attempts to hold the contraction, indicating a weak muscle. The bottom screen gives information from the surface sensors and shows a slight rise during the contraction, indicating that the woman is using her abdominal muscles (accessory) to assist in the contraction.

Photo by author.

3. On viewing the tracings, the women is assisted in how to modify her behavior and identify and isolate her PFM while keeping her accessory muscles quiet.
4. During the therapy session, the clinician provides verbal "biofeedback" regarding how well she identifies the correct muscles and use of incorrect muscles.
5. Goals are summarized in Table 38.4.
C. Requirements for insurance coverage of biofeedback
   1. Woman must be
      a. Physically capable of participating in treatment plan
      b. Motivated to comply with exercise regime at home.
      c. Trained on a one-to-one basis, with face-to-face involvement between patient and practitioner
      d. Most insurance will pay for up to six visits.

TABLE 38.4

GOALS
Identify and isolate the PFMs from the accessory muscles.
Increase pelvic muscle strength.
Ensure utilization of the correct muscles.
Avoid unwanted contraction of the accessory muscles.
Increase sensory perception and "muscle awareness."

D. Follow-up
   1. Visits every 1 to 3 weeks depending on woman's response and progress
   2. Often takes 2 to 3 weeks to learn how to develop muscle awareness and to isolate the pelvic floor
   3. Needs to practice the Kegel exercises at home as described above
   4. Daily exercise is the key to continued success and bladder control. Appendix 38.1 is a sample handout of exercises for the woman to practice at home.

Bibliography

Berghmans, L. C., Frederiks, C. M., de Bie, R. A., Weil, E. H., Smeets, L. W., van Waalwijk van Doorn, E. S., Janknegt, R. A. (1996). Efficacy of biofeedback when included with pelvic floor muscle exercise treatment for genuine stress incontinence. *Neurourol Urodyn, 15*(1), 37–52.

Bø, K., & Hilde, G. (2012). Does it work in the long term? A systematic review on pelvic floor muscle training for female stress urinary incontinence. *Neurourol Urodyn.* doi:10.1002/nau.22292

Gadel Hak, N., El-Hemaly, M., Hamdy, E., … Hamed, H. (2011, March). Pelvic floor dyssynergia: Efficacy of biofeedback training. *Arab Journal of Gastroenterology* (the official publication of the Pan-Arab Association of Gastroenterology), *12*(1), 15–19.

Goode, P. S., Burgio, K. L., Johnson, T. M. 2nd, … Lloyd, L. K. (2011). Behavioral therapy with or without biofeedback and pelvic floor electrical stimulation for persistent postprostatectomy incontinence. *The Journal of the American Medical, 305*(2), 151–159. doi: 10.1001/jama.2010.1072

Hay-Smith, J., Morkved, S., Fairbrother, K. A., & Herbison, G. P. (2008, October 8). Pelvic floor muscle training for prevention and treatment of urinary and faecal incontinence in antenatal and postnatal women. *Cochrane Database of Systematic Reviews* (4), CD007471.

Herderschee, R., Hay-Smith, E. J., Herbison, G. P., Roovers, J. P., Heineman, M. J. (2011). Feedback or biofeedback to augment pelvic floor muscle training for urinary incontinence in women. *Cochrane Database of Systematic Reviews* (7), CD009252.

Kegel, A. H. (1948). Progressive resistance exercise in the functional restoration of the perineal muscle. *American Journal of Obstetrics and Gynecology, 56,* 238–249.

Kincade, J. F., Dougherty, M. C., Busby-Whitehead, J., ... Rix, A. D. (2005). Self-monitoring and pelvic floor muscle exercises to treat urinary incontinence. *Urologic Nursing, 25*(5), 353–363.

Lukban, J., & Whitmore, K. (2002). Pelvic floor muscle re-education treatment of the overactive bladder and painful bladder syndrome. *Clinics in Obstetrics and Gynecology, 45*(1), 273–285.

Neumann, P. B., Grimmer, K. A., & Deenadayalan, Y. (2006). Pelvic floor muscle training and adjunctive therapies for the treatment of stress urinary incontinence in women: A systemic review. *BMC Women's Health, 6,* 11. doi: 10.1186/1472-6874-6-11

Sievert, K. D., Amend, B., Toomey, P. A., Robinson, D., Milsom, I., Koelbl, H., ... Newman, D. K. (2012). Can we prevent incontinence? ICI-RS 2011. *Neurourology and Urodynamics, 31*(3), 390–399.

Tremback-Bell, A., Levine, A. M., Dawson, G., & Perlis, S. M. (2012, September/December). Young women's self-efficacy in performing pelvic muscle exercises. *Journal of Women's Health Physical Therapy, 36*(3), 158–163. doi: 10.1097/JWH.0b013e318276f4a7

Tremback-Bell, A., Levine, A. M., Dawson, G., & Perlis, S. M. (2013, January/April). Young women's urinary incontinence perceived educational needs. *Journal of Women's Health Physical Therapy, 37*(1), 29–34. doi: 10.1097/JWH.0bo13e31828c1a94

APPENDIX

Pelvic Fitness in Just Minutes a Day!

Life events can weaken pelvic muscles. Pregnancy, childbirth, and being over-weight can also do it. When the muscles in your lower pelvis get weak, any event that puts pressure on the bladder, such as coughing, sneezing, or laugh-ing, can cause leakage of urine, often at inconvenient times. This is called *stress incontinence*. Fortunately, there are exercises you can do to help make your muscles strong again. Pelvic muscles are like any other muscle; the more you exercise them, the stronger they become. It is pure mechanics. The more you exercise the pelvic floor muscle, the more it "bulks up." The more it "bulks up," the more pressure it exerts on your urethra, and the more pressure and compression on the sphincter muscles of your urethra, the less possibility of leaking. Simple enough.

1. *What is the pelvic muscle?* Your pelvic muscle provides support to your bladder, the vagina, and the uterus. If it weakens, it cannot support these organs and their position can change. This change in position can cause problems with normal function. Keeping the muscle strong can help prevent unwanted urine leakage.

2. *Finding the pelvic muscle.* The pelvic floor muscle is a big strap that supports your lower abdomen. It extends from the pubic bone in front to the tailbone at the base of your spine. When abdominal forces (jogging, coughing) overcome the strength of the pelvic muscle to hold urine in, you will leak, as you well know.

There are two ways to find it.

Without tensing the muscles of your leg, buttocks, or abdomen, imagine that you are trying to control the passing of gas or pinching off a stool. Or imagine you are in an elevator full of people and you feel the urge to pass gas. What do you do? You tighten or pull in the ring of muscle around your rectum. You should feel a lifting sensation in the area around the vagina or a pulling in of your rectum. It is *not* a vaginal tightening.

Another simple way is to try to stop or interrupt the flow of urine when sitting on a toilet. If you can do it, then you are using the right muscles. Sitting on the toilet, however, is not a good place to practice because of the unnatural position. Do not be discouraged if you are unable to stop or change the flow. Slowing the flow is a good start. There is no need to do this start-and-stop test on a regular basis. It is not a helpful way to exercise the pelvic floor muscles but might help you judge how you are improving.

When you first begin your exercise program, check yourself frequently by looking in a mirror or by placing your hands on your abdomen and buttocks to ensure that you do not feel your belly, thighs, or buttocks move. Remember . . . no abs, hips, or butts! If there is movement, continue to experiment until you have isolated the correct muscles of the pelvic floor. This may take a few days but do not give up. Also do not feel discouraged that you may not have been practicing the Kegels correctly over the past few years. Research suggests that more than 60% of woman do not use the right muscles.

3. *Practice makes perfect.* You can exercise any time or any place. No one needs to know what you are doing with your pelvic floor while sitting in the beauty parlor or commuting to work. When practicing, it is a good idea to alternate among lying, sitting, and standing. Some women find it helpful to have a "trigger" to remember the exercises by. It may be stopping at a stop sign or turning on the hot water faucet. It is a good idea to do exercises before getting out of bed in the morning and before sleep in the evening.

Now that you have found the right muscles to squeeze, there are two types of exercise you will need to perform. The pelvic floor muscle consists of two types of muscle fibers: short and long. Both are very different and each needs to be exercised differently. Most people do not know this and only do one type of exercise. That is only half of it.

The first exercise works on the long fibers and measures the holding ability of the muscles (building a strong dam to hold back urine). It is done by slowly tightening, lifting, and drawing in the rectal muscles and holding them to a count of five, then relaxing for count of five. Squeeze and lift the rectal area (the vaginal area comes along with it) without tightening the buttocks or belly (abdomen). If you sense a "pulling," then you are using the right muscles. Remember, most of the muscles of the pelvic are contracted rectally, not vaginally. At first, you will probably notice that the muscles do not want to stay contracted or tightened very long. If you feel the contraction letting go, just retighten the muscles. In fact, in the beginning, you may only be able to hold the contraction for 1 to 2 seconds. In a week or two, you will notice an improvement in the control and holding power of the contractions. The goal is to be able to maintain the tightening or squeeze for 10 seconds, with a 10-second relaxation period.

To practice this exercise, totally relax your body, tighten and hold for 5 to 10 seconds, and relax for the same amount of time. Do 10 reps in a row, three times a day.

The second exercise is a quick contraction, known as a "quick flick." This exercises the short muscle fibers of the pelvic floor. They are found around the sphincter. The rectal muscles are quickly tightened, lifted up, and let go. This strengthens the muscles that quickly shut off the flow of urine (like a faucet).

You should quickly squeeze five times to 10 times in a row, three to five times a day. Be sure to relax completely between each contraction. You should also use triggers to remember to do these.

Other Hints

Avoid at all cost any activity that puts pressure on your pelvic floor, such as lifting weights or other heavy objects. Never lift your child as a dead weight. Stand near a table or chair and lift the child to a standing position on the chair. Squeeze your rectal muscles while doing so. From that position, you can lift them into your arms.

Avoid constipation. Never push hard to have a bowel movement—just sit and relax. Daily fish oil, one to two capsules, two to three times a day, should do it.

These exercises really work! This is *not* a quick cure. You have had this condition for a long time, so it will take a long time to see any improvement. If you practice as directed, your muscle strength should increase 10% every 2 to 3 weeks.

Good luck . . . and remember to *squeeze!*

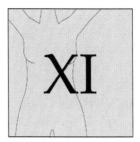

XI

Advanced Skills

Vulvar Cancer and Biopsy 39

Helen A. Carcio

I. **Vulvar cancer explained**
   A. Statistics
      1. Accounts for 0.7% of all female cancers, occurring in 1.8 per 100,000 women
      2. Is the fourth most common malignant tumor of the female genital tract
      3. It causes 500 deaths annually in the United States
   B. Occurrence
      1. Occurs most frequently in women older than 65 years
      2. Incidence is rising in younger women
      3. Usually diagnosed in the localized stage (about 60%)
   C. Surgery is the usual treatment.
   D. Most tumors are squamous cell in origin.
   E. Long-standing pruritus is the most common complaint.
   F. The most frequent site is the labia minora, in the middle or anterior portion.
   G. Risk factors
      1. History of herpes simplex virus type 2 (HSV2) or human papillomavirus (HPV)
      2. Multiple sexual partners
      3. Smoking, especially if history of HPV
      4. History of cervical cancer
      5. History of lichen sclerosus (LSA). Four percent of women who have LSA will later develop vulvar cancer.
   H. Early detection is key to reducing mortality rates.
   I. Indications
      1. All white lesions of the vulva must undergo biopsy study if short-term medical treatment is unsuccessful. Two thirds of the lesions appear acetowhite (white when vinegar is applied).
      2. Any suspicious lesions of any color and persistent ulcerations should be excised.

3. Visible lesion for which definitive diagnosis cannot be made on clinical grounds
4. Suspicion of possible malignancy
5. Visible lesion with presumed clinical diagnosis that is not responding to usual therapy

II. **Nonneoplastic epithelial disorders of the vulvar skin and mucosa**
   A. Squamous hyperplasia
      1. Proliferative response to an irritant or allergen that has become chronic
      2. The presenting symptom is pruritus, with or without vulvodynia.
      3. Suspect all substances that come in contact with the vulvar skin (see Box 39.1 for a list of vulvar irritants).
      4. Assessment includes
         a. Thick white patches caused by localized thickening of the epidermis (lichenification)
         b. Raised lesions, often bilaterally symmetric
         c. Vulva may appear dusky red in color.
         d. Vulvar skin thickened with prominent skin markings (Perdu's sign)
      5. Diagnosis
         a. Punch biopsy
         b. Histologic findings of acanthosis (irregular thickening of the malpighian layer), hyperkeratosis, and inflammatory infiltrate
   B. Lichen sclerosis
      1. Related to hormonal, genetic, and immunologic interactions
      2. Usually seen after a long period of self-diagnosis and treatment
      3. Symptoms include intractable itching, with or without vulvodynia
      4. Assessment includes
         a. Bluish-white papules, which progress to form thin white patches
         b. Tissue is friable and may develop petechiae.
         c. Skin is thin and wrinkles like parchment paper.
      5. Diagnosis
         a. Punch biopsy
         b. Histologic findings include loss of rete layers, homogenization, and inflammatory infiltrate
   C. Vulvar dermatologic manifestations that may be associated with systemic disease; may not need to be excised if the systemic condition is well documented
      1. Bechet's disease
         a. Small vesicles that ulcerate
         b. Systemic areas include oral ulcerations with uveitis and arthritis

---

┌─┐
│ │ **BOX 39.1** *Substances That May Cause Vulvar Irritation*
└─┘

- Laundry detergents/fabric softeners
- Chlorine bleach
- Fiberglass particles (residue in washing machine after washing fiberglass materials such as curtains)
- Propylene glycol in spermicides, lubricants, and vaginal medications
- Formalin found in the wool of permanent press fabrics
- Nylon (can give off formaldehyde vapors)
- Deodorant substances on sanitary pads and liners
- Vaginal sprays and douches
- Creams in topical antifungal agents
- Synthetic-fiber underwear
- Fabric dyes, especially in colored underwear
- Saliva
- Semen
- Bromine and chlorine compounds in hot tubs and swimming pools
- Prescribed medications such as antifungals, antibacterials, crotamiton

Note: The distribution of lesions may provide a clue to which agent may be responsible for the allergic reaction.

---

2. Pellagra
   a. A history of anorexia or poor dietary intake
   b. Hyperpigmentation and peeling of the vulva
   c. Systemic areas include dry scaly body skin with erythema of the mucous membrane.
3. Diabetes
   a. Chronic pruritus of vulva and erythema with a gray sheen
   b. Systemic areas include dry body skin and changes related to the kidney, retina, and heart.
4. Crohn's disease
   a. Knifelike slits in vulvar folds
   b. Associated with gastrointestinal problems of varying degree

III. **Differential diagnosis of other vulvar dermatoses**
   A. Table 39.1 compares and contrasts other dermatoses.
   B. A biopsy may be indicated because symptoms vary and may be cancerous.

IV. **Vulvar biopsy**
   A. Vulvar biopsy is a simple office procedure that is virtually free of complications and usually does not cause discomfort for the patient.

TABLE 39.1 Differential Diagnosis of Other Vulvar Dermatoses

CONDITION	CLINICAL CHARACTERISTICS	OTHER SKIN AREAS AFFECTED
Papulosquamous lesions		
Contact dermatitis	Pruritus, history of exposure to irritant or allergen, erythema and edema in contact areas	Other areas in contact with irritant/allergen, although vulvar skin more sensitive
Lichen simplex chronicus	Pruritus, history of chronic irritation, thickened, leathery skin with accentuated skin markings	Not common
Lichen planus	Pruritus, purplish plaques defined by cross-hatched skin lines	Flat-topped papules on wrist, lumbar back, thighs, lacey pattern on buccal mucosa
Seborrheic dermatitis	Usually pruritus, yellow or red lesions covered by greasy scales in areas of sebaceous glands	Face, scalp, particularly eyebrows and hairline
Psoriasis	Mild pruritus, red plaques or silvery scales with bleeding points beneath	Silvery plaques on scalp, knees, elbows, sacrum
Tinea curis	Variable, but usually dry, erythematous, annular lesions	May spread to buttocks and inner thighs
Vesiculobullous lesions		
Erythema multiforme	History of recent genital herpes or drug allergy, "iris-shaped" lesions	Target lesions, especially on palms and soles
Pemphigus	Blisters and erosion	Any other skin areas on body
Infections		
Folliculitis	Tiny, red papules with white pustular center punctured by hair shaft	Any other skin in hairy areas
Impetigo	Superficial ulcer with yellow crust	Usually spread from infection of other body parts

B. It is appropriate to use on lesions smaller than 0.5 cm. Refer larger lesions to a gynecologist.

C. The procedure takes approximately 15 minutes.

D. Excising all lesions, particularly fissures, ulcerations, or thick plaques, is mandatory because of the risk of cancer, no matter how small (only 1% to 2% risk).

E. Must be a full-thickness biopsy sample

F. Histologic findings are diagnostic

V. Assessment

A. Ask about other dermatologic conditions on other parts of the body because a condition such as psoriasis can occur on the vulva.

B. Carefully evaluate the vagina and cervix, remembering that discharge from these areas bathes the vulvar tissues.

C. Perform a vaginal wet mount (see Chapter 10, "Assessment of Menopausal Status") on any discharge.

VI. Indications

A. To differentiate between benign and malignant conditions: Women who smoke or who are infected with HPV 16 or HSV 2 are at higher risk for vulvar cancer.

   1. If the patient is seropositive, she is at even higher risk.

      a. Women with HPV seropositivity are three and a half times more likely to develop in situ disease and more than two and a half times more likely to develop invasive disease.

   2. The more a woman smokes and the longer she smokes, the greater the risk.

      a. Current smokers are at almost six and a half times the risk for in situ disease and at three times the risk for invasive disease.

B. Confirm histologic characteristics

VII. Patient preparation

A. Explain that discomfort during the procedure is usually minimal.

B. The reasons for the biopsy study should be explained and the technique should be outlined.

VIII. The procedure

A. Some comments

   1. It is important to have good lighting.

   2. Use of 5% acetic acid can greatly enhance identification of atypical areas such as intraepithelial neoplasia or HPV infection, which will often turn aceto-white a few minutes after application on the vulva.

   3. Toluidine blue dye is no longer used owing to the high rate of false-positive and false-negative results.

4. A large magnifying lens is essential to highlight abnormal areas for biopsy study.
5. Colposcopy may be used and is particularly helpful in diagnosing HPV infection (usually not available in primary care settings).

B. Equipment
   1. Hand magnifying lens (or colposcope)
   2. Betadine swabs
   3. Anesthetic agent
   4. A 25-gauge needle
   5. Syringe—0.3 mL
   6. Two- to 4-mm Keyes's punch biopsy (disposable)
   7. Iris forceps
   8. Fine scissors
   9. Monsel's paste or silver nitrate sticks
   10. Sterile gauze sponges
   11. Labeled pathology container of formalin
   12. Paperwork for lab requisition
   13. Acetic acid (vinegar)

C. Identify area to be biopsied. Multiple biopsy sites (two to three) may be indicated.

D. Anesthesia
   1. Local infiltration of 1% Xylocaine without epinephrine
   2. Inject anesthetic solution subdermally with fine-gauge needle (0.5–1 mL per site).
   3. A wheal (4–5 mm) is created, which facilitates the biopsy by raising the lesion above the dermas and promotes local vasoconstriction, minimizing blood loss.

E. The biopsy procedure
   1. Cleanse area using antiseptic solution or iodine-soaked swabs.
   2. The dermal punch is like a corkborer.
   3. Place the punch biopsy over the site, and rotate back and forth three or four times while holding the skin taut with the opposite hand (an assistant may be recruited to hold the skin)
   4. The epithelium and dermis should be cut until the proper thickness is obtained.
   5. Bore out in a circular manner.
      a. Depth comes with practice—too deep of a cut results in cutting large blood vessels, increasing bleeding.
      b. Too shallow a cut results in loss of an identifiable plug.
   6. Once a plug is made, remove the cutter.
   7. Grasp the plug with the forceps and separate from the skin. Snip dermal skin areas transversely to sever the base with scissors.
   8. If the plug is lifted off and remains in the punch, dislodge the plug from the punch using a toothpick.

F. Control bleeding
1. Bleeding is usually minimal because the dermis contains few blood vessels.
2. Pressure may be all that is required to stop any bleeding.
3. Use silver nitrate to cauterize area or put a drop of Monsel's solution over the site for hemostasis.
4. If bleeding persists, add a single suture using 4-0 Vicryl or Chromic.
5. A sanitary pad may be used for additional pressure.
G. Laboratory preparation
1. Gently place the sample in formalin and properly label the container.
2. Complete required forms.
3. Document biopsy site(s) and the procedure itself, including the patient's response.
4. If biopsy samples from different sites are obtained, place in separate containers and label with the site.

IX. **Follow-up**
A. Care of the biopsy site
1. The patient is instructed to keep the incision clean and dry.
2. Baths should be taken daily until any soreness is gone.
3. Blot dry. Be careful not to remove any healing scab.
4. Reassure the patient that the biopsy site will become practically invisible in 1 to 2 weeks.
5. Avoid intercourse for 2 or 3 days.
B. The patient is instructed to call if any redness or increasing discomfort occurs or the signs of infection develop such as pus formation.
C. Return to discuss results and recommendations for treatment.

X. **Complications: Rare bleeding or infection; occasional oozing from the site may persist.**

XI. **Teach vulvar self-examination**
A. Most vulvar malignancies are visible.
1. Vulvar examination should be performed monthly by women who are sexually active or who are older than 18 years of age.
2. The patient must recognize the importance of early detection of vulvar disease.
3. Understand the basic vulvar anatomy and function.
4. Learn the proper use of a handheld mirror to optimize viewing the vulva.
5. Perform the examination monthly between menses.
6. Report any new growths or changes.

Bibliography

American Cancer Society. (2013). *Cancer facts and figures 2013.* Atlanta, GA: American Cancer Society.

Carter, J. S., & Downs, L. S. Jr. (2012). Vulvar and vaginal cancer. *Obstetrics & Gynecology Clinics of North America, 39,* 213.

Darney, P. D., Horbach, N. S., & Kom, A. P. (2005). *Protocols for office gynecologic surgery.* Cambridge: Blackwell Science.

Elkas, J. C., Berek, J. S., & Goff, B. K. (2012). *Vulvar cancer: Staging, treatment and prognosis.* Retrieved August 1, 2012, from http://www.uptodate.com/index

Frequently Asked Questions. (2012). Gynecologic problems FAQ088. Disorders of the vulva. *American College of Obstetrics and Gynecology.* Retrieved August 1, 2012, from http://www.acog.org/For_Patients

Fuh, K. C., & Berek, J. S. (2012). Current management of vulvar cancer. *Hematology/ Oncology Clinics of North America, 26,* 45.

Goldstein, G. R., & Goldstein, A. T. (2009, May). Punch biopsy for the evaluation of vulvar dermatoses. *The Journal of Sexual Medicine, 6*(5), 1214–1217. [Medline]

Kaufman, R. (1997). Vulvar examination and biopsy. In M. J. Evans, M. P. Johnson, & K. S. Moghissi (Eds.), *Invasive outpatient procedures in reproductive medicine* (pp. 143–149). Philadelphia, PA: Lippincott.

Endometrial Biopsy

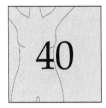

40

Helen A. Carcio

I. **Endometrial biopsy explained. Endometrial biopsy examination is used mainly to diagnose endometrial cancer and the presence of a luteal-phase defect (LPD).**
   A. It is a method of removing a sample of representative tissue from the endometrium.
      1. It provides a histologic specimen of glandular epithelium from the uterine endometrial wall.
      2. It may be referred to as endometrial sampling because of the negative connotations that arise with the use of the word "biopsy."
      3. It is inexpensive and usually well tolerated by the woman.
      4. It is relatively easy to perform and can be performed appropriately by a trained nurse practitioner, midwife, or physician assistant.
      5. Advances in pipelles have made the procedure relatively simple to perform in the office, without the need for general anesthesia.
      6. Although the technique is relatively easy to perform by the clinician, it is often viewed as invasive by the patient.
      7. Although it is a blind procedure, its accuracy rate in identifying endometrial hyperplasia is greater than 90%.

II. **Some comments concerning endometrial cancer**
   A. Incidence
      1. Cancer accounts for nearly 8% of all cancers in women.
      2. Most common gynecological malignancy
      3. American Cancer Society estimates 49,560 new diagnoses and 8,190 deaths in 2013.
      4. Incidence is higher in Black and Hispanic women than in White and Asian women.
      5. Most uterine cancers are adenocarcinoma of the endometrium.

B. Risk factors
   1. Age: The incidence of endometrial cancer increases with age, particularly in those older than 65 years.
   2. Rare in women younger than 45 years
   3. Obesity causes an increase in the presence of exogenous estrogens from peripheral conversions of estrogen in the fat cells.
      a. No progesterone is present to counterbalance the excess estrogen (unless on hormone replacement therapy [HRT]).
      b. Uterine cancer develops in women who are more than 50 pounds overweight 10 times more frequently than in women who are average weight.
   4. Hyperestrogenic state is possibly related to the following
      a. Polycystic ovarian syndrome
      b. Early menarche
      c. Late menopause
   5. Use of unopposed estrogen
      a. During the 1950s and 1960s, estrogen was given as replacement therapy without progesterone.
      b. This practice caused a dramatic increase in the occurrence of endometrial cancer.
      c. Clinicians are now aware of the need to use progesterone supplementation with estrogen replacement therapy or to monitor the endometrium in a woman unwilling or unable to take progesterone.
   6. Use of tamoxifen therapy as treatment for women with breast cancer
      a. It is antiestrogenic to breast tissue.
      b. It has an estrogenic effect on the lining of the uterus.
      c. It may contribute to endometrial stimulation, resulting in eventual hyperplasia and possible cancer.
      d. Its benefits in treating breast cancer probably outweigh the risk for development of endometrial cancer.
   7. Endometrial hyperplasia and endometrial polyps
   8. Previous breast or ovarian cancer
   9. Nulliparity
      a. The risk for endometrial cancer is twice as high than in a woman who has one child.
      b. The risk is three times as high than in a woman who has five children.
   10. A personal history of hypertension or diabetes
C. Protective factors: Progesterone use greatly diminishes hyperplasia of the endometrium. Oral contraceptives, particularly if used during the later reproductive years
D. Clinical features
   1. Abnormal uterine bleeding, particularly in postmenopausal women, including

a. Heavy menses
b. Intermenstrual bleeding
c. Frequent menstruation
2. The older the woman, the higher the level of suspicion should be.
3. Endometrial cells found on a Pap smear

III. **Some comments concerning LPD**
A. The condition exists when the corpus luteum secretes an inadequate amount of progesterone.
B. Three percent to 4% of infertile women have LPD.
C. LPD is suspected when the luteal phase (the interval between ovulation and menstruation) is less than 11 days.
D. Causes
1. Inadequate progesterone production by the granulosa cells of the ovary
2. Hyperprolactinemia, which can cause an abnormal luteal phase
3. Psychogenic stress, nutritional factors, and exercise can cause a deficiency in the luteinizing hormone (LH) pulse.
4. Kidney, liver, and immunologic diseases affect the corpus luteum cells.

IV. **Endometrial biopsy examination explained**
A. Historical perspective
1. Endometrial biopsy was first performed as early as the Ancient Greek era and was originally used as a treatment for abnormal uterine bleeding.
2. In the 1950s, the normal characteristics of the endometrium were established, which led to the ability to apply endometrial dating to help diagnose LPDs.
B. Relationship to dilatation and curettage (D&C)
1. Use of endometrial biopsy as a screen has replaced the need for D&C, which was previously the gold standard in many cases.
2. Recent studies found results were histologically similar between specimens collected by D&C and those obtained by endometrial biopsy.
3. Endometrial biopsy is more cost-effective and less invasive.

V. **Indications for biopsy study**
A. Complaints of uterine bleeding in any postmenopausal woman: The level of concern should increase with the patient's advancing age, particularly if the woman
1. Is obese
2. Is taking unopposed estrogen replacement therapy (ERT)
3. Has had no spotting or bleeding for 12 months or longer
4. The bleeding is excessive, prolonged, or irregular.
5. Is taking cyclic ERT with an increase in bleeding pattern

  B. Postmenopausal women in whom bleeding begins or increases (if previously present) with the initiation of hormone replacement therapy that does not resolve after 3 to 6 months of therapy

    1. Some providers perform endometrial biopsy before the initiation of ERT, but most do not consider it necessary.

  C. Monitoring endometrial response to hormonal influences of unopposed ERT in those women undergoing ERT who are unable or unwilling to take progesterone

    1. Progesterone protects the endometrium from the effects of unopposed estrogen.

      a. Women who are not taking progesterone are at increased risk for hyperplasia, which may lead to adenocarcinoma.

      b. Must monitor the patient yearly and document that the woman is aware of the increased risk for development of endometrial cancer

      c. Biopsy study is sufficient, but the woman may choose to undergo ultrsonography to measure the width of the endometrial stripe.

        (1) The uterine lining is seen as a thin line or stripe.

        (2) The width of the stripe determines whether the lining of the uterus has thickened due to hyperplasia.

          • Less than 5 mm: No hyperplasia

          • Between 5 and 10 mm: Gray zone

          • Greater than 10: Hyperplasia

  D. Endometrial cells found on a routine Pap smear, especially

    1. If taken more than 10 days from the first day of the menstrual period

    2. In any patient older than 40 years of age

    3. In the presence of irregular bleeding

  E. Infertile women with suspected LPD

    1. Documents endometrial response to progesterone

    2. Evaluates the luteal phase, for endometrial dating in an infertile woman suspected of having an LPD

      a. A discrepancy of more than 2 days between the woman's endometrial histologic stage and menstrual dating is diagnostically significant.

    3. Also obtains valuable information about the patency of the cervical os

  F. It is rarely performed before age 40 because 95% of cancers occur in woman older than 40 years of age. Box 40.1 lists the exceptions.

  G. Women who are undergoing tamoxifen treatment for breast cancer

  H. Follow-up of abnormal ultrasound if endometrial thickness (stripe) is greater than 5 mm

  I. Women in whom pelvic inflammatory disease (PID) is suspected (controversial)

> ## BOX 40.1 *Indications for Biopsy Study Before Age 40*
>
> Biopsy study before age 40 is only indicated if the following factors are present:
> - Obesity (may have higher levels of estrogen)
> - Long-standing anovulation or irregulär menstrual cycles
> - History of other adenocarcinomas such as of the breast or colon
> - Functional metrorrhagia with dysfunctional uterine bleeding

1. Endometritis is a fairly frequent cause of irregular bleeding in young women.
2. Endometritis often precedes and then accompanies salpingitis.
3. Offers an objective test in the diagnosis of PID to improve diagnostic accuracy
   a. Positive if histologic findings of plasma cell endometritis are found

VI. **Contraindications to biopsy study**
   A. Pregnancy or poorly involuted postpartum uterus (a sensitive pregnancy test can be performed before)
   B. Infection
      1. Any infection can be passed into the uterine cavity and tubes as the pipelle passes through the cervical os.
      2. Active or chronic cervicitis: Defer until treated.
      3. Active or chronic vaginitis: Defer until treated.
   C. Uterine abnormalities such as a large myoma displacing the uterus, making obtaining of sample impossible
   D. Blood dyscrasias or suspected bleeding disorder
   E. Woman is febrile. Note: If there is a history of valvular heart disease or rheumatic fever, bacterial endocarditis is a risk and antibiotic prophylaxis is appropriate.

VII. **Examination of the woman**
   A. Subjective information must include
      1. Date of last menstrual period (LMP)
      2. Use of contraception; discuss compliance issues
      3. Risk-evaluation for sexually transmitted diseases (STDs) and human immunodeficiency virus (HIV)
      4. History of any bleeding problems
      5. Presence of symptoms of vaginal or cervical infections
      6. History of heart disease, especially rheumatic heart disease or mitral valve prolapse
      7. Allergies, especially to lidocaine (Xylocaine) or povidone-iodine (Betadine)

8. Level of pain associated with previous Pap smears
9. History of vasovagal episode or hypoglycemia
10. Inquire about food eaten that day. Offer sweetened juice to prevent a vasovagal reaction.
B. Objective findings
   1. Obtain vital signs, including temperature.
   2. Perform pelvic examination to assess for any signs of infection.
   3. Perform laboratory tests, if indicated.
      a. Sensitive pregnancy test
      b. Hematocrit
      c. Wet mount examination (see Chapter 31, "Vaginal Miscroscopy")

VIII. **Supplies**
   A. Supplies
      1. Nonsterile gloves
      2. Vaginal speculum
      3. Tenaculum
      4. Aseptic solution (Betadine)
      5. Cotton rectal swab
      6. Sterile pipelle (two)
      7. Biopsy sample container (10% formalin or other fixative)
      8. Two percent to 10% viscous lidocaine gels and Hurricane gel
      9. Sterile lubricant
   B. Characteristics of the pipelle
      1. Advances in the pipelle have made the procedure relatively simple to perform in the office without the need for general anesthesia.
      2. Single-use, disposable, clear instrument with colored, graduated markings graded from 4 cm to 10 cm
      3. Flexible polypropylene
      4. Size: Small caliber, 3.1 cm (outside diameter) and 2.6 cm (inner diameter); 23.5 cm in length
      5. Use: Histologic biopsy of uterine mucosal lining or sample extraction of uterine menstrual content
      6. Negative pressure: Rapid movement of the piston creates a negative pressure within the lumen of the sheath, allowing for aspiration of the mucosal tissue through the curette opening and into the lumen of the tube as the curette scrapes against the endometrial walls while being moved within the uterine cavity. The piston cannot be fully pulled out.

IX. **Preparation**
   A. Timing in the evaluation of LPD
      1. Performed 1 to 3 days before the expected onset of menses (take average of previous cycles)

2. Menses may begin on the day of the scheduled biopsy procedure because the timing is close. If this occurs, the biopsy procedure must be rescheduled for the next cycle, but a day or two earlier.

B. Can schedule evaluation of abnormal uterine bleeding or endometrial monitoring at any time

C. Analgesia
   1. Many clinicians suggest the use of nonsteroidal antiinflammatory medication in the event that mild cramping occurs.
   2. Administer ibuprofen, 400 mg, 30 to 60 minutes before the scheduled visit.

D. Anesthesia: In patients who are very sensitive to pain, topical anesthesia such as 20% benzocaine (Hurricane) can be applied to the cervix a few minutes before the procedure.

X. Informed consent and education

A. The clinician must clearly explain
   1. How much pain to expect
   2. Reasons for the procedure
   3. Risks involved, including perforation of the uterus, failure to obtain tissue, and infection
   4. Overall safety
   5. Realistic expectation of what will occur during the procedure
   6. What the results may indicate

B. Verbal or written consent should be obtained and documented.

XI. The procedure

A. Position: The woman is asked to assume a comfortable dorsal lithotomy position.

B. Bimanual examination
   1. A bimanual pelvic examination is first performed to determine the position and size of the uterus and to assess for any pelvic tenderness.
   2. A rectal examination may be necessary if the uterus is retroverted.
   3. Helps determine the direction of insertion of the catheter
   4. It is important to assess the size of the uterus so that its proper depth can be determined.

C. Use of lubricant: A lubricant should not be used because it may prevent proper interpretation of cervical cytology tests.

XII. Technique

A. Put on gloves (sterile gloves are not necessary). Care should be taken not to touch the parts of the instruments that will come in contact with the cervix or the endometrial cavity.

B. The speculum is inserted into the vagina, and the cervical os is visualized.

    1. The cervix should be well positioned, facing directly outward, between the blades of the speculum. (This helps with the insertion technique.)

C. Inspection

    1. The vagina and cervix are inspected for the presence of any usual discharge.

    2. If an infection is suspected, a wet mount examination should be performed.

        a. If white blood cells are present, the condition should be diagnosed and treated.

        b. Reschedule biopsy surgery for the next cycle.

D. Cleansing the area

    1. Using a rectal swab, the cervix and upper vagina are next swabbed free of discharge and cleansed with an antiseptic such as Betadine.

    2. Any excess Betadine should be removed to prevent contamination of the specimen.

E. Use of a tenaculum for anteflexion or retroflexion

    1. A tenaculum is usually not necessary.

    2. It is only used 15% of the time.

    3. If it is used, a lidocaine gel should be placed at the site the tenaculum will grasp for 5 minutes, or 1% lidocaine (0.5–1.0 ml) should be injected at the tenaculum site via a spinal needle. Either method will significantly reduce the pain of tenaculum application.

    4. The tenaculum may be necessary to stabilize the cervix and straighten the uterus to facilitate passage of the pipelle if there is a marked degree of anteflexion or retroflexion.

        a. Anteflexion

            (1) Grasp the anterior upper lip of the cervix between 2 o'clock and 10 o'clock. (Warn the patient that she will feel a pinch.)

            (2) This technique should compress approximately 1 cm of cervical tissue. (The tissue immediately turns white.)

            (3) Gently pull the cervix forward to straighten the cervical canal.

            (4) Guide the curved tip along the anterior surface of the endocervical canal.

        b. Retroflexion

            (1) Grasp the posterior lip of the cervix.

            (2) Guide the curved tip along the posterior surface of the endocervical canal.

        c. Remember that the uterine artery runs laterally at 3 o'clock and 9 o'clock.

5. The clinician may manually curve the tip of the pipelle while it is in the sterile package to accommodate the curvature of the uterus.
6. If the tip is not curved, the straight tip may become embedded into the posterior or anterior wall of the canal.

F. Pipelle insertion
1. If a topical anesthetic is being used, instill it into the cervical os using a swab.
2. Once the position of the uterus has been assessed; the cervical os, positioned, a thin pipelle or catheter is passed through the cervix, into the uterus to the fundus.
3. The tip of the catheter can be bent manually for easier insertion to accommodate the natural curve of the endocervical canal.
4. However, the clinician must be aware that the rigidness of the catheter may slightly increase chances of accidental perforation.
5. It is usually not necessary to sound the uterus.
6. Hold the pipelle lightly with a grip similar to holding a pencil.
7. As the pipelle is inserted through the cervix, the resistance of the internal os is felt as the pipelle is passed through.
8. Slowly and gently advance the catheter the full depth of the endometrial cavity, until the resistance of the fundus is felt.
9. Never use force against digitally felt resistance.
10. Assess the length of the uterus by noting the centimeters marked on the pipelle.
   a. In premenopausal women, 6 cm or more
   b. Less than 6 cm in postmenopausal women
   c. The cavity has probably not been entered if only the 3 cm to 4 cm mark has been reached.
   d. The woman may feel mild uterine cramps at this point.
   e. Once the pipelle is fully inserted and the tip is positioned properly, release traction of the tenaculum, if it is used.

G. Aspiration
1. The pipelle should be stabilized with the nondominant hand, using the dominant hand to pull the plunger fully back.
2. Rapidly pull the piston firmly, using one full motion, as far toward the proximal end of the sheath as it will go. The piston cannot be pulled out completely.
3. Slow, irregular pressure, or incomplete withdrawal of the plunger will not supply the suction required for an appropriate sample.
4. Correct technique creates negative pressure inside the pipelle, which allows for aspiration of the endometrial tissue into the open tip of the pipelle.
5. Next, the pipelle should be rotated continuously 360 degrees by rolling or twisting it between thumb and index finger as it

is rapidly, but gently, advanced and withdrawn between the fundus and internal os (Figure 40.1).

6. Withdraw and advance the pipelle three or four times (for 30 seconds).
7. As the tube is rotated, a column of tissue is seen as it is drawn into the tube, often filling it completely.
8. This suction from negative pressure generally yields an adequate sample.
9. If the pipelle is withdrawn from the os, the suction is lost.
10. If this occurs, the pipelle should be reinserted.
11. Once enough of a sample has been aspirated, the pipelle is slowly removed and the contents placed directly in preservative and sent to the pathology department for analysis.
12. If the instrument does not touch the container, it can be reinserted, if necessary.

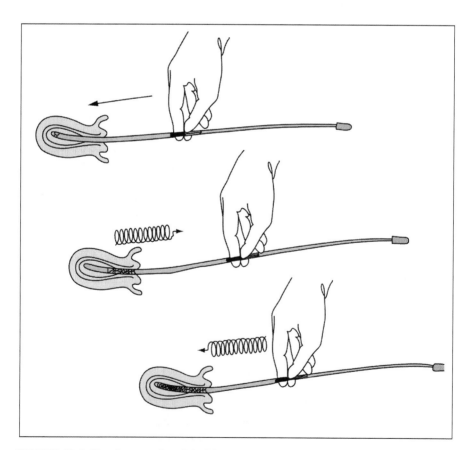

FIGURE 40.1 Simultaneously roll (twirl) sheath between fingers while moving sheath laterally and back and forth (in and out) between the fundus and internal os three or four times to obtain sample.

13. Record the depth, ease of insertion, and patient response.
14. Any bleeding from the tenaculum site usually abates rapidly.
15. The patient should remain supine for a few minutes until any pain or dizziness passes.
16. Supply the woman with a perineal pad.
H. Sampling
1. Recent studies suggest that the most representative samples are obtained from high in the corpus from both the anterior and posterior walls.
2. The samples should be superficial rather than deep because the deeper tissues often show less intense reactivity to progesterone.
3. If sufficient sample is not obtained, the procedure should be repeated at a later date.
4. The extent of the sample should correlate to the level of suspicion for malignancy.
5. For endometrial dating, only a single sample is necessary.

XIII. **Common problems**
A. Difficulty entering the os due to cervical stenosis
1. The cervix of a menopausal women is often tight. If this is the case, a smaller caliber (2 to 3 mm) pipelle should be used rather than the standard 4 mm.
2. If the flexible cannula bends in the middle with any pressure during attempts to pass through a tight cervical canal, grasp the cannula about 4 cm from its end with a ring or uterine dressing forceps. (This method minimizes the bending in the middle of the cannula as pressure is applied and eases its passage through the cervix.)
3. Additionally, the pipelle, with the tip curved, can be placed in a freezer to increase rigidity. Remember, this stiffness may slightly increase the risk of perforation.
4. A sterile lubricant can be placed on the pipelle to ease insertion in the elderly woman with a dry cervix.
5. Some clinicians recommend a 2-week course of vaginal estrogen before the biopsy sample is taken, to open the cervical os.
6. Refer if the os it still too tight or if the woman has severe atrophy, in which the external os may no longer be patent. The clinician should refer the patient to a gynecologist to open the os after the administration of paracervical anesthesia.
B. Minimal tissue obtained
1. Commonly seen in postmenopausal women evaluated for light spotting or bleeding

2. Consider the presence of a scant amount of tissue diagnostically sufficient if the following apply:
   a. The pipelle has passed at least 6 cm into the uterus.
   b. There is a clear sensation of having reached the fundus.
   c. The patient is not at high risk for endometrial cancer (due to factors other than age).

XIV. **After biopsy procedure**
   A. Preparing the specimen for analysis
      1. After the specimen has been obtained, clip off the tip of the cannula with scissors.
      2. Advance the piston so that the endometrial sample is expressed into a vial containing fixative.
      3. Fill out the paperwork and label the specimen, including information about the patient's clinical status.
      4. Indicate any hormone therapy the woman is receiving.
   B. Following the procedure observe the woman for
      1. Vasovagal response
         a. The woman should be closely observed for a vasovagal response.
         b. She should remain supine for a few minutes and then slowly be assisted to a sitting position.
         c. She should remain sitting until equilibrium is restored and any discomfort passes.
      2. Cramping
         a. Painful cramps usually subside rapidly and are well tolerated.
         b. If the cramps persist, an anti-inflammatory agent can be used.
   C. Referral
      1. Patient with contraindications
      2. Patient with a severely stenotic os
      3. Confer with supervising physician to discuss a patient at risk for bacterial endocarditis.

XV. **Complications (see Table 40.1)**
   A. The client should be advised to monitor any bleeding and to return should any of the following develop.
      1. Severe cramping or worsening discomfort or pain
      2. Heavy bleeding and clots or any bleeding lasting longer than 2 days
      3. Any foul-smelling discharge, with or without fever and chills
      4. Uterine perforation
         a. Is very rare
         b. Usually without serious sequelae

TABLE 40.1 Complications Associated With Endometrial Biopsy

COMPLICATION	RATE
Cervical stenosis	12/28
Excessive bleeding	5/28
Fever	4/28
Excessive pain	2/28
Vasovagal reaction	2/28
Uterine perforation	2/28
Interrupted pregnancy	1/28

    c. New catheters are very small and flexible, and carry little risk of perforation of the uterus.

    d. If perforation is suspected, the patient needs to be closely monitored for heavy bleeding.

  5. Interruption of a pregnancy when evaluating LPD

    a. There is a slight chance of disturbing an early pregnancy.

    b. Interruption of a pregnancy is rare, occurring in 1/1,500 biopsy procedures total, and in 1/500 biopsy studies for evaluating LPD. (The resulting miscarriage rate is 20%.)

    c. The woman may choose to use contraception during the cycle preceding surgery, or she may elect to continue trying to conceive because the risk is slight.

    d. Nothing is worse than disrupting an established pregnancy during an endometrial biopsy study in an infertile couple.

    e. A sensitive pregnancy test is recommended.

XVI. Follow-up

  A. LPD evaluation

    1. Ask the woman to call with the date that her next period begins.

    2. This information is essential for the accurate interpretation of results because they are based on the comparison of the histologic date to the day of menses.

    3. Normal results will confirm that ovulation has occurred and that there is adequate progesterone to support an early pregnancy.

  B. Results are usually available in 7 to 10 days.

  C. Have the client return in 2 weeks to discuss biopsy study results and any follow-up.

XVII. Diagnosis

    A. LPD

        1. LPD should be suspected if the endometrial tissue is "out of phase," demonstrating a lag of more than 2 days from the expected date of menses.

        2. The day of ovulation is counted forward to the date of the biopsy surgery.

        3. Additionally, the onset of the next menses is counted as day 28, counting back to the day of the biopsy surgery, and comparing it with the histologic date provided.

        4. A normal basal body temperature (BBT) or LH surge and an "in-phase" biopsy support the adequacy of the hypothalamic–pituitary–ovarian axis.

        5. If the biopsy is out of phase, further hormonal assessment is warranted.

    B. The case against the use of endometrial biopsy study in diagnosing LPD

        1. Endometrial biopsy examination is being used less and less because of the invasive nature of the test and the additional cost in both time and money.

        2. Some sources believe that there is a weak correlation between out-of-phase biopsy surgeries and infertility.

        3. Results are believed to be somewhat subjective, with different interpretations using the same sample.

        4. Other methods, such as the BBT, the over-the-counter ovulation predictor kit, and serum progesterone test, are accurate in documenting luteal function.

        5. Although a normal in-phase endometrial biopsy sample is strongly suggestive of an adequate luteal phase, an abnormal result does not always indicate LPD because 25% to 30% of abnormal biopsy samples are found in normally fertile women.

    C. Adenocarcinoma

        1. May note abundant friable fragments, which may appear as bits of rolled up tissue in the endometrial sample.

Bibliography

Bremer, C. (1992). Endometrial biopsy. *Female Patient, 17*(10), 15–28.

Clark, T. J., Mann, C. H., Shah, N., Khan, K. S., Song, F., & Gupta, J. K. (2002). Accuracy of outpatient endometrial biopsy in the diagnosis of endometrial cancer: A systematic quantitative review. *British Journal of Obstetrics and Gynecology, 109*, 313–321.

Katz, V. L. (2007). Diagnostic procedures: Imaging, endometrial sampling, endoscopy: Indications and contraindications, complications. In V. L. Katz, G. M. Lentz, R. A. Lobo, & D. M. Gershenson (Eds.), *Comprehensive gynecology* (5th ed.). Philadelphia, PA: Mosby.

Kaunitz, A. M. (1993). Endometrial sampling in menopausal patients. *Menopausal Medicine, 1*, 5–8.

World Cancer Research Fund International. (2013). *Cancer facts and figures: Endometrial cancer rates.* Retrieved January 20, 2013, from http://www.wcrf.org/cancer_statistics/cancer_facts/endometrial_cancer_rates.php

Zuber, T. J. (2001). Endometrial biopsy. *American Family Physician 63,* 1131–1135.

Acrochordonectomy

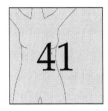

41

Helen A. Carcio

I. **Acrochordonectomy (removal of skin tags) explained**
   A. Acrochordonectomy is a good technique for the advanced practice clinician to master.
      1. Many women who are seen for their annual visit may complain of having a skin tag.
      2. Although not painful, women often find them unsightly and bothersome as they may snag on clothes or jewelry, particularly if they are seen around the face and neck.
      3. Because skin tags are harmless, often individuals elect to do nothing at all to get rid of them, but they may cause chaffing and irritation from the skin surfaces rubbing together, particularly in overweight individuals.

II. **Acrochordonectomy explained**
   A. An acrochordon is a flesh-toned, papillomatous, cutaneous lesion.
      1. If they are pedunculated, they are called cutaneous papillomas and soft fibromas.
      2. Histologically: The lesion is hyperplastic epidermis enclosing a dermal connective tissue stalk.
      3. Usually range in size from 2 mm to 5 mm, although they can grow quite large
      4. Commonly seen in the groin and armpits
      5. Generally speaking, skin tags are not painful and not associated with any other skin conditions.
   B. Causes
      1. A family history sometimes exists of acrochordons.
      2. Hormones during pregnancy
      3. Obesity
      4. High cholesterol

C. There are many products on the market or some women try to snip them off. Caution should be advised because the stalk contains blood vessels and may bleed or become infected.
D. The removal technique is easy and straightforward and can often be done during a routine physical examination.

III. **Removal**
   A. Technique 1
      1. Identify the lesion to be removed.
         a. Cleanse the lesion and surrounding area with an iodine swab.
         b. Rinse with sterile saline.
      2. A small amount of a numbing agent may be used.
      3. Apply a surgical clamp, such as a Kelly clamp, at the base of the acrochordon. The stalk is usually easily identified.
         a. Keep clamp in place for approximately 5 to 10 minutes to decrease blood flow
         b. Remove the clamp.
      4. Grasp the lesion with a small clamp and lift away from the skin.
      5. Excise the lesion using fine-bladed scissors (iris scissors).
      6. Cut in the middle of the approximately 2-mm compressed area left by the surgical clamp.
      7. A small circular adhesive bandage may be applied or the area may be left open.
      8. The skin usually heals smooth.
   B. Technique 2
      1. Identify the lesion to be removed.
      2. Apply petroleum jelly around the lesion, being careful not to cover the lesion itself with the petroleum jelly.
      3. Apply trichloroacetic acid (TCA) or bichloroacetic acid (BCA) or liquid nitrogen to the lesion until it turns white, being careful not to get any chemical on the surrounding skin. (The immediate area around it will turn red and a slight burning may occur, which usually subsides in a few minutes.)
      4. Inform the patient that the lesion will turn black and eventually fall off.
      5. There is a slight chance of scarring when and if some liquids make contact with healthy skin.
      6. If the lesion is larger than 2 mm, the client may have to return for a second chemical application.
      7. A lesion more than 5 mm should be referred to a dermatologist.
      8. Electrolysis destroys the lesion and the underlying skin.
   C. If the woman has many tags, only three or four should be removed at one time.

IV. Follow-up

A. The patient is advised to call should burning increase or signs of infection occur.

B. Return for removal of other lesions

Bibliography

Bolognia, J. L., Jarizzo, J. L., & Schaffer, J. V. (2012). *Dermatology* (3rd ed.). China: Saunders/Elsevier.

James, W. D., Elston, D. M., Berger, T. G., & Andrews, G. C. (2011). *Andrews' diseases of the skin: Clinical dermatology* (11th ed.). London, UK: Saunders/Elsevier.

Strother, G. D. (1998). Acrochordonectomy made easy. *Clinician Reviews, 8*(3), 75–83.

Cervical Polypectomy

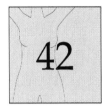

42

Helen A. Carcio

I. Polyps explained

  A. Description

    1. Polyps are the most common benign tumors of the cervix.

    2. They are found most often during the menstruating years. (Parous women in their fifth decade)

    3. Polyps are rare in young, non-menstruating women (6%).

    4. They are soft, pear-shaped (fingerlike), red to purple lesions and are usually pedunculated growths from the surface of the cervical canal (see Figure 42.1).

    5. They contain a large number of blood vessels, particularly near the surface.

    6. Diameter varies from several millimeters to 2 cm.

    7. They occur with overgrowth of one of the cervical folds.

    8. They are usually asymptomatic but may be friable and bleed with intercourse.

    9. Usually only one polyp is present but in rare cases, there may be two.

    10. Typically, polyps are not cancerous (benign) and are easy to remove. Polyps do not usually grow back. Women who have polyps once are at risk of growing more polyps.

    11. During a pelvic examination, the health care provider will see smooth, red, or purple finger-like growths on the cervix. A cervical biopsy will most often show cells that are consistent with a benign polyp. Rarely there may be abnormal, precancerous, or cancer cells in a polyp.

    12. Although most cervical polyps are not cancerous (benign), the removed tissue should be sent to a laboratory and checked further.

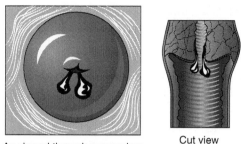

As viewed through a speculum   Cut view

FIGURE 42.1 Cervical polyps. Note how they are attached to a stalk.

    B. Microscopic analysis
        1. Loose vascular connective tissue covered by endocervical epithelium
        2. Stroma may be inflamed and edematous.
    C. Location
        1. Usually found in the lower endocervix; may protrude through the cervical os
        2. May be found at the squamocolumnar junction or portio vaginal.
    D. Cause
        1. Not completely understood
        2. May occur with
            a. An abnormal response to increased levels of estrogen
            b. Chronic inflammation
            c. Clogged blood vessels in the cervix
    E. Symptoms
        1. Abnormally heavy periods (menorrhagia)
        2. Abnormal vaginal bleeding
            a. After douching
            b. After intercourse
            c. After menopause
            d. Between periods
            e. Polyps may not cause symptoms.

II. **Polyps are easy to remove in the office at the time of the visit.**
    A. Technique 1
        1. Determine the site of origin.
        2. Grasp polyp with clamp.
        3. Twist until the polyp separates from the stalk.
        4. Apply silver nitrate or Monsel's solution for hemostasis.
    B. Technique 2 (if polyp is large; greater than 5 mm).
        1. Determine the site of origin.
        2. Clamp approximately 0.5 cm above the origin of the pedicle.

3. A surgical ligature is next tied between the clamp and the cervix.
4. Remove the clamp.
5. Using a pair of scissors with a fine blade, cut along the suture line to remove the polyp.
   a. Send specimen to the pathology department.
   b. All polyps should be sent to the pathology department because malignancy can occur in benign-appearing structures (0.2%–0.4% incidence).
6. It may be left attached to undergo infarction and slough.
C. Other methods
   1. Electrical current (LEEP) or laser therapy is used for any polyp greater than 5 mm.
   2. Traditional surgery to cut off and stitch close the polyp site
   3. Dilation and curettage, scraping the polyp off
D. Possible complications
   1. Bleeding and slight cramping for a few days after removal of a polyp
   2. Some cervical cancers may first appear as a polyp.
   3. Certain uterine polyps may be associated with uterine cancer.
   4. There is no need for special follow-up since polyps seldom recur after removal.

Bibliography

Centers for Disease Control and Prevention. (2012, May 30). Gynecologic cancers. Retrieved August 2, 2012, from http://www.cdc.gov/cancer/gynecologic

Katz, V. L. (2007). Benign gynecologic lesions: Vulva, vagina, cervix, uterus, oviduct, ovary. In V. L. Katz, G. M. Lentz, R. A. Lobo, & D. M. Gershenson (Eds.), *Comprehensive gynecology* (5th ed.). Philadelphia, PA: Mosby Elsevier.

National Library of Medicine—National Institutes of Health. (2012, February 26). Cervical polyps. Retrieved August 2, 2012, from http://www.nlm.nih.gov/medlineplus/ency/article/001494.htm

Incision and Drainage of Bartholin's Abscess

43

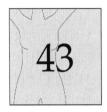

Helen A. Carcio

I. **Bartholin's glands explained**
   A. Bartholin's glands
      1. Located on each side of the opening of the vagina, on the lips of the labia
      2. Secrete a vaginal lubricating fluid during sexual stimulation
      3. Lubricating fluid normally travels from the gland down tiny ducts about 0.8 in.
      4. They are 2 cm long and drain into the lower part of the entrance to the vagina (see Figure 43.1).
      5. Protect vaginal tissue from irritation during sexual intercourse
   B. Bartholin's gland cyst is a fluid-filled swelling on one of the glands.
      1. Commonly occur in younger women who are sexually active
      2. Usually not an infection but cellulitis may occur in the area
      3. Not sexually transmitted but may be associated with gonorrhea
      4. About 2% of women will develop a Bartholin's gland cyst in their lifetime.
      5. Usually develop in only one of the two glands
      6. Ducts become blocked and fluid accumulates causing a cyst.
      7. Bartholin cysts/abscesses have a high rate of recurrence.
   C. Symptoms
      1. A woman may not even know she has it, and it may be picked up during a routine pelvic exam.
      2. May note a lump in the vagina
      3. Pain in the vaginal area especially during intercourse and movement
      4. Vulvar skin may be tender and red.
   D. Treatment may not be needed if a Bartholin's gland cyst is small and does not cause any symptoms. If the cyst does cause symptoms, treatment may be recommended.

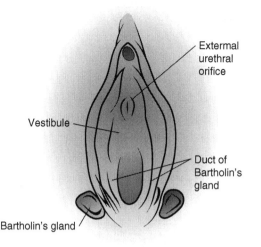

FIGURE 43.1 Position of Bartholin's glands at 5 o'clock and 7 o'clock around the vaginal oriface.

    E. Home care
       1. Sit in a warm bath a few times a day or applying a moist, warm compress
       2. Helps the fluid to drain from the cyst
       3. In many cases, home care may be enough to treat the cyst.

II. Treatment of Bartholin's gland abscess involves incision and drainage of cyst and insertion of Word catheter.
    A. Equipment
       1. 22-gauge needle
       2. 5-mL syringe (catheter inflation) with sterile water
       3. 25-gauge needle with 5-mL syringe (for application of anesthesia)
       4. 1% Xylocaine
       5. Scalpel with #11 blade
       6. Small hemostats (2)
       7. 4-x-4 gauze pads
       8. Antiseptic solution
       9. Bartholin gland drainage catheter (Word)

III. Preparation
    A. Position woman in lithotomy position.
       1. Cleanse area with antiseptic.
       2. Palate area to visualize location and size of the abscess.
       3. With needle bellow pointed upward, create a wheal by infiltrating the Xylocaine into the area of the duct.

IV. **The procedure**
  A. The incision
    1. Incise vaginal side wall and create a 3-mm incision through the mucosa into the cysts.
    2. Should be approximately 1 to 1½ cm long to fit the wound catheters
    3. Stab wound should be deep enough to allow for the flow of pus or mucus from the gland
    4. The catheter is put in place to drain the abscess and allow for re-epithelialization.
  B. Insertion of Word catheter
    1. Grasp the walls of the cysts with the hemostats to hold open.
      a. Stabilizes the walls
      b. Prevents creation of false tracts outside the cysts
    2. Using second hemostat, insert into stab wound and move around to break up any loculations
    3. Allow for cyst contents to drain and then irrigate cyst with 5 mL of saline.
    4. Test the balloon by filling with 3 mL sterile water and then deflate. (Do not use air.)
    5. With syringe and needle still attached, insert the balloon into the Bartholin gland through the incision.
    6. Inflate bulb with 2 to 3 mL of fluid through the sealed stopper.
    7. Inflate to the point to ensure that it will not fall out.
    8. Catheter should stay in place and comfortably fill the cavity
    9. Tuck catheter stem into the vagina.
      a. The catheter rests perpendicular to the perineum to avoid tension on the tissue due to bending of catheter stem.
      b. Catheter stem will not protrude out of the vagina, making it much more comfortable for the woman.

V. **Follow-up**
  A. Call should discomfort or signs of infection occur.
    1. Should return in 3 weeks to remove catheter once epithelialization occurs
    2. Catheter balloon is deflated and easily removed
    3. Antibiotic not normally required except if cellulitis is present around the vulvar opening of the duct
  B. Should refer to surgeon for marsupialization if the cyst recurs or the Word catheter does not resolve the abscess.
  C. Complications
    1. Continuous pain
      a. Bulb may have been overinflated in the cavity and can cause pain once the anesthesia wears off
    2. Infection at wound site

3. Catheter may fall out
   a. If stab wound opening is too large
   b. If bulb not sufficiently inflated
4. Catheter may deflate
   a. Stem of the catheter may be mistakenly punctured during insertion; catheter may gradually deflate and eventually fall out.

Bibliography

Chen, K. T. (n.d.). Disorders of Bartholin's gland. Retrieved March 6, 2012, from http:// www.uptodate.com/index

Cohen, S. D., Wright F., Hernandex E., & Dunton, C. J. (1990). Management of the Bartholin abscess. *American Journal of Gynecology Health, 4*(3), 42–44.

Goldberg, J. E. (1970). Simplified treatment for disease of Bartholin's gland. *Obstetrics and Gynecology 35,*109–110.

Mayo Clinic. (n.d). *Bartholin's cyst: Causes.* Retrieved November 1, 2013, from http:// www.mayoclinic.com/health/bartholin-cyst/DS00667/DSECTION=causes

Mayo Clinic. (n.d.). *Bartholin's cyst: Prevention.* Retrieved November 1, 2013, from http:// www.mayoclinic.com/health/bartholin-cyst/DS00667/DSECTION=prevention

Omole, F., Simmons, B., & Hacker, Y. (2003). Management of Bartholin's duct cyst and gland abscess. *American Family Physician, 68*(1),135–140.

Patil, S. & Sultan, A. H. (2007). Bartholin's cysts and abscesses. *Journal of Obstetrics and Gynaecology. 27,* 241.

Pundir, J. & Auld, B. J. (2008). A review of the management of diseases of the Bartholin's gland. *Journal of Obstetrics and Gynaecology, 28,* 161.

University of Maryland Medical Center. (n.d). *Bartholin's cyst or abscess.* Retrieved November 1, 2013, from http://umm.edu/Health/Medical/Ency/Articles/Bartholins-cyst-or-abscess

University of Michigan Health System. (n.d.). *Bartholin's gland cyst.* Retrieved November 1, 2013, from http://www.uofmhealth.org/health-library/tw2685#tw2688

Wechter, M. E., Wu, J. M., Marzano, D., & Haefner, H. (2009). Management of Bartholin duct cysts and abscesses: A systematic review. *Obstetrical and Gynecological Survey, 64,* 395.

Wood, B. (1964). New instrument for office treatment of cysts and abscesses of the Bartholin's gland. *Journal of the American Medical Association, 190,* 777.

Intrauterine Insemination 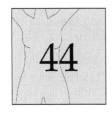 44

Carol Lesser

I. **Intrauterine insemination (IUI)**

    A. Indications for IUI

      1. Ejaculatory problems requiring masturbation and insemination of either a fresh or frozen specimen

      2. If male partner is unavailable at midcycle, frozen sperm can be inseminated.

      3. Certain fertility medications

        a. Clomiphene citrate may reduce midcycle secretions after several cycles. This is not an issue with other fertility medications.

      4. Reduced sperm parameters

        a. If a couple is not ready for in vitro fertilization (IVF), IUI may improve outcome.

      5. Cervical stenosis

        a. A relative problem

        b. Not an absolute indication for IUI

        c. If significant cervical surgery has been performed, IUI may be beneficial, especially if the patient notices an absence of cervical secretions, although this is rare.

      6. Avoid HIV or other sexually transmitted disease (STD) transmission. Affected partner's sperm may be sequestered, processed, and stored separately for future IUI or assisted reproductive technologies (ART).

      7. Male fertility preservation in the case of a cancer diagnosis or when gonadotoxic therapy or surgery may be planned

      8. Unexplained infertility or those not ready for IVF

      9. If using donor sperm

      10. Retroversion or retroflexion of the uterus is not an indication for IUI.

BOX 44.1 *Factors That Impact Success of Intrauterine Insemination*

- Age
- Unilateral or bilateral tubal patency
- Total motile sperm count
- Fertility medications versus natural cycle

    11. Previous vasectomy
        a. It is advised to bank sperm in case the need for it arises in the future.
        b. In these cases IUI or ART would be recommended to optimize sperm performance after cryopreservation.
  B. Technique
    1. Fresh IUI: Obtaining the specimen
        a. The specimen is most often obtained via masturbation into a sterile container that has been tested to be nontoxic to sperm.
        b. Can be collected at home or office if there is a private collection room
        c. Generally it is recommended to collect at home for privacy and a more relaxed atmosphere, which may improve the specimen.
           (1) Try to transport specimen within 1 hour.
           (2) When transporting, body warmth provides the best temperature if possible.
           (3) Avoid excessive heat, like the heater of the car, or excessive cold.
        d. Proper specimen identification is required. A driver's license is usually best.
        e. Once the specimen is identified and dropped off, it will require processing before the IUI can be performed.
           (1) Ask couple to return at the appointment time.
           (2) Processing usually takes at least 45 minutes.
           (3) If specimen is placed in an incubator, it will retain its motility for several hours in case there is a delay in the insemination.
        f. If male has performance anxiety or will be out of town at midcycle
           (1) Specimen can be frozen for future use.
           (2) If male has performance anxiety on the day of the IUI, be supportive and recommend going home and attempting intercourse later that day.

        (3) Provide Viagra if needed.

        (4) Consider rescheduling to the next day if not postovulatory.

  2. If frozen specimen is used, woman must properly identify

C. Preparing the woman

  1. Have the woman empty her bladder for comfort.

  2. Ensure that her last menses was normal and that her midcycle surge has been detected.

    a. IUI is performed up to and including day of ovulation.

    b. The day of ovulation predictor kit (OPK) color change as well as the next 2 days are good choices.

  3. A single insemination is adequate unless the specimen or timing proves to be suboptimal.

  4. If any symptom or concern for a vaginal or pelvic infection, do not proceed. In the case of a monilial infection, it is okay to proceed if tolerated by the patient.

  5. Some offices encourage gentle music or anything that encourages a more relaxed and less impersonal environment.

D. Insemination technique

  1. Bring prepared or thawed specimen into the room with catheter in sterile wrapper. Name should be visible. Draw up specimen when patient has identified the sperm source as her partner's.

  2. Partner may be present. If partner is uncomfortable watching procedure, have the partner stand at head of table to offer support.

  3. Review the procedure and what can be expected. Emphasize the process takes only a few minutes and is usually painless.

  4. Record specimen parameters, especially the total motile number of sperm if provided by the lab.

  5. Document whether fertility medications have been used and the menstrual cycle day.

  6. Document method of ovulation detection used. Most women use an OPK that detects a luteinizing hormone (LH) surge or another monitoring method that includes blood and ultrasound (see Table 44.1).

  7. Review potential complications and symptoms to report

    a. Rare occurrence of bleeding or cramping

    b. Prostaglandin reaction or vasovagal response

TABLE 44.1 Timing of IUI

OPK or urinary LH kit	Day of, or up to 2 days after, color change Most centers suggest day after
Ultrasound	If mature follicle (18–20 mm diameter) is seen: 24–36 hours later

8. Obtain written consent.
   a. Many states require written consent from both partners.
   b. Usually completed before the first insemination is performed and may need to be updated annually or if any change in relationship status
   c. Consents should be prepared and properly worded for single, heterosexual, and same-sex couples.
9. Help women into the lithotomy position.
   a. Use of stirrups is optional, as long as speculum placement is efficient and comfortable.
   b. Use non-latex gloves if known latex allergy
10. Assess the uterine size and position.
11. Insert speculum.
12. Assess cervical appearance.
    a. Note cervical secretions.
    b. Swab cervical secretions if copious to enable better access to os for catheter placement.
    c. Not necessary to examine the cervical mucus under the microscope because the patient is periovulatory
    d. Cervical secretions are a healthy sign of impending ovulation. Cervix is wiped with a large cotton scopette.
13. A variety of catheters exist for the purpose of IUI.
    a. Use the narrowest gauge for patient comfort.
    b. Catheters with "memory" can be bent to follow uterine flexion.
14. Thread the preloaded syringe through the os.
    a. Do not force.
    b. Once fundus is felt, pull back to prevent bleeding and trauma.
    c. This brings sperm closer to the tubal ostia.
15. Avoid a tenaculum except if entry is difficult as in the case of severe ante or retroversion of the uterus, as it can cause cramping.
16. If the cervix is stenotic, use the narrowest gauge possible.
    a. Tom cat catheters work well and are cost-effective. Otherwise, narrow catheters with memory can work well.
    b. Occasionally dilatation with a narrow dilator or os finder will help guide passage for the catheter to follow.
17. Patient should feel no more than mild cramping but not pain.
18. Slowly inject the sperm over 30 to 60 seconds to avoid cramping or retrograde flow.
19. Any excess specimen should be allowed to collect near the os.

20. Leaving the catheter in place or removing it if there is no backflow is acceptable.
21. Bleeding
    a. Friable cervices often bleed on contact.
    b. This should not affect the success of an IUI procedure.
    c. Bleeding from the tenaculum also is external bleeding and should not affect success.
    d. Avoid heavy bleeding with catheter placement.
22. Remove catheter in a way that avoids spillage.
23. Remove speculum sideways so any excess specimen will collect in the vagina.
24. Resting after IUI is controversial. It may be pleasant for the patient but is not medically necessary.
    a. Best not to rush the patient and give her a choice
    b. Some centers like to make the experience as relaxed as possible and encourage or provide music during the IUI.
25. A rare complication is a prostaglandin reaction.
    a. This was more common in the past when unwashed sperm was used for IUI.
    b. For vasovagal and prostaglandin reaction, do not leave the patient unattended.
    c. She will benefit from nonsteroidal anti-inflammatory drugs (NSAIDs) and reassurance that this will pass. Acetaminophen is generally not helpful.
    d. In rare cases with vasovagal reactions, patients can lose consciousness or have a mild seizure. (This is true for all gynecologic procedures when the cervical os is traversed.)
    e. Occasionally ammonium salts or even atropine will be administered.
    f. Monitor vital signs and discharge once stable and symptom free.
    g. When frozen sperm is used, the volume tends to be very low and incidence of prostaglandin reaction is also low.
    h. However, when this occurs, it is similar to a vasovagal reaction and the patient can be in extreme pain with cramping.
26. Instruct patient to call if fever, chills, unusual discharge, or bleeding develops.
27. Single versus double IUI is frequently debated. Single IUI is cost-effective and studies suggest comparable success rates. Couples can supplement with intercourse when able.
28. Instruct her to schedule or check for pregnancy in 2 weeks.

Bibliography

Goldstein, M., & Schlegel, P. N. (Eds.). (2013). *Surgical and medical management of male infertility*. New York, NY: Cambridge University Press.

Gordon, J. D., Rydfors, J. T., & Druzin, M. L. (2001). *Obstetrics, gynecology and infertility: Handbook for clinicians-resident survival guide* (5th ed.). Arlington, VA: Scrub Hill Press.

Lebovic, D., Gordon, J. D., & Taylor, R. (2013). *Reproductive endocrinology and infertility: Handbook for clinicians* (2nd ed.). Arlington, VA: Scrub Hill Press.

Lipshultz, L. I., Howards, S. S., & Niederberger, C. S. (Eds.). (2009). *Infertility in the male* (4th ed.). New York, NY: Cambridge University Press.

Percutaneous Tibial Nerve Stimulation

45

Leslie Saltzstein Wooldridge

I. Percutaneous tibial nerve stimulation (PTNS) defined: An office-based neuromodulation system designed to deliver retrograde access to the sacral nerve through percutaneous electrical stimulation of the tibial nerve. It is a minimally invasive procedure that acts indirectly (mechanism is not exactly known) via a central afferent impulse from the tibial nerve that targets the sacral nerve plexus in the spinal cord influencing reflexes via the pudendal nerve among the bladder, urethral sphincter, and pelvic floor, and is designed to alter aberrant bladder signals. Hence, controls overactive bladder.

A. Preparing the patient
   1. Review the treatments, including frequency and length.
   2. Discuss expected effects
      a. General efficacy
      b. Voiding changes
      c. Potential adverse effects of PTNS
      d. Reasonable patient goals
   3. Continued commitment to behavioral treatments
   4. Continuation/weaning of bladder medications

B. Procedure
   1. Equipment
      (a) A 34-gauge needle and lead wires that are connected to the stimulator to transmit current from the stimulator to the tibial nerve via the needle electrode
   2. Patient should be comfortably seated on a chair with leg comfortably elevated and foot exposed (see Figure 45.1).
   3. The insertion site: The needle electrode insertion site is on the inner leg, approximately 2 inches above the medial malleolus and 1 finger-width toward the back of the leg.

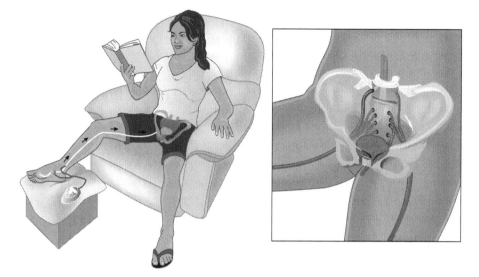

FIGURE 45.1 Position of a woman during PTNS. Note how the impulses travel from her tibial nerve to her pelvic girdle.

4. Therapy can be delivered independently by a trained nurse practitioner (NP), by an RN, or a physician assistant (PA) under physician's direction (need physician order).
5. Needle is to be inserted at a 60-degree angle.
6. After insertion of needle electrode
   a. Connect the lead wire to the stimulator (Figure 45.2).
   b. Attach the surface electrode to arch of foot.
   c. Attach the needle electrode clip to needle.
   d. Test patient response, including the presence of a toe flex and/or heel or foot vibration.
   e. Stimulate the patient for 30 minutes.
   f. When alarm goes off, disconnect and properly dispose of the components.
7. Documentation
   a. Consent form
   b. History and physical that includes bladder symptoms
   c. Treatment log
   d. Ongoing therapy
   e. Bladder records

II. Indications
   A. Overactive bladder (OAB) and associated symptoms of urgency, frequency, and urge incontinence
   B. Nocturia
   C. Patients refractory to more than two OAB medications
   D. Patients intolerant of drug side effects

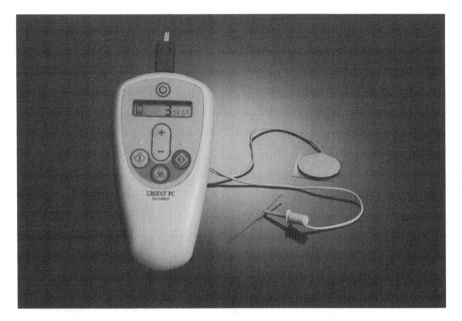

FIGURE 45.2 An Urgent PC stimulator.

E. Patients unable to take drugs orally
F. Patients unwilling to take drugs
G. Patients who already are taking drugs with anticholinergic effects and adding an OAB drug may be too much
H. According to the American Urologic Association (AUA)/ Society of Urodynamics, Female Pelvic Medicine and Urogenital Reconstruction (SUFU) Urology and Genito-Urinary Reconstruction Guidelines for OAB, PTNS is generally used on patients who are refractory or intolerant to treatment with medications and other behavioral interventions. At least 20% of patients are refractory to conservative treatment. Up to 80% of patients stop taking drugs within the first year of their prescription.
I. PTNS can also be used in conjunction with other treatments for OAB, including pelvic floor therapy and medications as needed to achieve patient goals.
J. The International Classification of Diseases ICD-10 codes that support medical necessity (www.wpsmedicare.com/j8macparta/ policy/updates/revised/index.shtml)
   1. R32 Urinary incontinence unspecified
   2. N39.41 Urge incontinence
   3. N39.46 Mixed incontinence (male) (female)
   4. N39.498 Other urinary incontinence
   5. R35.0 Urinary frequency
   6. R39.15 Urgency of urination

    K. Current procedural terminology code (CPT code): 64566 posterior tibial neurostimulation, percutaneous needle electrode, single treatment, includes programming

III. OAB statistics
- **A.** Who is affected by OAB
  1. 34 million adults in the United States
  2. Affects men and women almost equally: 16% and 16.9%
  3. Women more likely to have urinary urge incontinence than men: 9.3% to 2.6%
  4. Incidence increases with age
  5. Only 40% of those with symptoms seek treatment

IV. Contraindications
- **A.** Pregnancy or planning to get pregnant while being treated
- **B.** Pacemaker or implantable defibrillator
- **C.** Prone to excessive bleeding
- **D.** Nerve damage that could impact either the tibial nerve or pelvic floor function

V. Treatment efficacy
- **A.** 60% to 80% of patients respond positively
- **B.** Provides clinically significant reductions in
  1. Daytime voiding frequency
  2. Nighttime voiding frequency
  3. Leaking episodes
  4. Urgency
- **C.** Published literature shows effectiveness
  1. Head to head with anti-cholinergics—comparable changes in voiding parameters
  2. Against a sham-PTNS effect is not due to placebo effect
  3. Long term (3-year study) with ongoing therapy shows sustained symptom improvement
  4. Quality-of-life surveys have shown improvement with all studies.

VI. Treatment frequency
- **A.** 12 initial PTNS treatments
  1. Typically once a week
  2. Occasional treatment, as necessary, to sustain symptom improvement. Studies have shown about monthly treatments.
     a. After initial 12 treatments, slowly increase time between treatments.
     b. If symptoms reappear or increase in severity, return to treatment frequency that provides efficacy for your patient.
     c. Be sure to follow recommendations and payment schedules of local insurance companies, Medicare, and Medicaid plans as coverage differs from plan to plan.

VII. **Response to treatment**
  A. Patient may see improvement after five to six treatments.
  B. Patients respond differently.
  C. Despite response, it is recommended that all 12 initial treatments be completed before determining effectiveness.
  D. Baseline objective measurement is important for comparison outcome measurement. Use of bladder diaries gives the most objective data. Bladder records completed at baseline, after six treatments and after the twelfth treatment give the best indication of improvement in all areas of OAB.

VIII. **Risks of treatment: Low**
  A. Side effects
    1. Transient moderate pain at or near the stimulation site
    2. Transient, mild pain or skin inflammation at or near the stimulation site
    3. Transient mild bleeding at needle insertion site

IX. **Important issues to keep in mind**
  A. PTNS is a proven effective noninvasive therapy for OAB symptoms.
  B. Patient selection is key.
  C. Practitioner technique is important.
  D. As with any therapy, the desired result is not guaranteed. Keep expectations realistic.

X. **See Appendix for a sample worksheet to evaluate a woman for PTNS.**

Bibliography

American Urologic Association (AUA). (2012). *Treatment guidelines for overactive bladder 2012*. Retrieved from http://www.aua.org

Coyne, K. S., Payne, C., Bhattacharyya, S. K., Revicki, D. A., Thompson, C., Corey, R., & Hunt, T. L. (2004). The impact of urinary urgency and frequency on health-related quality of life in overactive bladder: Results from a national community survey. *Value in Health, 7*(4), 455–463.

Finazzi, Agrò E. (2006, September 27–30). Percuteneous tibial nerve stimulation (PTNS): Results at long term follow-up. *SIUD Congresso Nationale*. Rome, Italy.

MacDiarmid, S. A., Peters, K. M., Shobeiri, A., Wooldridge, L. S., et al. (2010). Long-term durability of percuteneous tibial nerve stimulation for the treatment of overactive bladder. *Journal of Urology, 183*, 234–240.

McGuire, E. J., Zhang, S. C., Howinski, E. R., & Lytton, B. (1983). Treatment of motor and sensory detrusor instability by electrical stimulation. *Journal of Urology, 129*, 78–79.

Peters, K. M., Carrico, D. J., Perez-Marrero, R. A., Wooldridge, L. S., et al. (2010, April). Randomized trial of percutaneous tibial nerve stimulation versus sham efficacy in the treatment of OAB: Results from the SUmiT trial. *Journal of Urology, 183,* 1438–1443.

Peters, K. M., Carrico, D. J., Wooldridge, L. S., Miller, C. J., & MacDiarmid S. A. (2013). Percutaneous tibial nerve stimulation for the long-term treatment of overactive bladder: Three-year results of the STEP study. *Journal of Urology, 189,* 2194–2201.

Peters, K. M., MacDiarmid, S. A., Wooldridge, L. S., Leong, F. C., Shobeiri, S. A., Rovner, E. S., ... Feagins, B. A. (2009). Randomized trial of percutaneous tibial nerve stimulation versus extended-release tolterodine: Results from the overactive bladder innovative therapy trial. *Journal of Urology, 182,* 1055–1061.

Stewart, W. F., Van Rooyen, J. B., Cundiff, G. W., et al. (2001). Prevalence and burden of overactive bladder in the United States. *World Journal of Urology, 20,* 327–336.

Urgent PC. (2013). *Uroplasty patient education materials.* Retrieved from http://www.urgentpcinfo.com

van Balken, M. R., Vergunst, H., & Bemelmans, B. L. (2006). Prognostic factors for successful percutaneous tibial nerve stimulation. *European Urology, 49,* 360–365.

van der Pal, F., van Balken, M. R., Heesakkers, J. P., Debruyne, F. M., & Bemelmans, B. L. (2006). Percutaneous tibial nerve stimulation in the treatment of refractory overactive bladder syndrome: Is maintenance treatment necessary? *BJU International, 97,* 547–550.

APPENDIX 45.1

Percutaneous Tibial Nerve Stimulation Worksheet

ONSET OF SYMPTOMS: (Date) _____

PREVIOUS TREATMENTS TRIED

- ☐ Kegel exercises
- ☐ Behavior modification
- ☐ Pelvic floor therapy

       Biofeedback......Yes ☐   No ☐   How long? _____
                                                    Dates

       E-Stim..............Yes ☐   No ☐   How long? _____
                                                    Dates

MEDICATIONS TRIED AND FAILED OR NOT TOLERATED

	Dose	Dates of Treatment—Reason for discontinuing
☐ Ditropan (oxybutynin)	_____	_____
☐ Detrol LA (tolteradine)	_____	_____
☐ Sanctura XR (trospium)	_____	_____
☐ Enablex (darifenicen)	_____	_____
☐ Vesicare (solifenicen)	_____	_____
☐ Oxytrol (oxybutynin)	_____	_____
☐ Toviaz (fesoterodine)	_____	_____
☐ Gelnique (oxybutynin)	_____	_____
☐ Other	_____	

PRESENCE OF CONTRAINDICATIONS

Pacemaker..........................   Yes ☐   No ☐

Implantable defibrillator.........   Yes ☐   No ☐

Prone to excessive bleeding.....   Yes ☐   No ☐

Nerve damage......................   Yes ☐   No ☐

Pregnant.............................   Yes ☐   No ☐

Other _____   Yes ☐   No ☐

CHRONIC ILLNESS

Diabetes........................   Yes ❑   No ❑

Neuropathy....................   Yes ❑   No ❑

Other _____

PATIENT GOALS

❑ Decreased urgency

❑ Decreased frequency

❑ Decreased episodes of urinary incontinence

❑ Sleep through the night

❑ Stay dry all day

❑ Void every _____ hours

❑ Avoid embarrassing social moments

❑ Other:

PRECAUTIONS EXPLAINED TO PATIENT

❑   Discomfort

❑   Bleeding at stimulation site

_____

_____

Date

_____

Date

Pessary Insertion

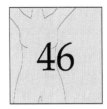

46

Helen A. Carcio

I. **Pessary**
   A. Historical perspectives
      1. Pessaries frequently appear in both Greek and Latin literature.
      2. The term usually refers to a mechanical device, such as a ball, wool, or lint soaked in medicine. They were very dissimilar from the modern pessary. The earliest pessaries were stones.
      3. Most pessaries had string attachments to facilitate removal.
      4. More than 200 different types of pessaries have been used throughout history.
      5. Now pessaries are made of polyvinyl plastic or medical-grade silicone, replacing the traditional red rubber material.
         a. Nontoxic silicone does not absorb vaginal secretions or odors.
         b. Material is biologically inert; allergic reactions are rare.
         c. This type of silicone material should not be confused with the silicone gel found in breast implants.
         d. The material can be autoclaved or boiled, or sterilized in Cidex.
      6. Ten to 20 years ago, use of the pessary was replaced by vaginal surgery.
      7. Pessaries are now increasing in use as baby boomers are aging and experiencing prolapse.
      8. The pessary offers a viable alternative to surgery.
      9. Different devices are often used to treat the same problem in different patients.
      10. The satisfaction rate with pessary use is high, with 72% to 95% reporting symptom relief.
      11. Pessary fittings and the device itself are reimbursed by Medicare.

B. Purpose
  1. To support the pelvic organs in close alignment to their proper anatomic position in the treatment of second- through fourth-degree prolapse
  2. To restore continence by stabilizing the bladder base
     a. Anchored between the pubic notch and the posterior vaginal fornix
     b. Ring or knob of the pessary compresses the urethra and increases the closing pressure.
     c. Provides a sling to support the redundant tissue of the prolapse
  3. To support an anterior-pointing cervix during pregnancy (Hodge pessary)
  4. To support and correct retrodisplacement of the uterus in early pregnancy
  5. To provide an alternative treatment for women who are at a high risk for surgical repair of the prolapse
  6. Note: Pessaries should only be inserted into a well-estrogenized vagina (see Chapter 12, "Atrophic Vaginitis, Vulvovaginal Atrophy")

C. Cornerstone of therapy for genital prolapse
  1. The number of women 65 and older will double in the next 20 years.
  2. Demand for pessary use is expected to grow by 45% in the next 30 years.

D. Proper management of a pessary is significantly less invasive and is safer than its surgical counterpart.
  1. Women have an 11% chance of surgery for prolapse or incontinence by age 80.
  2. Many women would prefer a conservative approach.
  3. Is a "low-tech" nonsurgical alternative to a high-tech surgery
  4. Satisfaction rate is high with pessary users: 72% to 90% report symptom relief.
  5. Pessary use does not preclude surgery at a later point.

E. Goals
  1. Can be used as a temporary measure for relief of symptoms while a patient delays surgery until a more opportune time, or until she decides whether to have surgery
  2. Used as a permanent alternative to prolapse surgery, particularly in elderly women who are at surgical risk
  3. Used as a diagnostic aid to determine whether there is relief of symptoms with prolapse replacement. It serves as a useful predictor of a successful outcome from surgical management.
     a. Can uncover urinary incontinence, which is masked by obstruction of the urinary outflow tract

F. Some comments related to the role of the advanced practice clinician

1. When selecting a pessary, a clinician may be overwhelmed by the choices of pessary size and style, and may feel insecure regarding which to choose for which condition.
   a. The three or four sizes in the middle are most commonly used.
   b. Most pessary wearers do well with the most common sizes.
   c. No need to recreate the anatomy
2. Modern use is a function of the clinician's experience and training, along with the availability of the device.
3. With knowledge and practice, an advanced practice clinician can become adept at fitting and caring for the supportive vaginal pessary.
4. As the population of older women increases, knowledge and skill in the use of pessaries in lieu of or as an adjunct to surgery should be considered.
5. Most pessaries come with printed material from the manufacturer that gives instructions regarding the insertion and care of a specific device.
6. Clinicians soon develop favorite types that they become familiar with.

G. Coitus
1. Coitus is possible with many pessaries that are not vaginally occlusive.
2. The woman must have the dexterity to remove and reinsert the pessary.
3. Never assume that because a patient is elderly she is not sexually active.
4. Sexual intercourse is not possible with the following types of pessaries:
   a. Gellhorn
   b. Doughnut
   c. Shatz
H. Pessaries are available in various sizes, shapes, and materials.
I. Uterine prolapse is the most common gynecologic problem that is corrected by pessaries.
J. If a pessary is made of latex rubber, the clinician needs to determine whether the woman has a sensitivity to latex before fitting. Very few pessaries are made of latex anymore.
K. Not all women can use a pessary. Box 46.1 lists reasons for discontinuing use of a pessary.

II. General principles for fitting a pessary
A. Some comments
1. Pessaries are generally fit by trial and error.
2. The pessary retention test: Insert two fingers in vagina and extend to both fornices. With fingers thus extended, pull hand

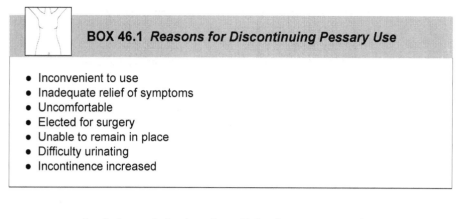

BOX 46.1 *Reasons for Discontinuing Pessary Use*

- Inconvenient to use
- Inadequate relief of symptoms
- Uncomfortable
- Elected for surgery
- Unable to remain in place
- Difficulty urinating
- Incontinence increased

back through the introitus. If the fingers stay in the original extended position then it is unlikely that the woman will be able to retain a pessary because the vaginal introitus is too wide.

3. Preparation of the woman
   a. Have her arrive with her rectum as empty as possible. There is no need for an enema.
   b. Large amounts of stool in the rectum may alter the fit of the pessary.
4. To measure for a pessary, once again insert the first two fingers deep into the vaginal canal. Fold thumb against the forefinger where it touches the introitus or use forefinger from other hand to measure. Withdraw hand and measure against the pessary or the fitting kit (Figure 46.1).

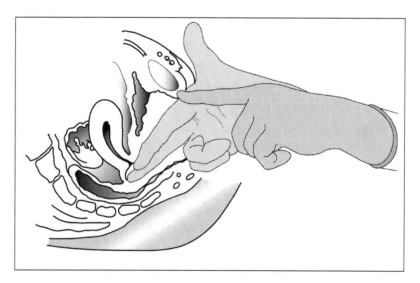

FIGURE 46.1 Measuring the vaginal canal for a pessary.

5. Inform the woman that two or three pessaries may be tried before proper fit is achieved.
   a. The pessary should fit comfortably behind the pubic bone.
   b. Once the proper size is found, the patient should be completely comfortable.
6. Have at least three sizes (often middle sizes) of a given pessary available during the fitting process.
7. A pessary fitting kit is available but is usually not necessary because they only give an approximation.
8. Many pessaries are difficult for the patient to remove and insert correctly, and she needs to receive routine follow-up care from her clinician.
9. Factors related to an unsuccessful fitting
   a. Woman's lack of understanding regarding the pessary or commitment
   b. A short vaginal length (less than 6 cm)
   c. Wide vaginal introitus (greater than 4 finger breaths)
   d. Previous pelvic surgery
   e. Obesity (abdominal pressure may force pessary out)
   f. The fitting process is a "trial and error" and usually two to three pessaries will be tried before a correct fit is achieved.
10. Recommendations for follow-up vary. After initial visit, recommend
    a. Routine return in 12 to 72 hours
       (1) Do not fit a pessary on a Thursday or Friday because the woman may run into problems over the weekend.
    b. Must return sooner if
       (1) Urination or defecation is difficult.
       (2) The pessary is uncomfortable in any way.
       (3) The pessary falls out
          • Reassure patient that this is a common event and to just clean the pessary, put in a plastic baggie, and return with it.
          • Will most likely occur during the straining of a bowel movement
    c. Return visit is important to
       (1) Recheck the size.
       (2) Question the patient regarding urination and defecation to assess status.
       (3) Observe for a tissue reaction such as discharge, irritation, or ulceration.
       (4) Reassure and support the woman.
       (5) Determine the presence of any discomfort. (If it is fit properly, the pessary should not be felt.)
11. Every woman with a pessary must be followed up closely by her clinician if she is not able to perform self-care.

    a. It is possible to forget or neglect a pessary. A list of pessary users within a given office must be kept and followed closely.

      (1) Suggest an older woman wear a medic alert bracelet or have a card stating that she is wearing a pessary.

    b. Patient or clinician must routinely observe for any ulcerations or irritation from undue pressure (this is minimized by vaginal estrogen use).

    c. Return every 4 to 6 weeks (never more than 12 weeks) depending on individual considerations.

      (1) May alter follow-up plan: If odor develops at 12 weeks, the patient needs to return earlier for next visit.

      (2) Remember that a pessary is a foreign body and that there are limited nerve endings in the vagina and cervix. Therefore, a woman may not sense that any ulcerations are occurring.

12. A pessary should not be used in a noncompliant patient or a woman unable to care for herself unless her caregivers are well aware that the pessary is in place and that the patient will receive routine follow-up care.

13. Because many pessary users are elderly, it is important to keep in mind that a woman's status may change over the years (e.g., due to a stroke).

    a. Caregivers (such as nursing home personnel) may not be aware that a pessary is in place.

    b. A list should be kept with the expected routine for follow-up; contact the patient if visits are missed.

14. Estrogen therapy (see Chapter 12, "Atrophic Vaginitis, Vulvovaginal Atrophy").

    a. Recommend estrogen therapy, preferably via the vaginal route, 1 to 2 weeks before the necessary fitting in order to

      (1) Nourish the vaginal tissues

      (2) Mature squamous epithelial tissues

      (3) Increase pliability of submucosal connective tissue

      (4) Improve perineal muscle tone

    b. Routinely recommend as an adjunct to pessary use

      (1) May not be necessary in the postmenopausal woman receiving estrogen replacement therapy

      (2) May be in the form of estrogen cream, suppositories, or estradiol vaginal ring (Estring)

      (3) If Estring is used, insert before the pessary and change every 3 months.

15. If any vaginal conditions are present

    a. Perform a wet mount and treat diagnosed condition.

    b. If ulcerations are present, local estrogen therapy is recommended.

BOX 46.2 *Contraindications to Pessary Use*

- Active vaginitis
- Abnormal Pap smear
- Acute pelvic inflammatory disease
- Endometriosis (research varies)
- Noncompliant patient
- Woman with dementia without possibility of reasonable follow-up

---

16. There are very few contraindications for pessary use (Box 46.2).
    a. After seeing the various types of pessaries, some women have an aversion to such a "foreign-looking object" being inside of them.
    b. Most patients view the pessary as a godsend.
17. Use the largest pessary a patient can accommodate comfortably.
18. Fit ring-and-lever pessaries snugly behind the symphysis pubis, posterior to the cervix.
19. If the pessary fits properly, the examiner should be able to sweep the tip of the finger around the pessary and the vaginal wall. This prevents the breakdown of tissue.
20. Many women who have had a hysterectomy are in need of a pessary.
    a. Although most pessaries fit up against the cervix, a cervix is not necessary to anchor the pessary.
    b. The vaginal wall works as well.
B. General insertion technique
    1. Ask the patient to empty her bladder and rectum, and to position herself as mentioned earlier.
       a. If a large cystocele is present, the woman may need to be straight catheterized, and the bladder emptied.
       b. With incontinence pessaries, it is imperative that the woman void before leaving the clinical site because the knob of the pessary may obstruct the urethra. Some clinicians do not recommend voiding before fitting, to ensure that the woman has urine to void following the fitting.
    2. Wear gloves; an unlubricated glove makes handling of the pessary easier.
    3. Perform a pelvic examination to determine the size, shape, and position of the uterus and associated structures.
    4. Pessary retention test
       a. Insert two fingers in vagina and extend fingers to either side of the vaginal fornices.
       b. Keep fingers thus extended and pull back through the orifice.

   c. If you pull hand straight through without having to collapse the fingers, it is unlikely that a pessary will fit because the introitus is too wide.
5. Approximate size by using fingers to determine the length and depth of the vaginal vault (generally can predict within one size either way).
   a. May use lubricant for a narrow or small introitus
   b. May cause the pessary to be slippery and difficult to bend or hold
   c. Best to lubricate only the entering edge
6. Spread the labia, and pull downward with the nondominant hand.
7. Ask patient to bear down.
8. Grade prolapse
9. Displacement of a prolapse
   a. Insert two fingers into the vagina, push the uterine corpus out of the cul-de-sac, and anteflex it into or above the long axis of the vagina.
   b. With the opposite hand on the anterior abdominal wall, elevate the fundus and hold it in place while inserting the pessary into the vagina.
10. Fit for various pessaries as described under each section below.
11. Begin fitting with the largest size that will fit comfortably, allowing room for the fingertip to sweep around.
12. After insertion
   a. Separate the labia, observing the introitus.
   b. Ask the patient to stand and bear down while being examined.
   c. The pessary should descend and become visible at the introitus but ascend with relaxation.
   d. The presence of the pessary should not be apparent to the user.
   e. Ask the patient to walk around the room, to sit, or to even use the toilet.
   f. Reassess fit.
   g. If the pessary has shifted, try a larger size.
13. A larger size may be necessary after using the pessary for a few weeks, due to an enlargement of the vault with the pessary in position.

III. **Description of the various types of pessaries**
   A. The ring pessary (the incontinence ring; Figure 46.2).
      1. Indications
         a. First- and second-degree uterine prolapse
         b. The administration of estrogen is advocated to improve tissue circulation and regain vaginal mucosal integrity.

    c. The folding ring pessary is especially useful for a patient who is sexually active because it can easily be inserted and removed, or it may remain in place during intercourse (as with a diaphragm).

    d. If a cystocele or rectocele is present, use the ring with support.

2. Description: Comes with a porous diaphragm for additional support

    a. Membrane helps support a mild cystocele that accompanies a prolapse.

    b. It is usually made of medical-grade silicone.

3. Insertion technique

    a. Fit similar to a diaphragm

    b. Measure the length of the vaginal canal against the examining finger, measured against the pessary.

    c. Bend pessary in half at the notches.

    d. Insert the pessary with the folded arc concavity facing downward.

    e. Direct downward past the cervix into the posterior fornix.

    f. Place in the posterior fornix, allowing ring to spring open once it is in the vagina.

    g. Give a quarter turn to secure in position to prevent the pessary from falling in on itself and coming out of the vagina.

    h. When the pessary is placed properly, it will take up redundant vaginal tissue, forming a sling that will support and elevate the uterus, to flatten and support the cystocele (Figure 46.3).

4. Removal

    a. Palpate the notch, and rotate a quarter turn, gently pulling down and out to remove. It is nearly impossible to refold while it is inside the vagina.

    b. It is much easier to insert a pessary than to remove one.

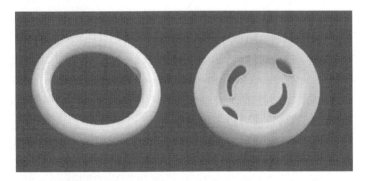

FIGURE 46.2 Ring with and without support.
Photo courtesy of PersonalMed.

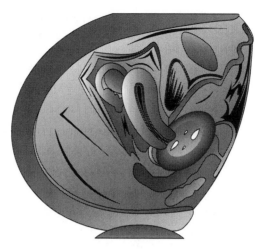

FIGURE 46.3 Vaginal placement of the ring pessary.

5. Available sizes
   a. Available in 14 sizes, numbered 0 to 13
   b. Correlate to a diameter of 4.44 cm to 12.7 cm
B. The lever pessary called Hodge or Smith
   1. Indications
      a. Uterine retroversion: Posteriorly displaces the cervix and the uterus is anteverted.
      b. Incompetent cervix in pregnancy
      c. Mild uterine prolapse with retroversion
      d. Diagnostic evaluation of patients with large cystocele or urinary stress incontinence demonstrates support of the anterior vagina.
      e. Provides support to the proximal urethra, promoting increase in urethral function length and closing pressure without causing obstruction
      f. Useful for stress urinary incontinence, with or without prolapse
      g. If it is properly fitted, sexual intercourse is possible.
   2. Insertion technique
      a. First, manually elevate a retrodisplaced uterus.
      b. Fold the device along the long axis, with the curved end oriented toward the vaginal introitus.
      c. Push into the vagina by the index finger, advancing the posterior bar into the posterior vaginal fornix.
      d. Keep pressure on the posterior bar during insertion.
      e. Anchor the anterior bar under the symphysis pubis (similar to diaphragm insertion).
      f. Note: The long arm of the pessary should face anteriorly, so that the device straddles the rectum.

3. The Smith pessary has a narrower anterior limb for use in a patient with a deep symphysis and a well-defined, narrow pubic arch.
4. The Hodge pessary
   a. Border anterior limb prevents the pessary from turning.
   b. Used when there is minimal pubic support and the symphysis is somewhat shallow
   c. The anterior notch prevents urethral impingement and obstruction.
   d. It comes with a support for correction of a concomitant cystocele.
   e. It is especially useful for patients with stress in continence.
   f. Establishes a diagnostic means of predicting which patients would be responsive to surgical correction
   g. The Hodge pessary with support is indicated for women with stress urinary incontinence, with a mild cystocele, and a very small introitus.
5. Risser pessary
   a. Modification of the Hodge pessary
   b. The Hodge pessary has a wider bar and a deeper notch, which allows a larger weight-bearing region with a lesser likelihood of soft tissue pressure necrosis.
6. Available sizes
   a. Ten available sizes (0–9), measuring width and length
   b. Recommend stocking fitting sizes 2 through 4
C. Gehrung pessary
   1. Indications: Correction of a cystocele and rectocele
   2. Description
      a. Provides support to the anterior vaginal wall; arms or heels rest flat on the vaginal floor
      b. Avoids pressure on the rectum while supporting the bladder
      c. Does not interfere with douching or coitus
      d. Arclike, flexible plastic
      e. Bars may also flatten out a rectocele.
      f. May be underused
   3. Insertion: Creates a bladder bridge
      a. The unusual shape of the pessary may make the clinician uncomfortable with insertion.
      b. It is relatively simple to insert.
      c. Fold with the arch convexity oriented upward, with both heels parallel to the pelvic floor, left heel first.
      d. Hold the device on its side, and insert the lateral bar over the perineum and into the vagina.
      e. When it is positioned intravaginally, push one heel back and the other forward to complete a 90-degree rotation, so that the convex curved portion lies against the anterior vaginal wall.

      f. The back arch should be positioned over the cervix in the anterior fornix, and the front arch should be positioned behind the symphysis.

      g. Both heels should be resting on the pelvic floor, with the arches and cross-support forming a bridge to raise the bladder.

   4. Available sizes

      a. Choice of 10 sizes (0–9)

      b. Recommended stocking sizes: 3, 4, and 5

D. Gellhorn pessary (Figures 46.4 and 46.5)

   1. Indications: Provides support of a third-degree uterine prolapse and procidentia. (Note: Gellhorn comes with both a short and long stem.)

   2. Description

      a. Most commonly used pessary for uterine prolapse (ring and doughnut pessaries also commonly used).

      b. Available

         (1) Flexible silicone

         (2) 95% rigid acrylic

      c. Silicone can be boiled or autoclaved; acrylic should not be autoclaved or boiled because heat can alter the shape.

         (1) Needs to be disinfected in Cidex

         (2) Never use alcohol because it will give the acrylic a shattered appearance.

      d. Provides less support for a rectocele because it fits superiorly and anteriorly, with less surface area to support the posterior segment.

      e. May be difficult to insert in women with a narrow introitus (e.g., virginal).

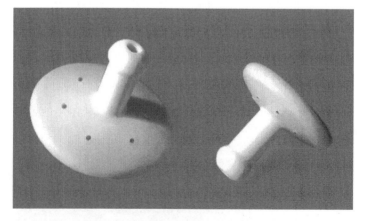

FIGURE 46.4 Gellhorn pessary. Note holes for drainage of vaginal discharge. The stem comes in two sizes, long and short. The disk compresses the urethra at the bladder neck and the stem helps anchor the pessary in place.
Photo courtesy of PersonalMed.

    f. Cervix rests against the flat base of the pessary, with the stem extending to the vaginal orifice.

       (1) The base of the pessary is large enough to support the tissue proximal to it, and rests above the levator muscles.

       (2) Its concave shape provides suction, helping to prevent spontaneous expulsion.

       (3) Stem fills the vagina, preventing the device from turning (requires a capacious vaginal vault).

    g. It is useful with intact (not lax) perineal body. If the patient is not successful, may progress to a cube.

3. Insertion

    a. The main method of determining the proper size of the Gellhorn pessary is by trial and error.

    b. Lubricate the edge of the round disc.

    c. Insert sidewise, with the disc portion held parallel to the introitus.

    d. Apply downward pressure on the perineum with the non-dominant hand.

    e. Be careful to avoid the urethral opening while the perineum is pushed downward.

    f. Push the pessary into the vagina using a corkscrew-like motion until the disc lies transversely beneath the cervix.

    g. Once the large disc is inside the vagina, push forward until the end of the stem slips within the orifice (Figure 46.5).

4. Removal

    a. Fill a 20-mL slip tip syringe with warm water. Insert tip through the hole in the stem of the Gellhorn. Flush the fluid through the hole to release the suction behind the Gellhorn.

    b. Grasp the knob and gently pull disc toward introitus.

    c. If it is difficult to grasp the knob, insert a clamp through the hole and gently pull downward.

    d. The clinician may have to reach behind disc with the non-dominate hand and bend forward to break any seal caused by suction (may be difficult).

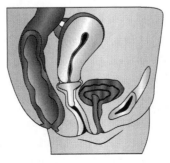

FIGURE 46.5 Gellhorn pessary (note the base holds up the cervix).

      e. Use fingers to spread labia and turn the disc so that it is nearly parallel to the introitus.

      f. Push downward on the perineum to ease the pessary out of the vagina.

  5. Available sizes

      a. Comes in varying sizes of disc diameter, from 1½ to 3½ inches, increasing in quarter-inch increments.

      b. Choose from sizes 1 to 9.

      c. The recommended fitting size includes 2¼, 2½, 2¾.

E. Doughnut (Figure 46.6)

  1. Indications: Occludes upper vagina and supports a uterine prolapse

      a. Mass of the inflated pessary must be greater than the defect in the levator sling.

      b. It provides no support for the proximal urethra and can actually increase incontinence.

      c. Good for prolapse of the vagina after hysterectomy

  2. Description

      a. Useful for uterine prolapse, some recommend for third- to fourth-degree cystocele or rectocele

      b. The hollow ring comes in two models of medical-grade silicone.

      c. Coitus is not possible with the pessary in place.

  3. Insertion technique

      a. Similar to the ring pessary, but there is no notch, so internal rotation is not necessary.

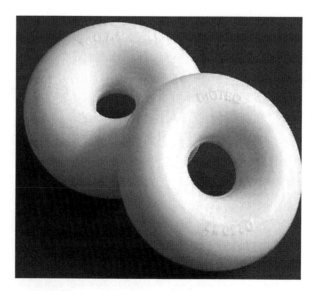

FIGURE 46.6 Donut pessary, which fills the vaginal space to support a prolapse.
Photo courtesy of PersonalMed.

      b. Once the labia is separated with nondominant hand, compress the doughnut. (It is somewhat rigid, so it does not compress too much.)

      c. With two fingers of the nondominant hand pressing down on the peritoneum, hold the pessary parallel, angle slightly, and slip past introitus into vagina.

   4. Removal technique

      a. Hook finger inside on the center of the pessary (will not fit through hole, however).

      b. Compress the doughnut using the thumb and middle finger, and bring them parallel.

      c. Gently pull down and out through introitus. (The clinician may have to lubricate the pessary to remove it.)

   5. Available sizes

      a. There is a choice of six sizes, ranging in diameter from 2 to 3 ¾ inches.

      b. Recommended stocking size 2 and 3.

F. Cube

   1. Indications: Third-degree prolapse, cystocele, or rectocele, with or without vaginal tone

      a. Often, this is the only satisfactory support for patients with complete prolapse complicated by cystourethrocele.

      b. It is excellent for vaginal wall prolapse in that it keeps the vaginal wall from collapsing by using six pressure points.

   2. Description

      a. Each side of cube has concave suction cups that adhere to the vaginal walls, helping to restore the anatomic vaginal support of the pelvic organs (see Figure 46.7).

      b. Moist vaginal mucosa invaginates into the concavities owing to a slight negative pressure.

      c. Needs to be removed daily or requires regular follow-up care initiated by clinician or patient

         (1) Requires highly motivated patient with good dexterity

         (2) Difficult to remove (action of suction), so it may not be possible to be removed by the older client

         (3) Remember that the longer the cube is left in place, the stronger the negative pressure and thus the more difficult it is to remove.

         (4) The cube completely fills the vagina and blocks off drainage of any secretions.

      d. Some clinicians recommend its use in younger women who have incontinence with exercise.

         (1) It can be inserted before vigorous exercise in young women to eliminate leakage.

         (2) Other clinicians would recommend the ring with support for this condition.

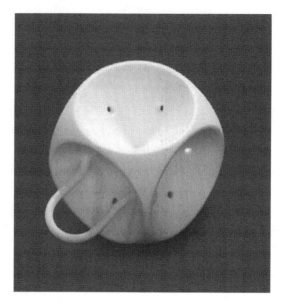

FIGURE 46.7 Cube pessary. Note the six concave sides. The holes are for drainage.
Photo courtesy of PersonalMed.

3. Insertion
    a. It requires the compression of the cube before placement into the vagina.
    b. The string should be oriented toward the vagina.
        (1) Some clinicians recommend that the string be removed because it may be irritating.
        (2) It should never be used to pull the pessary out because it may cause vaginal tears of the fragile mucosa.
    c. Insert by compressing the cube as much as possible.
    d. Spread the labia with the nondominant hand.
    e. Push the compressed cube through introitus.
    f. Place as high in the vagina as possible.
4. Removal
    a. Removal may be difficult because of the suction that has been created.
    b. Suction must be broken before removal.
    c. Do not pull on the string to remove.
    d. Slide the fingertips between the vaginal mucosa and the pessary to break the seal.
    e. Compress the pessary and remove.
    f. If the woman is not able to remove the pessary, she needs to see her clinician immediately. If the pessary is firmly suctioned to the vaginal wall, the following technique may be necessary:
        (1) Insert 5 mL of lidocaine jelly.
        (2) Sweep the fingers around the cube to dispel the jelly.

       (3) Visualize the pessary.

       (4) Grasp the pessary with ring forceps.

       (5) Apply gentle traction, and pull down and out.

  5. Available sizes

    a. Eight sizes (0–7)

    b. The sizes correspond to 1 inch and 2 inches (25 mm to 50 mm).

    c. Recommend stocking sizes 2 to 4; need a minimum of four sizes to fit a patient properly

G. Inflatoball pessary

  1. Description: Used to be made of latex but is now available in silicone

    a. Support is adjusted by varying air pressure via the two-way valve.

    b. The patient can easily remove and clean this device herself; even with a stenotic introitus, it can be inflated and reinflated.

  2. Indications

    a. Genital prolapse

    b. Extreme degrees of uterine prolapse

    c. Prolapse of the vagina following a total hysterectomy

  3. Insertion

    a. Approximate size by using fingers to determine the vaginal vault width.

    b. With the pessary deflated, hold it compressed between the thumb and forefingers.

    c. While it is deflated, insert the metal part of the bulb into the air vent.

    d. Insert the deflated pessary into the vaginal vault.

    e. Inflate the ball by squeezing the bulb to the desired pressure.

    f. Inflate the ball to a diameter large enough so that one finger can pass around the pessary and the vaginal wall.

  4. Removal

    a. Deflate the pessary.

    b. Gently pull the deflated pessary through the introitus (do not pull on the stem).

  5. Available sizes

    a. Small, medium, large, and extra large

    b. Corresponding to ball diameter of 2 to 2.5 inches

    c. Recommended stocking fitting sizes medium and large

H. Incontinence ring pessary (Figure 46.8)

  1. Description

    a. Designed to stabilize the urethra and the urethrovesical junction

    b. Woman must void following insertion before leaving the office to make sure the urethra is not obstructed

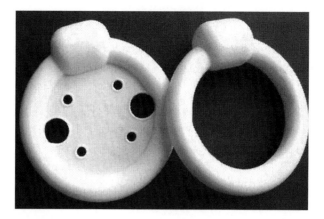

FIGURE 46.8 Incontinence ring pessary with knob. Note: It comes with or without support. The holes allow for drainage of vaginal discharge. The knob applies pressure against the bladder neck and compresses the urethra.
Photo courtesy of PersonalMed.

2. Indication
   a. Stress incontinence
   b. Diagnostic test to assess the surgical outcome
3. Insertion technique
   a. Similar to the ring pessary without support
   b. Must fit properly because if it is too small, the knob may not remain in proper position, and if it is too large, it may obstruct the urethra and cause urinary retention.
   c. Fold the pessary in half. The knob is in the middle of the concave.
   d. Push the pessary up and behind the cervix.
   e. Insert a gloved hand into the vagina and rotate the knob from its position on the side of the vagina to the front of the vagina with the knob resting behind the pubic bone.
4. Incontinence dish
   a. Variation of the incontinence ring
   b. It is indicated for stress urinary incontinence associated with a mild first- or second-degree prolapse.
   c. It is available in sizes 55 mm to 85 mm, in increments of 5 mm.
   d. Insert end without knob first. It is fitted with the knob behind the pubic bone.
5. Incontinence dish with support (Figure 46.9)
   a. Variation of dish with flexible membrane to support a mild cystocele
   b. It is indicated for stress urinary incontinence in conjunction with a first- or second-degree prolapse, or a mild cystocele. (Some clinicians recommend this type of pessary for second- or third-degree cystocele because it provides additional support for the cystocele.)

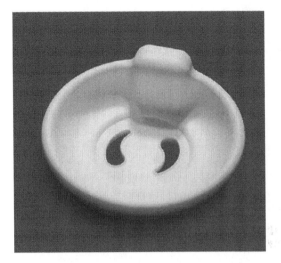

FIGURE 46.9 Incontinence dish. Bowl shape allows for support of a cystocele. Has large holes for drainage of vaginal discharge.
Photo courtesy of PersonalMed.

    c. It is available in sizes 55 mm to 85 mm, in increments of 5 mm.
    d. It is fit with the knob behind the pubic bone to further compress the urethra to decrease urine loss.

IV. Follow-up
    A. Must continuously monitor the woman for as long as the pessary is in place: Although it is inert, it is still considered a foreign body.
    B. Keep a list of all pessary users to make sure they are seen every 2 to 3 months. A forgotten pessary can cause serious complications. The woman can obtain a medic alert card at www.medid.com/phorm/phorm.php
    C. The pessary may require sizing alterations or a complete change in style at subsequent visits.
    D. Discuss with the patient any possible problems.
        1. Coital discomfort (if intercourse is allowable)
        2. Disturbance in bowel or urinary function
        3. Whether or not it remained in place
        4. Overall comfort
        5. Presence of any odor
        6. Change in discharge
            a. A yellow or white, or mild to moderate, discharge is usually present.
            b. If the discharge increases during subsequent visits, question the patient's compliance with the vaginal care routine.
            c. The discharge should never be foul smelling.
                (1) Perform a wet mount, and treat any infection.
                (2) Replace the pessary after the infection is resolved.

E.   At this point, one may discuss the possibility of the woman cleaning her own pessary.
   1.   Particularly if she is used to touching her own genitals
      a.   Older women are not as familiar
      b.   If the woman has previously used a diaphragm, it may be easy for her to learn how to use a pessary.
      c.   Observe dexterity
      d.   Evaluate compliance issues and ability to perform self-care.
   2.   Most pessaries are difficult to insert and remove, so a woman must not feel that she has failed if she is unable to do it herself.
   3.   Do not even raise the possibility if it is obvious that the woman is unable to manage the pessary.
F.   Provide instructions regarding
   1.   Use of lubricant to ease insertion
      a.   Nonpetroleum-based lubricants are not caustic and can be used.
   2.   Douching
      a.   No consensus has been presented as to its effectiveness.
      b.   The woman should always consult with her clinician first.
      c.   Mild vinegar may help to acidify the vagina.
   3.   Use of estrogen
      a.   Vaginal estrogen, unless contraindicated, is recommended over systemic estrogen.
         (1)   Vaginal creams or pill is inserted twice weekly.
         (2)   Estring should be replaced every 3 months (should be inserted before pessary).
      b.   May be used in conjunction with systemic preparations
      c.   The patient may have difficulty using the applicator and inserting the cream. (Many patients are older and have limited experience with devices such as tampons.)
      d.   Will mature vaginal epithelium and improve perineal muscle tone
   4.   Use of Trimo-San
      a.   This is a cleansing, deodorant gel with a pH of 4 used to maintain antibacterial acid environment.
      b.   The patient should use one-half applicator two times per week.
      c.   The active ingredient is oxyquinoline sulfate.
G.   Pessary care and cleaning
   1.   If the patient is unable to remove the pessary, it should be removed and the patient should be observed for any excoriation, ulceration, or foul discharge.
   2.   Clean the pessary in warm, soapy water; rinse thoroughly; and reinsert.
   3.   Irrigate the vagina using a 20-mL syringe with an irrigating tip using warm water. A weak solution of betadine or vinegar may be used.

4. Document type and amount of solution used and note character of discharge.
5. Replace the pessary if the old one shows signs of physical defects.
   a. It may become discolored but does not need to be replaced.

H. Complications
   1. Increase in vaginal discharge
   2. Odor
   3. Cytologic atypia from inflammatory changes that may occur
   4. Poorly fitted or improper schedule of cleaning may cause ulcerations and excoriation.
   5. Incarceration: The cervix and uterus may herniate through the center of a poorly fitted ring pessary and become strangulated.
   6. In a neglected pessary, tissue may grow around it.
   7. There should be no evidence of serious problems with long-term wear of a well-maintained pessary.

I. Maintenance visits
   1. Slight bleeding may be seen during removal of pessary; question the patient's compliance with estrogen therapy.
   2. If using the Estring, replace the ring every 3 months during the 3-month cleaning visit. Insert before the pessary.
   3. Refit pessary if there has been a gain or loss of 20 pounds or more (discuss diet).
   4. If heavy discharge
      a. Perform wet mount to check for infection.
      b. If no infection is present, recommend vinegar and water douche.
         (1) One-quarter cup vinegar to 1 quart of warm water
         (2) Douche once to twice weekly.
   5. Reinforce use of Kegel exercises (see Chapter 38, "Pelvic Floor Rehabilitation").
      a. Compliance is the key.
      b. Success rate of over 80% resolution of incontinence can be achieved in 4 to 8 weeks.
   6. Offer support groups.

J. Monitor urination
   1. Ask the woman to keep a voiding diary.
      a. Keep the diary for 1 week.
      b. Include frequency and quality of fluids
      c. Note quantity and frequency of urination.
      d. Record which type of activities cause leaking.
   2. Note use of pads.
      a. Brand name
      b. How often has to wear (continuous versus intermittent)
      c. How often has to change if continuous

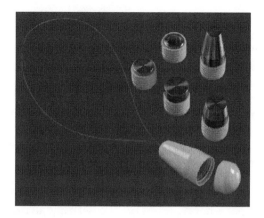

FIGURE 46.10 Vaginal weights. Note how the cones become progressively larger. *Photo courtesy of PersonalMed.*

    3. Kegel exercises
       a. Inquire whether the patient has done them in the past.
       b. Was she successful?
    4. Kegel exercise cones (Figure 46.10)
       a. These cones were designed as an aid to locating and identifying the correct pelvic floor muscle.
       b. Five interchangeable cone-shaped plastic weights ranging from 1 to 3 ounces
       c. Smooth, hypoallergenic
       d. Used in conjunction with a home exercise program
       e. Begin by attaching the lightweight cone to the plastic insertion device.
       f. Ask the woman to walk around doing routine activities.
       g. The pelvic floor reflexively tightens to retain the smooth, slippery cone.
       h. Once she is able to retain the cone for 15 minutes, she should progress to the next heavier size.
       i. Patients with a prolapse or pessary cannot use cones because the pressure will force the cone to be expelled.

VI. Pessaries in the 21st century
    A. Newer devices to manage pelvic organ prolapse
       1. Uresta
         a. Uniquely shaped pessary that allows a woman to self-manage; easy to remove and insert
         b. The tissues compress the urethra and may reduce leakage.
         c. May soon be available as an over-the-counter option
       2. Colpexin Sphere
         a. Round plastic sphere that is placed intravaginally above the levator ani muscle
         b. Space-occupying properties allow support of the prolapse.

c. Reflectively causes contraction of the pelvic floor muscle in an attempt to retain the sphere

3. Urethral inserts: FemSoft insert

   a. The single-use disposable device—made of soft silicone—is a tube with a balloon-like tip. Encasing the tube is a sheath filled with mineral oil.

   b. The device is inserted into the urethra and up into the neck of the bladder with an applicator.

      (1) Most of the mineral oil in the device then flows into the balloon tip.

      (2) Because the balloon tip is soft and filled with fluid, it conforms to the shape of your bladder neck, creating a seal that prevents urine from leaking out.

      (3) When a woman needs to urinate, simply removes the insert. Urethral inserts are small, tampon-like disposable plugs that a woman inserts into her urethra to prevent urine from leaking out.

      (4) Urethral inserts are generally worn before engaging in activities that might result in stress urinary incontinence; they may be worn throughout the day.

      (5) Urethral inserts are not meant to be worn 24 hours a day.

      (6) Urethral inserts are available by prescription.

4. Poise Impressa Bladder Support (Figure 46.11)

   a. An over-the-counter, nonabsorbent, disposable intravaginal device that physically supports the urethra to help prevent stress urinary incontinence (SUI) leaks.

   b. Inserted with an applicator and removed by the pull of a string.

   c. Women may wear it for up to 8 hours within a 24-hour time period.

   d. Women can use the bathroom normally without having to remove the device.

   e. Provides support to the urethra whenever pressure is transferred from the abdomen to the pelvic floor.

   f. Normal urinary flow and vaginal secretions remain unaffected.

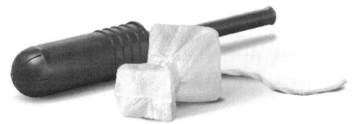

FIGURE 46.11 The Poise Impressa with applicator.
Photo courtesy of Kimberly Clark.

Bibliography

Abdool, Z., Thakar, R., Sultan, A. H., & Oliver, R. S. (2011). Prospective evaluation of outcome of vaginal pessaries versus surgery in women with symptomatic pelvic organ prolapse. *International Urogynecology Journal, 22,* 273.

Carcio, H. A. (2003). Comprehensive continence care. *Advance for Nurse Practitioners, 12*(10), 26–35.

Carcio, H. A. (2004). The vaginal pessary: An effective yet underused tool for incontinence and prolapse. *Advance for Nurse Practitioners, 12*(10), 47–48, 50, 52–54, 56.

Clemons, J. L., Brubaker, L., & Falk, S. J. (n.d.) Vaginal pessary treatment of prolapse and incontinence. UpToDate. http://www.uptodate.com/contents/vaginal-pessary-treatment-of-prolapse-and-incontinence

Culligan, P. J. (2012). Nonsurgical management of pelvic organ prolapse. *Obstetrical & Gynecological, 119*(4), 852–860.

Friedman, S., Sandhu, K. S., Wang, C., Wang, C., & Megdy, S. (2010). Factors influencing long-term pessary use. International Urogynecology Journal, 21, 673.

Hagen, S., Stark, D., Maher, C., & Adams, E. (2006, October 18). Conservative management of pelvic organ prolapse in women. *Cochrane Database of Systematic Reviews, 4,* CD003882.

Handa, V. L., Whitcomb, E., Weidner, A. C., Nygaard, I., Brubaker, L., Bradley, C. S., (2011). Sexual function before and after non-surgical treatment for stress urinary incontinence. *Female Pelvic Medicine & Reconstructive Surgery, 17,* 30.

Lone, F., Thakar, R., Sultan, A. H., & Karamalis, G. (2011). A 5-year prospective study of vaginal pessary use for pelvic organ prolapse. *International Journal of Gynaecology and Obstetrics, 114,* 56.

National Institute for Health and Clinical Excellence (NICE). (2006, October). Clinical Guideline 40. *Urinary incontinence: The management of urinary incontinence in women.* Retrieved May 2013, from http://www.nice.org.uk

Tam, T., & Davies, M. (2013, December). Pessaries for vaginal prolapse: Critical factors to successful fit and continued use. *OBG Management, 25*(12), 42–44,48–52, 59.

UpToDate. http://www.uptodate.com/contents/vaginal-pessary-treatment-of-prolapse-and-incontinence. Updated February 8, 2013.

Index